# ATLAS OF SPINE SURGERY

ROBERT B. WINTER, M.D.
JOHN W. LONSTEIN, M.D.
FRANCIS DENIS, M.D.
MICHAEL D. SMITH, M.D.

Minnesota Spine Center, Minneapolis, Minnesota

*With contributions by Joseph Garamella, M.D., and David M. Arnold, M.D.*

W. B. SAUNDERS COMPANY
*A Division of Harcourt Brace & Company*
PHILADELPHIA  LONDON  TORONTO  MONTREAL  SYDNEY  TOKYO

**W. B. SAUNDERS COMPANY**
*A Division of Harcourt Brace & Company*

The Curtis Center
Independence Square West
Philadelphia, Pennsylvania 19106

**Library of Congress Cataloging-in-Publication Data**

Atlas of spine surgery/Robert B. Winter . . . [et al.] ; with contributions by Joseph Garamella and
    David M. Arnold.—1st ed.
        p.  cm.
    ISBN 0-7216-2958-X
    1. Spine—Surgery—Atlases.  I. Winter, Robert B.
    [DNLM: 1. Spine—surgery—atlases.  WE 17 A88063345 1995]
    RD768.A86  1995
    617.3′75059—dc20
    DNLM/DLC                                                                94-29593

ATLAS OF SPINE SURGERY                               ISBN  0-7216-2958-X

# Preface

This atlas brings together the commonly used techniques for spine surgery. We have made the decision to limit the techniques to those that are established and appear to stand the test of time. This atlas emanated from the frustrations of our residents, fellows, and postgraduate spine surgery visitors in being able to find illustrated techniques for the many different spinal procedures currently available. It required researching a dozen textbooks and an equal number of scientific articles to locate drawings related to these procedures. Therefore, it seemed only a matter of common sense to pull them together into one resource. No attempt has been made to delve into the historic origins of any given procedures, and for this reason, we have chosen not to list any bibliography.

Spinal instrumentation is an area that is in an enormous state of flux, with new systems being added almost monthly. Consequently, we have chosen to illustrate instrumentation that is used on a daily basis in our practice, has stood the test of time, and represents the basic principles that will remain true regardless of more minor changes in instrument design. For example, in the section on the lumbar spine dealing with internal fixation using pedicle screws, we have chosen to portray a generic screw insertion so as to not favor one implant over another. It is clearly obvious that whichever pedicle screw device is used, it may fail if the surgeon does not find and insert the pedicle screws properly.

Furthermore, this is an atlas and not a textbook. It is beyond the scope of this book to discuss the indications or contraindications for any given operative procedure. It is understood that the surgeon will use intelligence, common sense, and the widespread published literature both in textbooks and scientific articles that deals with indications and contraindications for any given procedure.

There are many people to thank for this book. All of us owe a great debt of gratitude to Andy Grivas, our medical illustrator, for his tremendous skills. To Lynn Gilsrud, we owe great thanks for her manuscript typing and the endless redrafts and revisions that can be so frustrating. To the staff of W. B. Saunders, our thanks for their production of a high-quality book.

Finally, this book is dedicated to the memory of Dr. Aydin Bilgutay, a thoracic surgeon with whom we worked for many, many years. His early and untimely death from cancer not only kept him from significant participation in the writing of the section on anterior exposures, but also denied us the enormous clinical skills of this wonderful surgeon. We miss him greatly.

ROBERT B. WINTER

JOHN E. LONSTEIN

FRANCIS DENIS

MICHAEL D. SMITH

# Contents

# CONTENTS

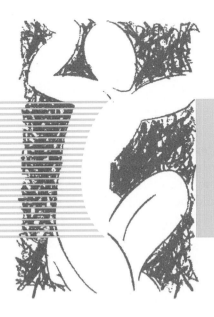

# ANTERIOR UPPER CERVICAL PROCEDURES

# Transoral

The patient is placed in a semireclining position with the head secured to prevent excessive skull motion. A halo ring, or neurosurgical temporary head holder, is a valuable but not essential adjunct to head immobilization. The neural pressure points on the arms and legs should be well-padded to prevent compression neuropathies (Fig. 1–1).

A soft rubber catheter is placed through the nostril and looped about the uvula to facilitate its cephalad retraction (Fig. 1–2A). Nasotracheal intubation with a reinforced airway is preferred, although elective tracheostomy can be used if prolonged postoperative mechanical ventilation is anticipated (Fig. 1–2B).

A fully articulated and adjustable, self-retaining retractor system facilitates upward retraction of the hard and soft palates and downward on the tongue. Dilute epinephrine solution is injected into the midline posterior pharyngeal tissue (Fig. 1–2C).

A midline transmucosal dissection is performed, starting slightly cephalad to the anterior tubercle of C1 and carried distally atop the body of C2. Slow and deliberate dissection is necessary to preserve a stout pharyngomucosal flap, required for later closure (Fig. 1–3).

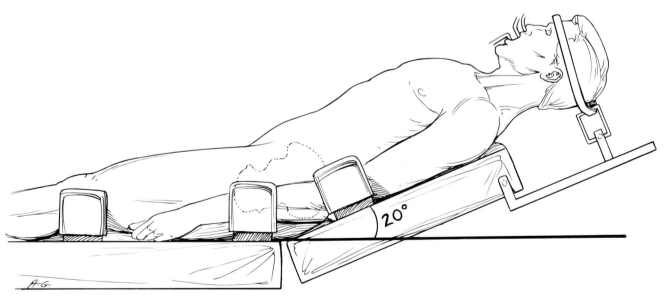

*Figure 1–1*

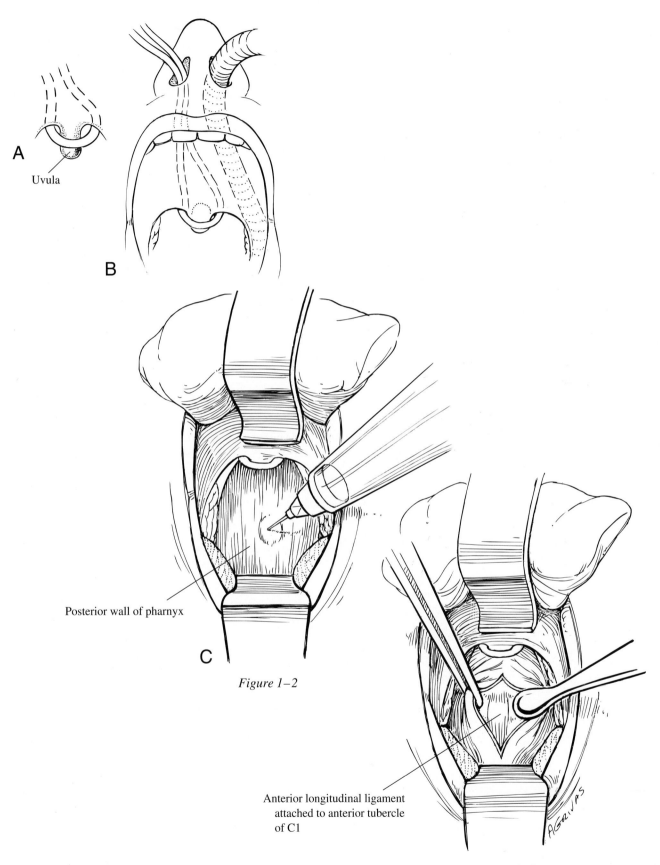

A

Uvula

B

Posterior wall of pharnyx

C

*Figure 1–2*

Anterior longitudinal ligament
attached to anterior tubercle
of C1

*Figure 1–3*

3

# ANTERIOR UPPER CERVICAL PROCEDURES

Additional laterally directed, malleable retractors are placed after suitable proximal and distal exposure has been obtained. The anterior arch of C1, from the midportion of the lateral masses bilaterally, is now exposed (Fig. 1–4).

The anterior arch of C1 can then be removed using a high-speed carbide burr or bone rongeurs (Fig. 1–5).

The pannus and dens are then removed, which exposes the dura. The decompression is complete when the dura bulges freely into the decompression defect and the medial aspect of the lateral masses, bilaterally, are visible (Fig. 1–6).

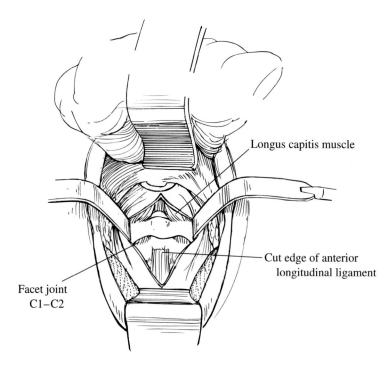

Longus capitis muscle

Cut edge of anterior
longitudinal ligament

Facet joint
C1–C2

*Figure 1–4*

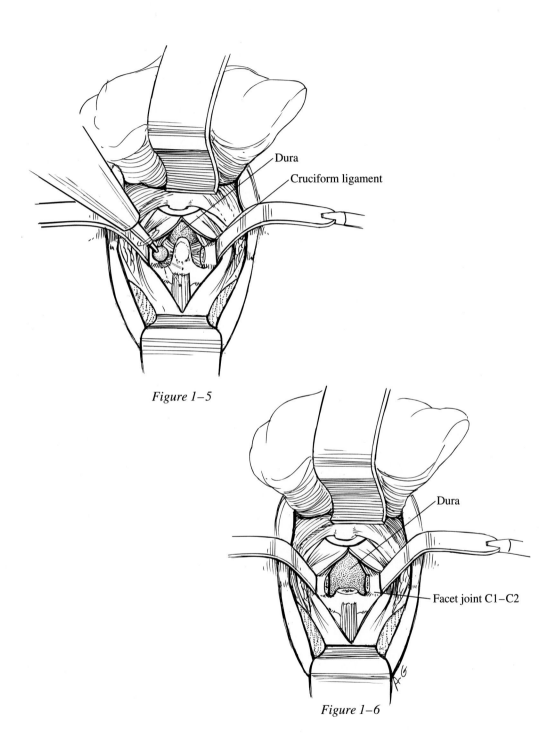

Dura

Cruciform ligament

*Figure 1–5*

Dura

Facet joint C1–C2

*Figure 1–6*

5

# ANTERIOR UPPER CERVICAL PROCEDURES

It is imperative for the surgeon to keep an appropriate midline orientation during the performance of the anterior C1–C2 decompressions. The anterior tubercle is an important surgical landmark and aids in the initiation of a midline decompression (Fig. 1–7). Once a thorough anterior exposure of the ring of C1 has been carried out so that the medial edge of the anterior aspect of the C1–C2 facet joint is visible, the anterior ring can be quickly removed using hand instruments or a high-speed carbide burr. Surgical loupes and a headlight, or a microscope, speed the dissection and improve the overall safety of the procedure (Fig. 1–8). Once the anterior arch has been removed, the dens can then be removed with fine curettes. Additional pannus can be resected and a satisfactory spinal decompression should then be achieved (Fig. 1–9).

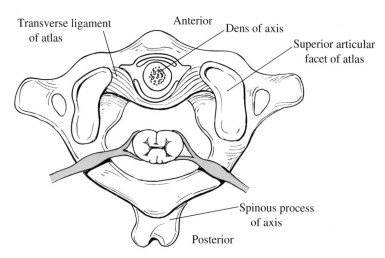

Normal Anatomy

*Figure 1–7*

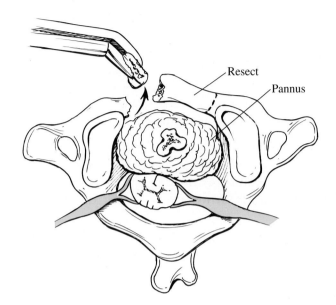

*Figure 1-8*

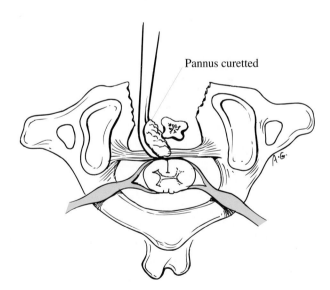

*Figure 1-9*

# Anterior Retropharyngeal Approach

The patient is supine with the head turned to the left. A transverse roll is placed beneath the shoulder blades to provide for mild neck extension. Pad all potential peripheral neural compression points. A small Kirschner wire is inserted percutaneously through the anterior aspect of the mandible, and skeletal traction is applied to elevate the mandible and facilitate proximal surgical exposure. A transverse submandibular incision is used (Fig. 1–10).

This approach requires thorough knowledge of the complex proximal cervical anatomy. Injury to the marginal mandibular branch of the facial nerve can lead to troublesome and painful neuromas, whereas injury to the hypoglossal or superior laryngeal nerve can result in tongue or speech difficulties, respectively (Fig. 1–11).

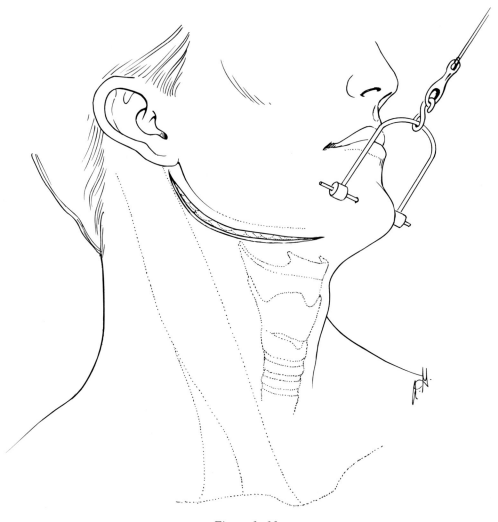

*Figure 1–10*

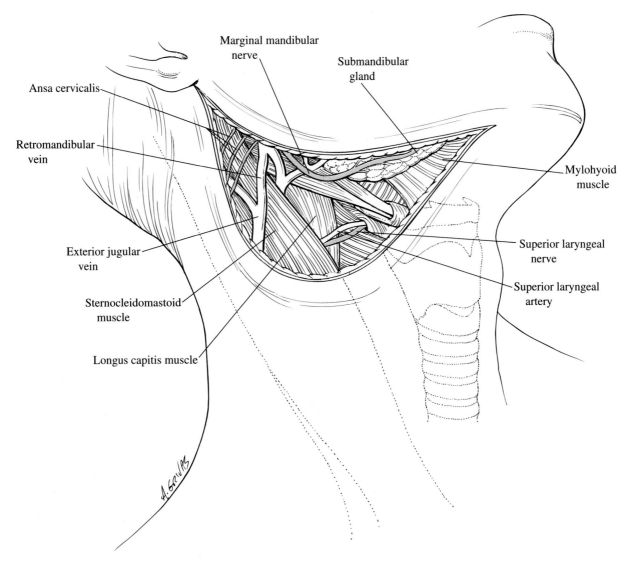

Ansa cervicalis

Retromandibular
vein

Exterior jugular
vein

Sternocleidomastoid
muscle

Longus capitis muscle

Marginal mandibular
nerve

Submandibular
gland

Mylohyoid
muscle

Superior laryngeal
nerve

Superior laryngeal
artery

*Figure 1–11*

9

Numerous descending submandibular and superficial cervical veins are divided between ties. The hypoglossal nerve is gently protected throughout the entire procedure, and excessive retraction on the digastric muscle is avoided to prevent the possibility of a postoperative facial nerve paralysis (Fig. 1–12).

Once the hypoglossal nerve is protected, the opening between the common carotid neurovascular structures laterally and the trachea and esophageal structures medially is then developed by blunt digital dissection. The pretracheal and the prevertebral fascia, layers of the deep cervical investing fascia, are then split longitudinally, exposing the anterior and anterolateral aspects of the vertebral bodies of C2 and C3. Surgical loupes and headlight illumination greatly facilitate dissection (Fig. 1–13).

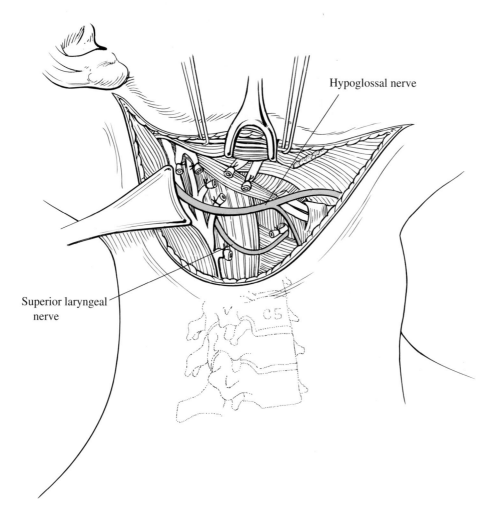

Figure 1–12

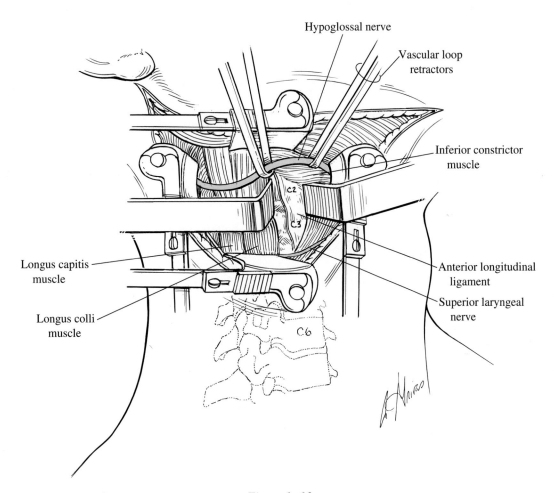

Hypoglossal nerve

Vascular loop retractors

Inferior constrictor muscle

Longus capitis muscle

Longus colli muscle

Anterior longitudinal ligament

Superior laryngeal nerve

C2

C3

C6

*Figure 1–13*

A thorough C2–C3 diskectomy is initiated by sharply incising the disk annulus (Fig. 1–14A,B).

A high-speed carbide burr, with intermittent water irrigation, is used to perform the initial subtotal medial corpectomy (Fig. 1–15).

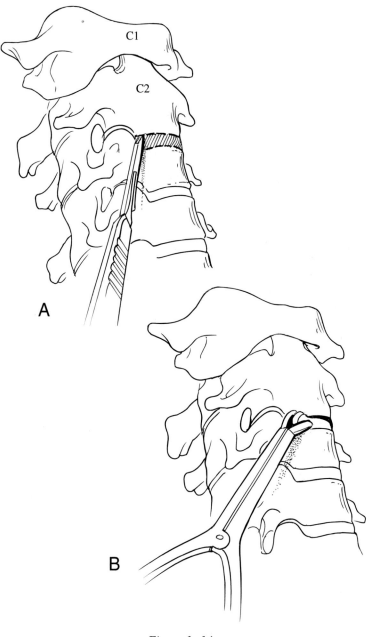

*Figure 1–14*

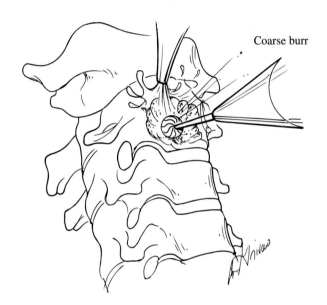

Coarse burr

*Figure 1–15*

The resection of bone, utilizing the high-speed carbide burr, is made in an anteroposterior direction. The posterior vertebral cortex is cautiously approached (Fig. 1–16).

A high-speed diamond burr, along with continuous water irrigation, is used to thin and perforate the vertebral cortex along the lateral aspects of the spinal canal bilaterally (Fig. 1–17A).

Once the posterior vertebral cortex has been perforated, a detached island of bone and disk material is gently pulled away from the spinal canal completing the spinal canal decompression (Fig. 1–17B).

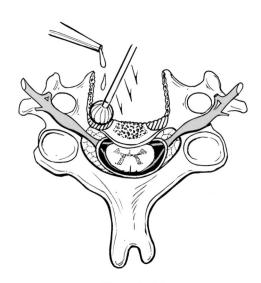

*Figure 1–16*

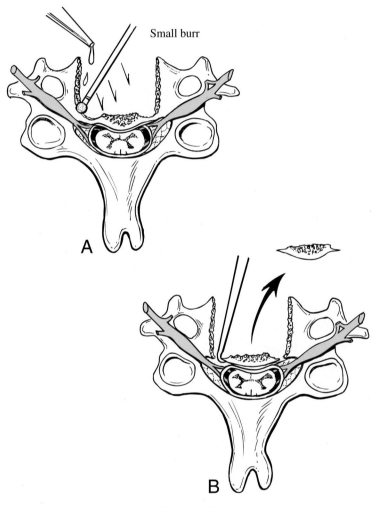

Small burr

A

B

*Figure 1–17*

# ANTERIOR UPPER CERVICAL PROCEDURES

A tricortical cancellous strut is harvested from the ilium. This should be done with an oscillating saw to prevent stress risers, which occur from the use of impact tools (Fig. 1–18).

A larger radius carbide burr is used to fashion a circular seating hole in the superior aspect of the remainder C3. The dens (if still present) is then notched to obtain a sculptured graft. Skeletal traction is increased transiently to provide increased distraction of the upper cervical spine for easier insertion of the graft (Fig. 1–19).

The graft is gently impacted and the interstices grafted with additional cancellous bone (Figs. 1–20, 1–21A,B). A standard layer anatomic closure over a suction drain is used.

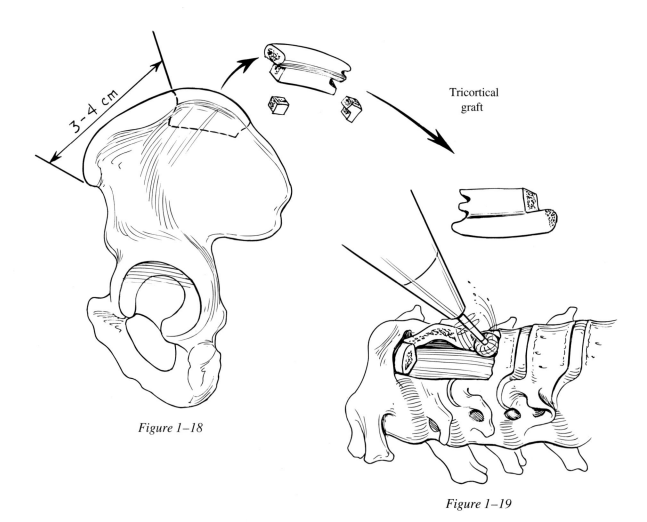

3–4 cm

Tricortical graft

*Figure 1–18*

*Figure 1–19*

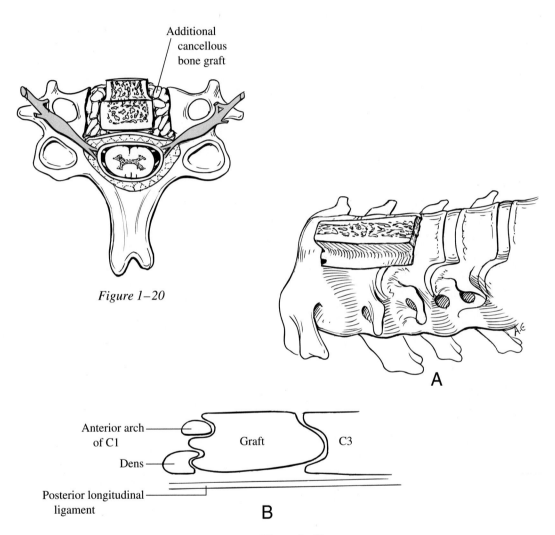

Additional
cancellous
bone graft

*Figure 1–20*

A

Anterior arch
of C1

Dens

Posterior longitudinal
ligament

Graft

C3

B

*Figure 1–21*

17

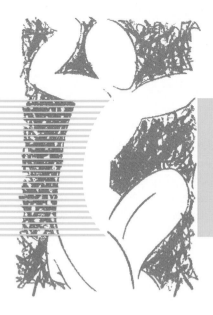

2

# POSTERIOR UPPER CERVICAL PROCEDURES

# Positioning

The patient is in the prone position, which provides free access to the posterior cervical region and the airway. There should be no pressure on the forehead or orbits. To accomplish this, suspend a halo ring from a sturdy ether screen with multiple loops of twisted surgical wire and stabilizing tapes from each side of the ring. In addition, using adhesive tape to draw the shoulders downward and away from the operative field will provide an accessible and extensile surgical exposure and ability to obtain intraoperative radiographs (Fig. 2–1).

# Procedures

Most upper cervical procedures require a midline exposure starting at its most cephalad extent about the inion and carried distally as needed. Presurgical injection with dilute epinephrine solution aids in hemostasis (Fig. 2–2).

Once the superficial tissues have been incised, the ligamentum nuchae is identified. It is imperative to stay within this meandering ligament to decrease blood loss and to have a stout tissue layer for closure (Fig. 2–3).

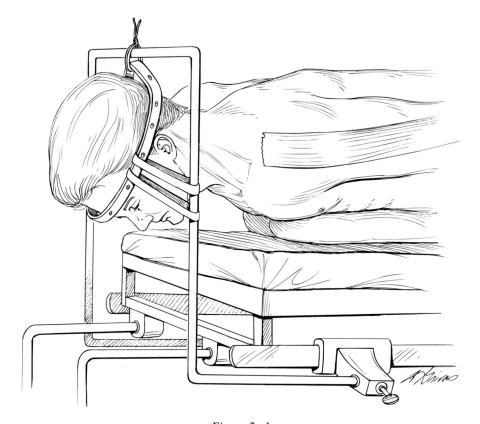

*Figure 2–1*

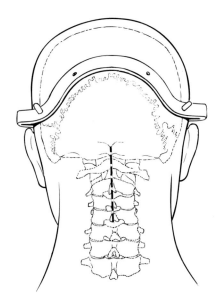

*Figure 2–2*

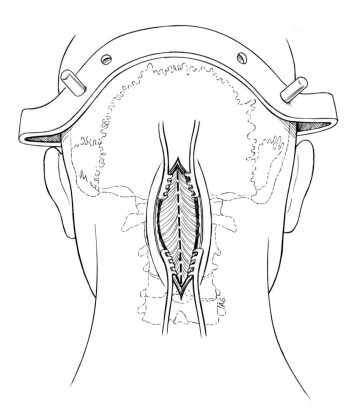

*Figure 2–3*

# POSTERIOR UPPER CERVICAL PROCEDURES

Strong, self-retaining retractors keep the tissues under tension, aid in hemostasis, and facilitate dissection. With care, subperiosteal detachments of the strong muscular attachments of the erector spinal muscle on C2 and the converging fibrous origins of the short skull rotators on the posterior tubercle of C1 are made (Fig. 2–4).

Lateral exposure is limited owing to the presence of the vertebral artery, approximately 1.5 cm lateral to the midline of C1. Once the greater occipital nerve is encountered and the fragile venae comitantes of the paravertebral venous plexus are exposed, further lateral dissection endangers the vertebral artery. Wandering into this artery inadvertently can have disastrous complications (Fig. 2–5).

Deep, single-pronged, Gelpe-type retractors aid in maintaining a good, deep surgical exposure (Fig. 2–6).

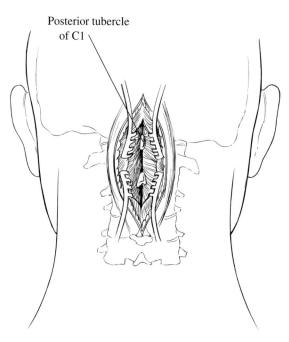

Posterior tubercle
of C1

*Figure 2–4*

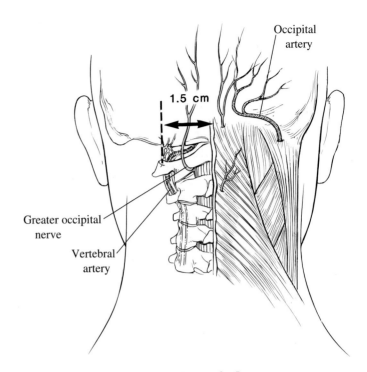

Occipital
artery

1.5 cm

Greater occipital
nerve

Vertebral
artery

*Figure 2–5*

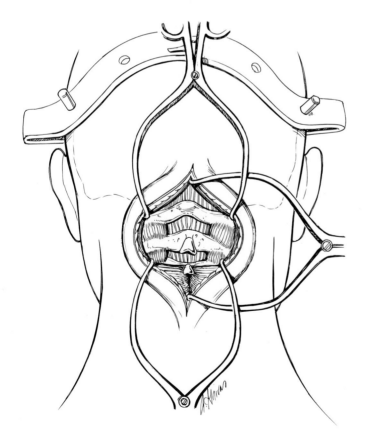

*Figure 2–6*

23

# POSTERIOR UPPER CERVICAL PROCEDURES

Occipitocervical arthrodesis requires further proximal subperiosteal exposure of the skull base (Fig. 2–7).

The inion is thicker at its prominence near the ridge. Bone is cautiously removed adjacent to the ridge using a high-speed diamond burr with continuous water irrigation or, alternatively, small curettes. The midline ridge is preserved. A single strand of 20-gauge stainless steel wire is passed through the base of this ridge of thick cortical bone. This wire secures bone grafts to the base of the skull (Fig. 2–8A).

A sublaminar wire at C1 is passed through the ridge in an inferior to superior direction using the blunt end of a heavy suture on a short radius needle. The suture is then tied to a doubled-over monofilament wire and, using the suture as a guide, pulled underneath the C1 lamina. This is a rapid and atraumatic method of passing the wire under the ring of C1. If marked instability is present, the ring may be grasped with Kocher clamps to stabilize it (Fig. 2–8B,C).

A wire is passed through C2 and circles the inferior aspect of C2 for stable bone graft fixation (Fig. 2–8D).

Thick iliac crest bone grafts containing both cortical and cancellous bone are harvested using osteotomes. The grafts are securely affixed to the base of the skull and the exposed and decorticated posterior elements of C1 and C2 using the previously passed wires in a horizontal mattress suture technique (Fig. 2–9).

In situations where additional stability is needed, a rectangular metal ring device may be necessary. This is formed by securing the ring to multiple sublaminar wires passed at C1, C2, and C3 and through burr holes at the base of the skull. Most occipitocervical fusions do not require this device. The rectangular ring must be carefully formed to accommodate junctional occipitocervical lordosis (Fig. 2–10).

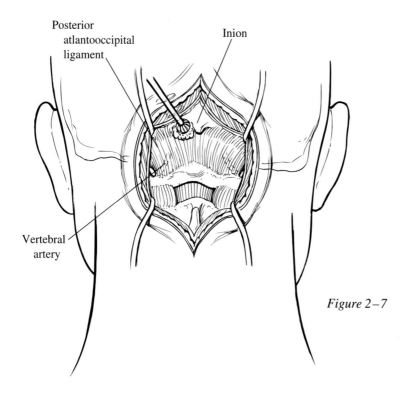

Posterior atlantooccipital ligament

Inion

Vertebral artery

*Figure 2–7*

24

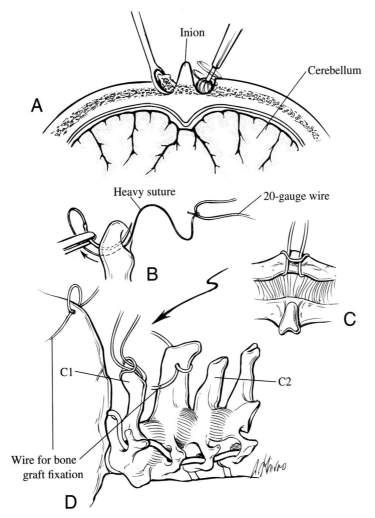

*Figure 2–8*

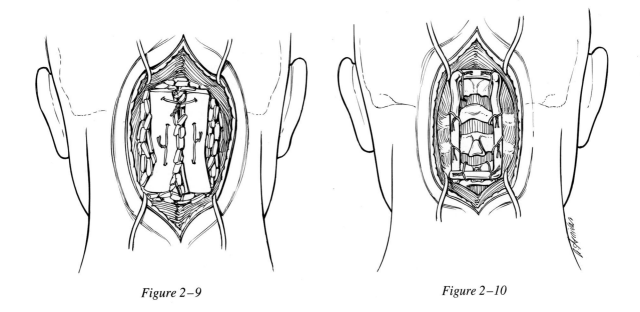

*Figure 2–9*

*Figure 2–10*

# POSTERIOR UPPER CERVICAL PROCEDURES

Occasionally, deficiencies of the posterior elements, particularly hypoplasia or the presence of a bifid ring of C1, require alternative fusion techniques. A distally based occipital periosteal flap is turned down and suture-secured to the superior portion of the arch of C2 (Fig. 2–11). Additional massive cancellous grafting over the denuded occipital and remaining posterior elements of C2 is then performed. A standard anatomic closure is used (Fig. 2–12).

In select circumstances, plate fixation may be needed. A wide bilateral exposure and sufficiently strong bone without osteopenia is necessary for this technique to work. Using a depth-controlled drill, holes are made in the occipital bone. Contoured malleable plates are fastened to the bone with lateral mass screws. The screws are typically 10 to 12 mm in length (Fig. 2–13).

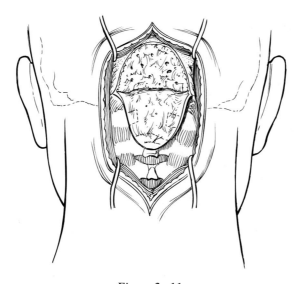

*Figure 2–11*

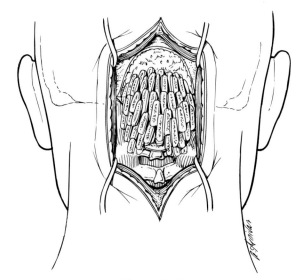

*Figure 2–12*

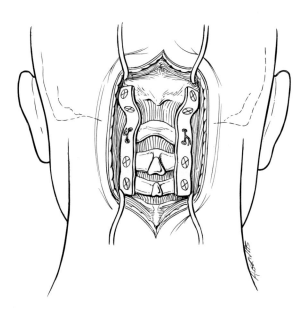

*Figure 2–13*

27

# C1–C2 FUSIONS

There are a variety of well-accepted and clinically utilized arthrodesis techniques for the C1–C2 area. The occipitocervical arthrodesis was described earlier. The Brooks technique utilizes four monofilament 20-gauge sublaminar wires at C1 and C2 over separate sculpted iliac corticocancellous grafts (Fig. 2–14).

The Gallie technique uses a single sublaminar wire at C1 passed around the base of C2 and around a sculpted interposed corticocancellous iliac crest bone graft. The graft is included in the mechanical device (Fig. 2–15).

The midline technique utilizes an 18-gauge sublaminar wire at C1 and a transspinous process wire at C2. Additional cancellous grafting is placed around the decorticated posterior elements of C1 and C2 (Fig. 2–16).

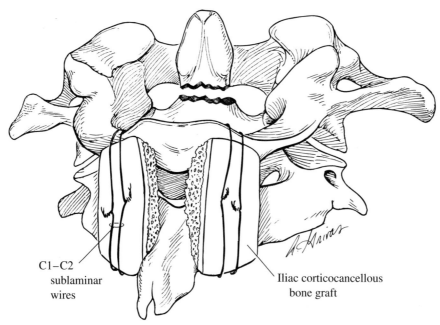

C1–C2
sublaminar
wires

Iliac corticocancellous
bone graft

*Figure 2–14*

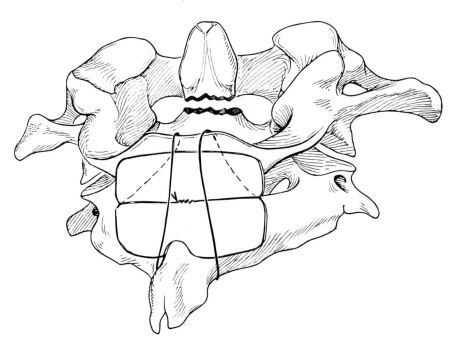

*Figure 2–15*

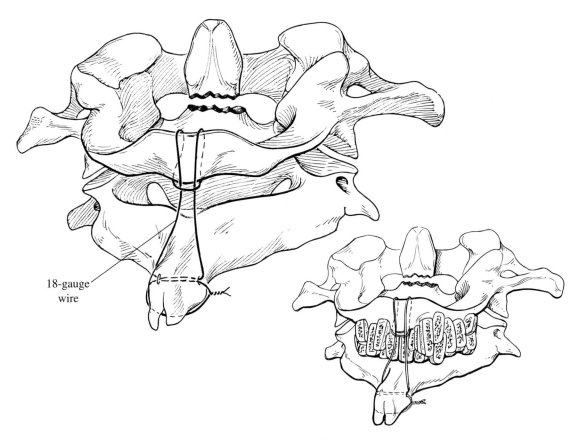

18-gauge
wire

*Figure 2–16*

29

# POSTERIOR UPPER CERVICAL PROCEDURES

The lateral mass screw technique utilizes a single screw placed in each lateral mass through the C1–C2 facet joint. The C1–C2 articulation is curetted prior to screw insertion. Avoid perforation of the spinal canal medially, injury to the vertebral artery laterally, or inadvertent perforation of the screw through the lateral mass anteriorly. Although this technique provides superior mechanical properties, there are hazards associated with it, and it should be reserved for special circumstances. The angle of insertion varies according to each patient's anatomy. The appropriate vertical inclination of the drill and length is determined fluoroscopically. The lateral spinal canal is palpated with a fine instrument; this serves as a guide to prevent medial perforation. The angle of drill placement and screw insertion is of critical importance in the C1–C2 area. The vertebral artery occupies the lateral and superolateral quadrants of the facet joint. Therefore, the screw should be positioned in the inner and upper aspects of the pedicle and laminar junction of C2, directed at an angle approximately 45° relative to the vertical, and in a nearly straight anteroposterior direction. Image-enhanced radiography performed during drilling and screw insertion aids in accurate screw placement (Fig. 2–17A,B,C).

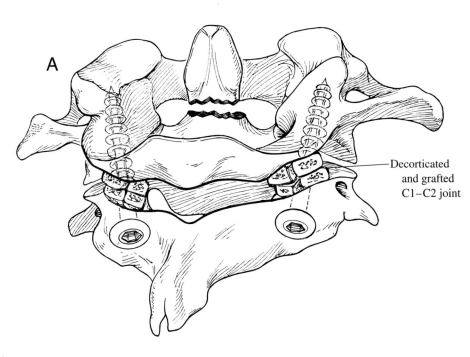

A

Decorticated
and grafted
C1–C2 joint

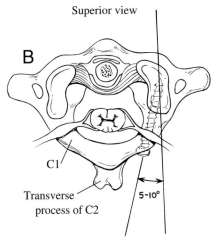

B

Superior view

C1

Transverse
process of C2

5-10°

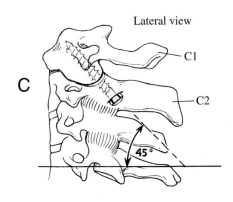

C

Lateral view

C1

C2

45°

*Figure 2–17*

31

# POSTERIOR UPPER CERVICAL PROCEDURES

The Clark technique utilizes a sculpted interposed one-piece C1–C2 graft secured with four sublaminar double-twisted 24-gauge wires at C1–C2. Although a bit more tedious, it can provide better rotational and translational control than other wire techniques (Fig. 2–18).

Supplemental polymethyl methacrylate (PMMA) applied to the posterior aspect of the wire and bone graft device can provide increased mechanical fixation. Its routine use must be tempered because of the potential complications of methyl methacrylate implantation in the posterior cervical spine. Excessive bulk of PMMA can make wound closure difficult and predispose to postoperative dehiscence (Fig. 2–19).

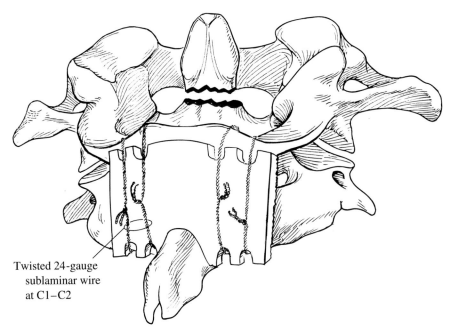

Twisted 24-gauge
sublaminar wire
at C1–C2

*Figure 2–18*

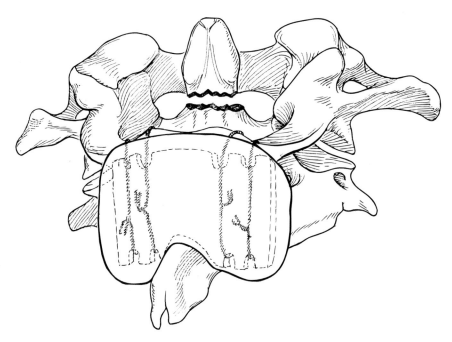

*Figure 2–19*

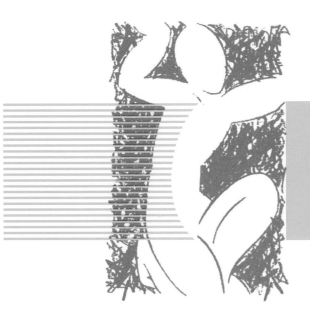

# 3

# APPLICATION
# OF A HALO

# APPLICATION OF A HALO

Anatomic studies of the human skull have shown that the optimal position for pin insertion is in the anterolateral and posterolateral aspects of the skull. Maximal thickness of the cortical bone of the skull is present at these locations (Fig. 3–1).

The anterolateral pins are placed lateral to the supraorbital notch, located in the midportion of the superior aspect of the orbit. This is a safe location and prevents penetration of the frontal sinus or the supraorbital nerve. Insertion of the pins within the substance of the temporalis muscle predisposes the patient to pin site infections or pain with mastication (Fig. 3–2A). In many patients, placement within the hairline is possible, thus reducing the visible scar (Fig. 3–2B).

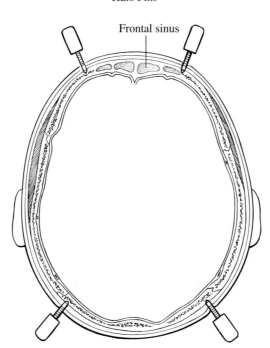

Halo Pins

Frontal sinus

*Figure 3–1*

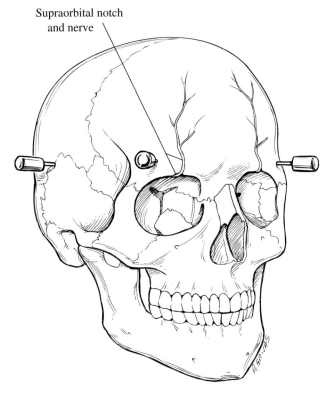

Supraorbital notch
and nerve

*Figure 3–2A*

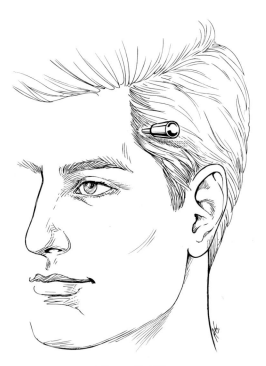

*Figure 3–2B*

37

# APPLICATION OF A HALO

Optimal placement of the halo ring, in the normocephalic individual, is below the equator of the skull, slightly above the superior margin of the brow, and approximately 1 cm above the tip of the pinna bilaterally. If the inferior margin of the ring is projected posteriorly, it is approximately 1 cm above the palpable inion protuberance. Great care should be used to assure that the ring is symmetrically placed in the anteroposterior, lateral, and rotational planes (Figs. 3–3, 3–4, and 3–5).

A halo head holder, shaped like a large spoon, is used to support the head, while simultaneously allowing free access to the entire perimeter of the skull. This narrow head support is placed under the patient's head, and the weight of the patient's torso stabilizes the support. This position permits thorough preparation of the pin sites and hair shampooing prior to ring application (Fig. 3–6).

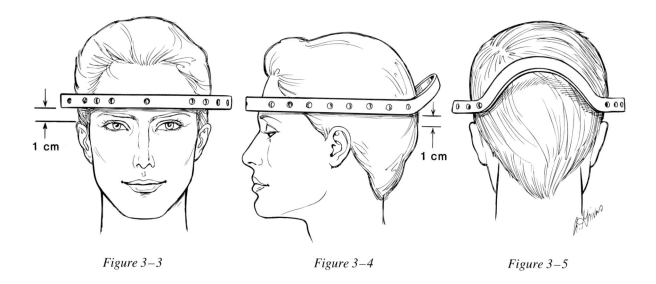

*Figure 3–3*          *Figure 3–4*          *Figure 3–5*

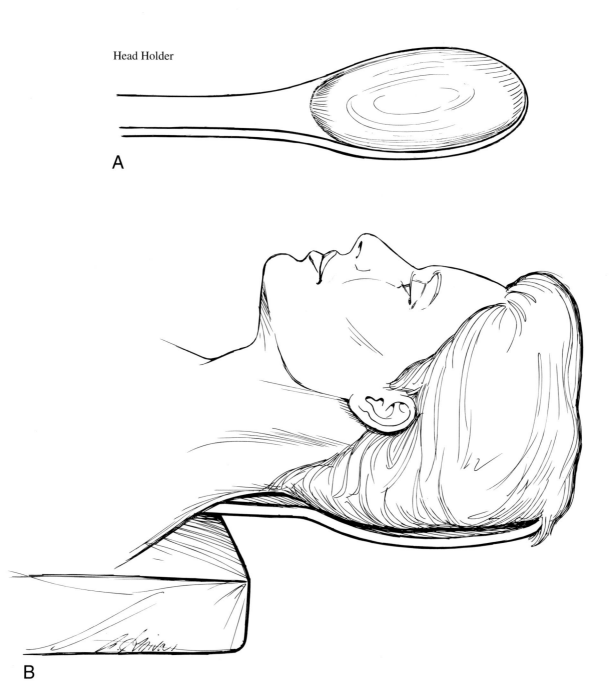

Head Holder

A

B

Figure 3–6

# APPLICATION OF A HALO

Strict asepsis should be maintained during ring application. The eyes are protected with multiple layers of cotton sponges and are gently taped shut. If the eyes are open during ring application, possible tethering of the eyelids in a semi-open position will likely require reapplication of the ring. Suitable clearance of the ring to the skull (2–3 cm) allows for easier access to the pin sites, pin care, and hair hygiene. Routine shaving of the posterior pin sites is not employed (Fig. 3–7).

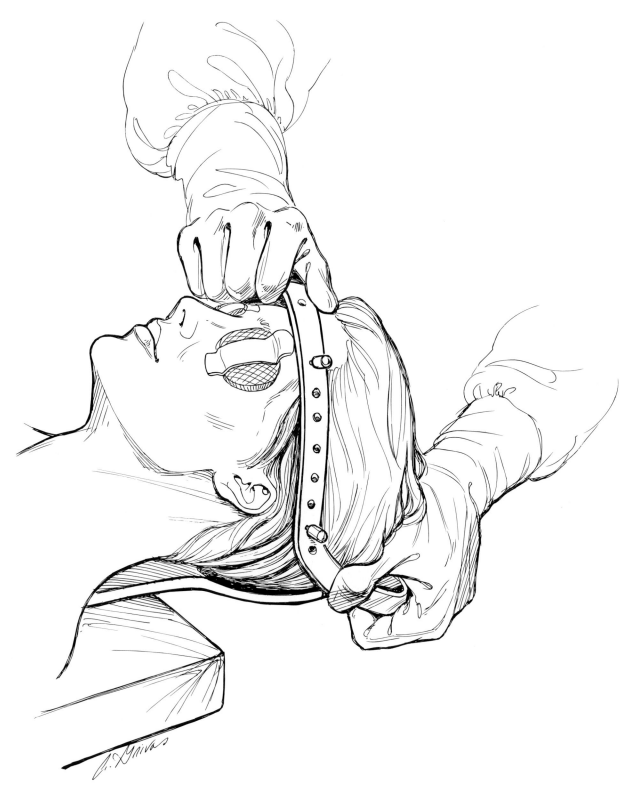

*Figure 3–7*

# APPLICATION OF A HALO

The pins are placed gently in the appropriate four quadrant locations and tightened in an alternating catty-corner fashion using finger-tight tension. Once solid pin-bone contact is obtained in all four pins, a sequential torquing routine (first to 2, then to 4, then to 6 in/lb) is applied. A careful two-hand technique is used to hold the screwdriver on the pins. This is to prevent the potential disastrous complication of a disengaged screwdriver lacerating the orbital contents (Fig. 3–8).

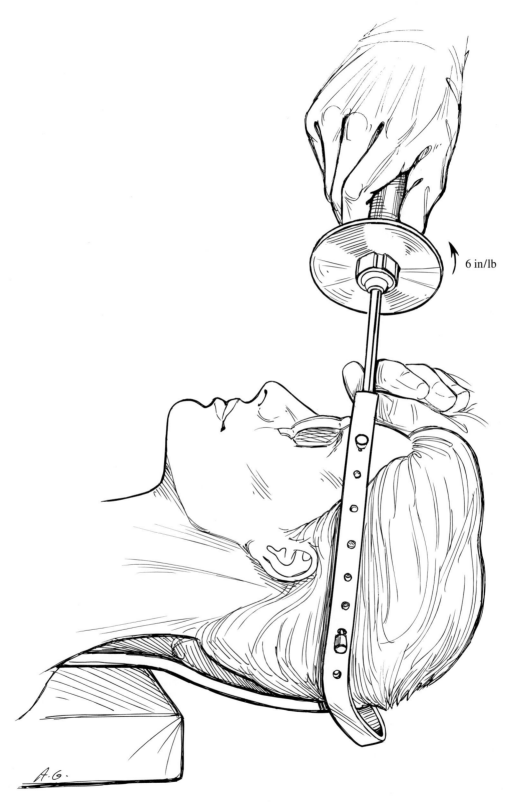

6 in/lb

*Figure 3–8*

43

# APPLICATION OF A HALO

Numerous commercially available halo-vest combinations are available; however, we have observed that a well-fashioned and well-molded halo cast provides the best clinical occipital and upper thoracic immobilization. In order to be effective, careful application of the cast with molding of the plaster to conform to the patient's torso and iliac crests is essential. If possible, the supporting upright structures are placed as far as possible from the midlateral axis to allow freer access to the cervical spine for radiography (Fig. 3–9).

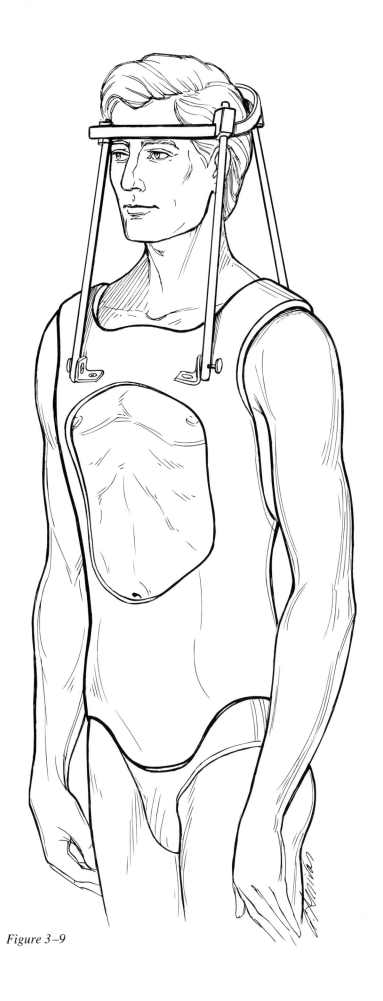

Figure 3–9

45

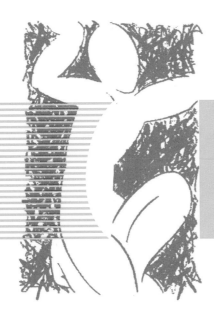

# 4

# ANTERIOR LOWER CERVICAL PROCEDURES

# Anterior Exposure (C3–T1)

For degenerative, post-traumatic, and neoplastic lesions of the cervical spine, the anterior approach is widely used. Proper positioning is essential. The head is rotated away from the incision site. The occiput is padded with a circular foam pillow with a center cutout, which cradles the skull and provides better stabilization. A rolled bath towel is placed transversely underneath the shoulders to slightly extend and stabilize the posterior shoulder musculature. Extremes of cervical extension (i.e., no more than what can be demonstrated by the awake patient preoperatively) should be carefully avoided to prevent increased spinal cord compression under anesthesia. Use adhesive tape to gently retract the shoulder to allow more thorough access to the lower cervical and cervical thoracic region (Fig. 4–1).

The carotid tubercle, a lateral extension of the transverse process of C6, is an important surgical landmark. The cricoid cartilage is often palpable and is located at the C6 level as well. The location of the transverse incision for anterior exposure of the anterior cervical spine based on finger widths above the clavicle (2 fingerbreadths for C6–7 disk space, 2 1/2 for the C5–6 level, and 3 for the C4–5 level, the three most common areas necessary for anterior cervical surgery) tends to be less reliable in patients with short, heavy necks; excessive obesity; or thoracic hyperkyphosis (Fig. 4–2).

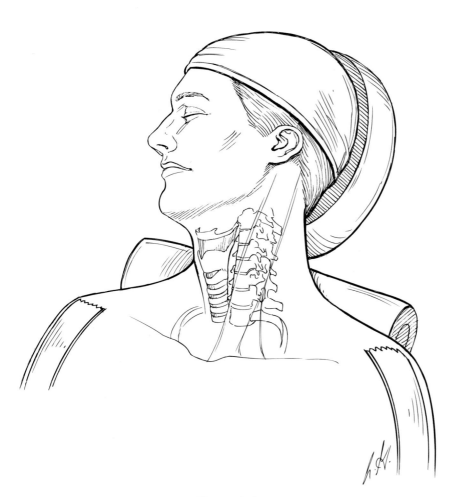

*Figure 4–1*

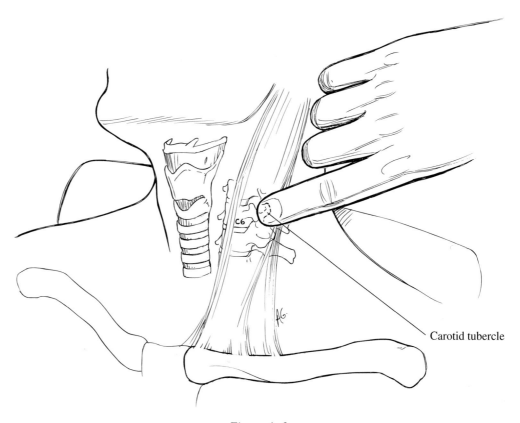

Carotid tubercle

*Figure 4–2*

49

# ANTERIOR LOWER CERVICAL PROCEDURES

Transverse incisions in line with naturally occurring wrinkles or skin creases yield the best cosmetic results. The incision should be carried slightly beyond the midline of the sternocleidomastoid muscle. Extension of the incision beyond the lateral border of the sternocleidomastoid does not appreciably increase the overall exposure. The subcutaneous tissue is divided in line with the skin incision. The platysma muscle can be divided along the axis of the incision or its fibers bluntly dissected and its medial lateral divisions retracted (Fig. 4–3).

The superficial layer of the cervical fascia, which contains the platysma muscle, is then split in line with the skin incision. This usually exposes one or two large branches of the anterior jugular venous system. These can be moved and protected with retractors or divided between ties. The invaginating fascia on the anterior border of the sternocleidomastoid muscle is then released proximally and distally to allow for further lateral retraction (Fig. 4–4).

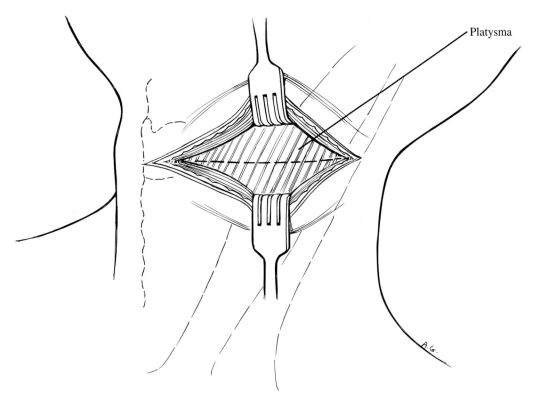

Figure 4–3

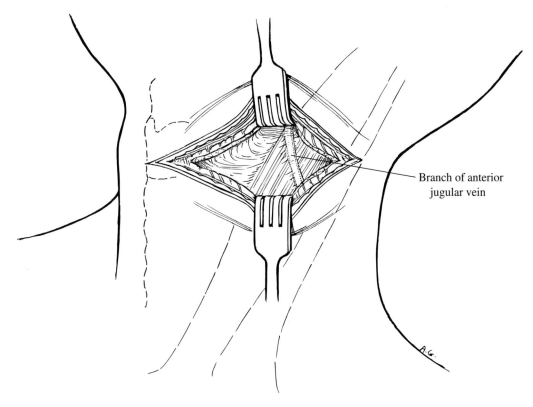

Figure 4–4

51

# ANTERIOR LOWER CERVICAL PROCEDURES

Using blunt digital dissection, the common carotid neurovascular structure is palpated and gently retracted laterally with the surgeon's index finger. A smooth right angle retractor is used to retract the tracheoesophageal structures medially, which causes tension to the middle layer of the deep cervical fascia. The fascia is dissected in a linear longitudinal fashion. Transverse dissection endangers the traversing superior or inferior thyroid arteries. In asthenic individuals, this dissection can often be done digitally (Fig. 4–5).

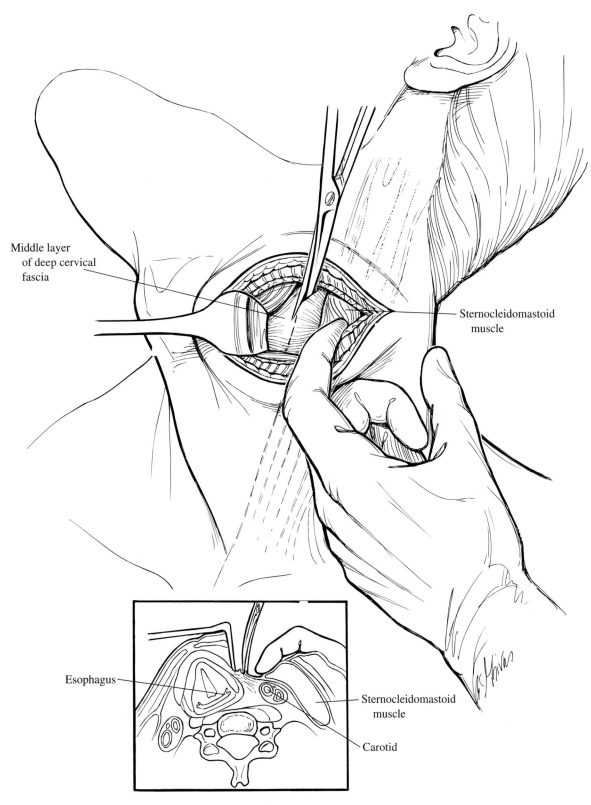

Middle layer
of deep cervical
fascia

Sternocleidomastoid
muscle

Esophagus

Sternocleidomastoid
muscle

Carotid

*Figure 4–5*

# ANTERIOR LOWER CERVICAL PROCEDURES

Once the middle layer of cervical fascia has been divided, the pretracheal and the prevertebral layers of deep cervical fascia can be seen overlying the anterior cervical spine. These are split longitudinally to allow for direct exposure and surgical access to the vertebral body and disk spaces. The anterior longitudinal ligament is incised with an electric cautery pencil, or a small periosteal elevator can be used but may promote active emissary vein bleeding (Fig. 4–6).

The inserting longus colli muscle is dissected in a medial, bilateral fashion and retracted laterally until the anterior surface of the vertebral body is seen to curve posteriorly. Further dissection laterally can compromise the vertebral artery traversing through the foramen transversarium or damage the sympathetic plexus (Fig. 4–7).

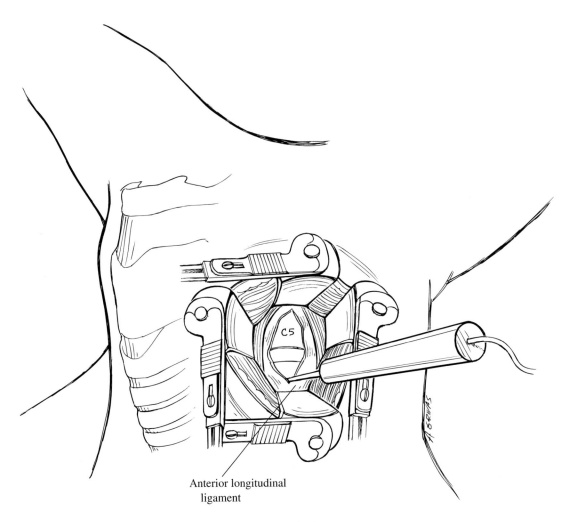

Anterior longitudinal
ligament

*Figure 4–6*

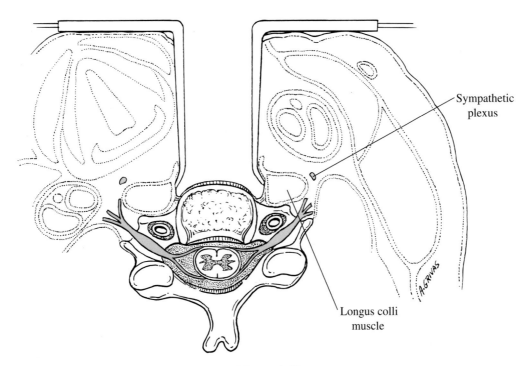

Sympathetic
plexus

Longus colli
muscle

*Figure 4–7*

# *Anterior Diskectomy and Spur Removal*

A surgical headlight and magnifying loupes can improve the visibility and the safety of the diskectomy and nerve root decompression. The disk annulus is sharply incised throughout the lateral width of the exposed disk anteriorly (Fig. 4–8). The disk is removed piecemeal using a combination of pituitary rongeurs and curettes. Care is used to preserve the cortical end plate because perforation of that structure can lead to occasional bone bleeding, particularly in osteoporotic individuals. Also, with an intact cortical end plate the intervertebral disk space spreader can be placed on a strong resilient surface (Fig. 4–9A). The posterior longitudinal ligament is cautiously approached and all disk material thoroughly removed. The removal of disk material is not complete until the uncinate joints (joints of Luschka) are well visualized bilaterally (Fig. 4–9B).

In cases in which it is advisable to remove a large osteophyte, a small high-speed carbide burr is used to thin the majority of the osteophyte. The posterior longitudinal ligament is then cautiously approached. Once the bone is sufficiently thinned, a small, straight or angled curette is used to pry away the remaining thin shelf of bone. Osteophyte removal is not necessary in the majority of routine cervical spine diskectomies (Fig. 4–10).

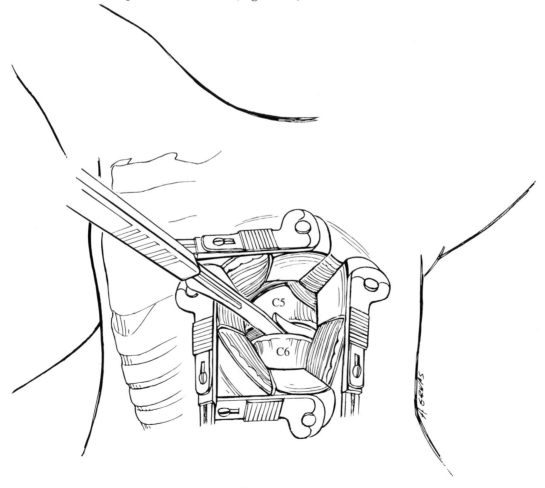

C5

C6

*Figure 4–8*

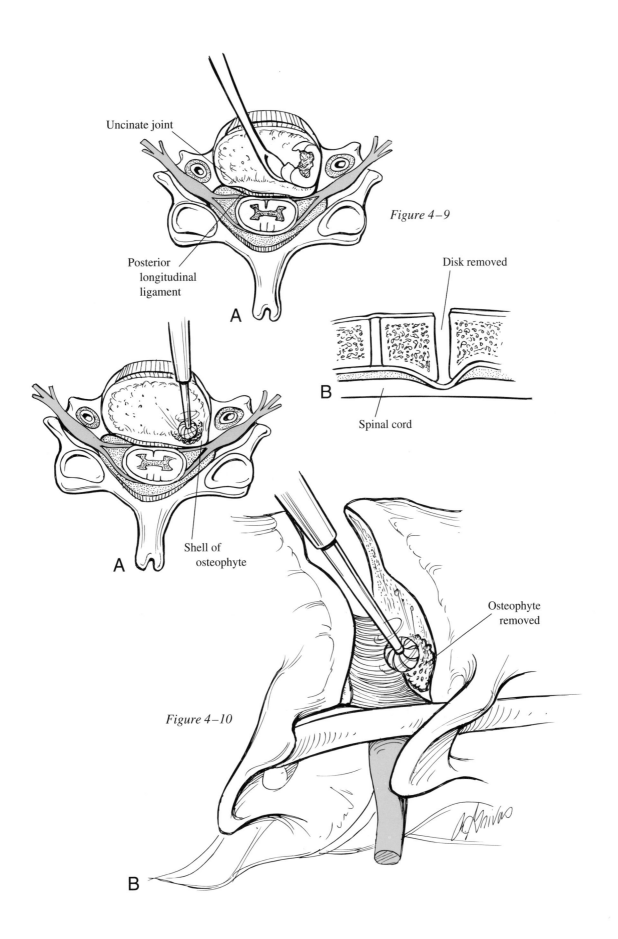

Uncinate joint

Posterior
longitudinal
ligament

A

*Figure 4–9*

Disk removed

B

Spinal cord

Shell of
osteophyte

A

*Figure 4–10*

Osteophyte
removed

B

57

# Anterior Diskectomy and One Level Fusion

## Tricortical Graft (Smith–Robinson) Technique

When performing an anterior fusion with a tricortical graft (Smith–Robinson) technique, an elliptical or straight-side cutting carbide burr is used to decorticate the end plate and create a planar bone grafting surface on the superior and inferior end plates. This provides an ideal fusion surface, optimizes the area for arthrodesis by decortication, and allows for easier insertion of the graft (Fig. 4–11).

The disk space is then gently distracted by manual axial traction of the head by the anesthesiologist or with a mechanical disk space spreader. The graft is inserted without undue impaction caused by the use of a drift. A drift, and hammering, could cause stress risers in the graft with the potential for graft collapse in the postoperative period (Fig. 4–12).

The graft should nearly span the entire disk space, be of sufficient height to gently distract the disk space, and be of sufficient depth so that the cortical margin of the graft is recessed slightly below the anterior cortical margin of the inferior and superior disk spaces. Graft extrusion should rarely occur if the graft is of appropriate length and is inserted without undue mechanical tension (Fig. 4–13).

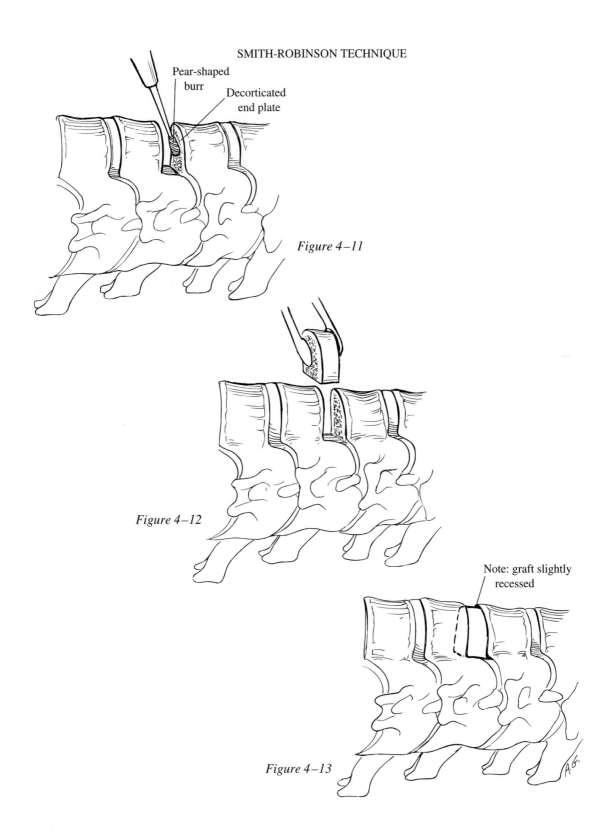

Pear-shaped
burr

Decorticated
end plate

*Figure 4–11*

*Figure 4–12*

Note: graft slightly
recessed

*Figure 4–13*

## HOLE AND DOWEL (CLOWARD) TECHNIQUE

With a hole and dowel (Cloward) technique, a bicortical graft is harvested from the anterior iliac crest with a slightly oversized hole saw. After gentle distraction of the disk space, the graft (plug) is inserted into a slightly undersized drill hole at the disk level to be fused. The Cloward technique is not as biomechanically sound as the other reconstruction because the relatively cancellous grafts are placed within the softer midvertebral cancellous bone. In osteoporotic individuals, fusions are prone to collapse and cause kyphosis (Fig. 4–14).

## KEYSTONE (SIMMONS) TECHNIQUE

In the keystone (Simmons) technique, a slightly trapezoid-shaped, cortical cancellous strut is gently impacted into an angulated recess in the vertebral bodies above and below the area of diskectomy. This technique provides good mechanical interdigitation of the graft and has a theoretically decreased risk of graft extrusion (Fig. 4–15).

## CLOWARD TECHNIQUE

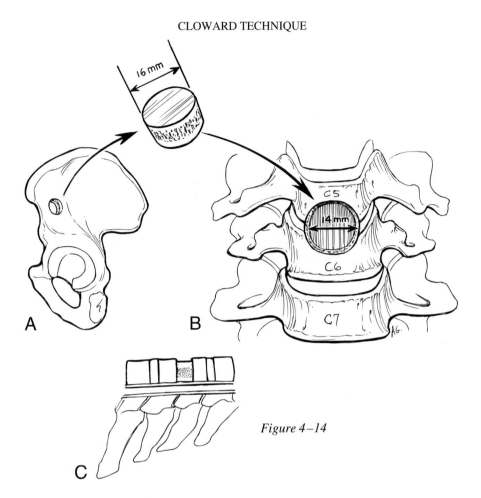

*Figure 4–14*

## SIMMONS TECHNIQUE

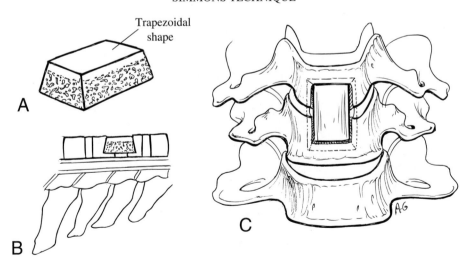

*Figure 4–15*

61

# Anterior Vertebrectomy with Decompression

A standard anterolateral approach to the cervical spine is carried out. The appropriate vertebral body levels are identified radiographically and clinically. The longus colli bilaterally is subperiosteally dissected laterally in order to positively identify the lateral and the posterior descent of the vertebral bodies. This identifies the lateral extent of dissection (Fig. 4–16A; see also Figs. 4–1 through 4–7).

If self-retaining retractors are used, they should be carefully placed under the longus colli muscle. The placement of toothed retractors should be done under direct vision. A thorough diskectomy involving all the disks around the decompression is carried out. After removal of the disks, a Leksell rongeur is used to quickly remove the anterior 5/8 of the vertebral body (Fig. 4–16B). A coarse high-speed burr is used to thin and expediently remove the next 1/4 of the vertebral body until the posterior cortex is seen (Fig. 4–17).

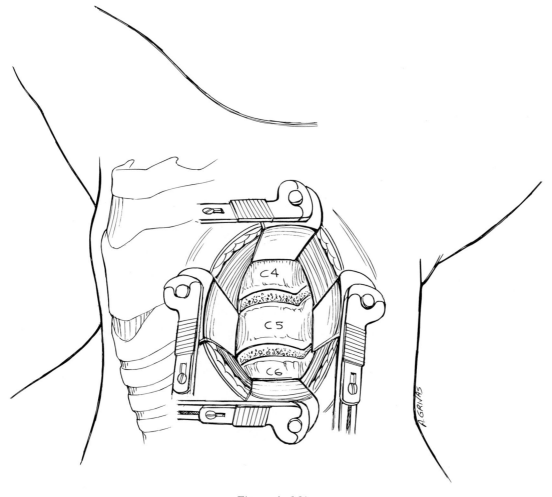

*Figure 4–16A*

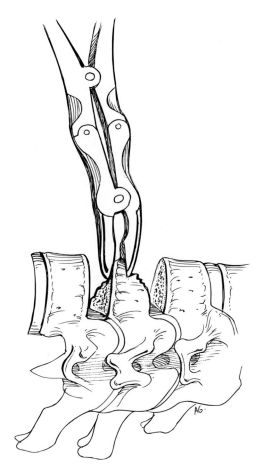

Figure 4–16B

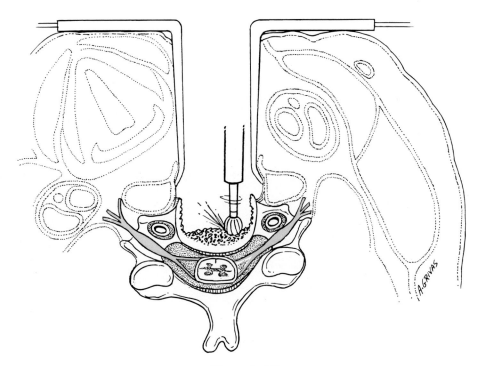

Figure 4–17

63

# ANTERIOR LOWER CERVICAL PROCEDURES

The removal of bone, osteophyte, and disk material must be done in a strictly anteroposterior direction (Fig. 4–18).

Following this, a high-speed diamond burr under continuous water irrigation is used to thin and perforate the posterior cortex. The vertebral artery runs approximately in the mid-third of the height of the vertebral body and care is used for undermining with a small (1 or 2 mm) diamond burr laterally. Injury to the vertebral artery can cause a difficult surgical problem and usually requires ligation for control (Fig. 4–19).

The posterior cortex can then be removed with small curettes pulling the thinned cortex into the surgically created trough (Fig. 4–20).

If needed, additional decompression of the uncinate joints at the levels of the lateral recesses can be carried out with a small diamond burr. This must be done carefully to avoid vertebral artery laceration (Fig. 4–21). The base of the pedicle can often be palpated, which serves to indicate that the lateral extent of decompression has been achieved.

The width of the decompression is determined from the width between the medial aspect of the uncinate joints bilaterally.

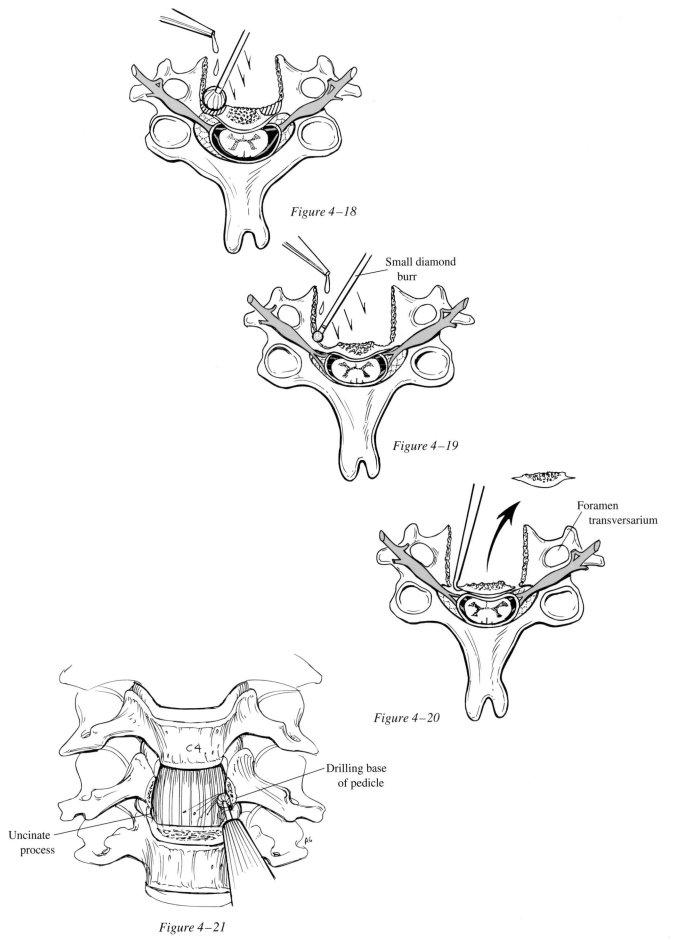

*Figure 4–18*

Small diamond
burr

*Figure 4–19*

Foramen
transversarium

*Figure 4–20*

C4

Drilling base
of pedicle

Uncinate
process

*Figure 4–21*

# ILIAC STRUT RECONSTRUCTION

After completing a single level or two-level vertebrectomy, a tricortical iliac crest strut reconstruction is often suitable. A tricortical iliac strut is harvested with a power saw under continuous water irrigation (Fig. 4–22A).

Small depressions in the inferior and superior vertebral body endplates (approximately the radius of an index fingertip) are made with either curettes or a large carbide burr (Fig. 4–22B).

The graft is tamped in (with deliberate control using small drifts and gentle mallet strokes). This is the most uncontrolled portion of the procedure and requires great care. The cortical margins are inserted posteriorly. The superior end of the graft is inserted and tamped superiorly to lock it into the upper endplate depression. The inferior lip of the graft is then driven posteriorly. Strong skeletal traction, via a halo ring or Gardner–Wells bow, is temporarily increased to 40 or 50 lb to aid in cervical spine distraction and ease the graft insertion. If impacted too vigorously, the graft will fracture in osteoporotic individuals and increase the likelihood of iatrogenic neurologic injury (Fig. 4–22C).

After the graft is seated, the traction is discontinued and a radiograph is taken immediately to verify appropriate graft positioning.

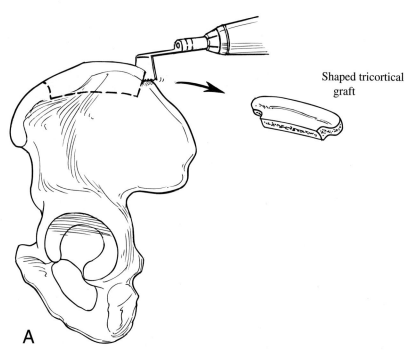

Shaped tricortical graft

A

*Figure 4–22*

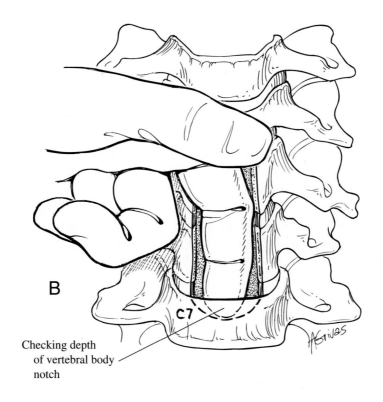

B

Checking depth
of vertebral body
notch

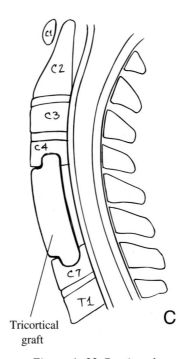

Tricortical
graft

C

*Figure 4–22 Continued*

# FIBULAR STRUT RECONSTRUCTION

A tricortical graft from the pelvis generally can span two spinal segments but not much more because of a curvature mismatch between the cervical spine lordosis and the iliac crest contour. Therefore, for more than two and one-half levels, a mid-diaphyseal fibular graft is necessary. This may be either an allograft, which saves operative time and bone graft donor site morbidity, or an autograft, which may be obtained under tourniquet control (see Chapter 15, Section B). If somatosensory-evoked potentials are being used during the decompression, sterile electrodes facilitate positioning, patient preparation, and draping of the lower extremity. A drill hole in the graft along its edge aids in precise graft insertion (Fig. 4–23A). The sequence of graft introduction and insertion is similar to the ilial strut placement (Figs. 4–23B and 4–24). Additional cancellous grafting around the strut can be added as needed for arthrodesis (Fig. 4–25).

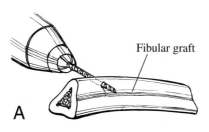

Fibular graft

A

*Figure 4–23*

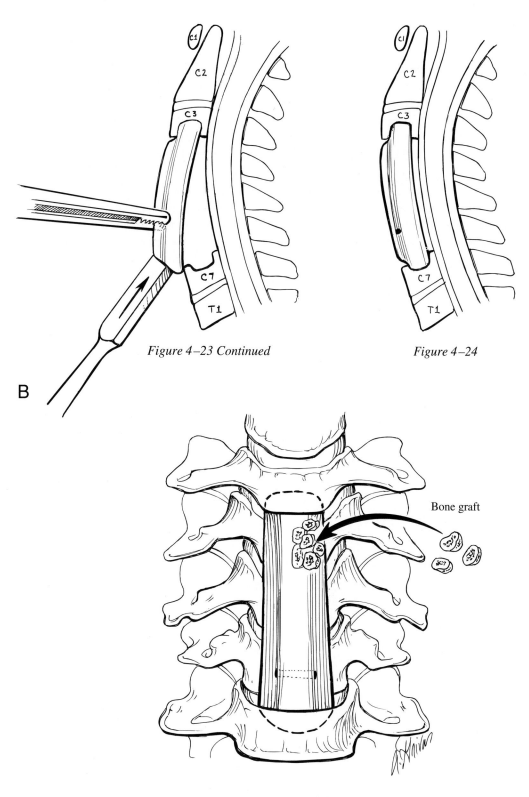

B

*Figure 4–23 Continued*

*Figure 4–24*

Bone graft

*Figure 4–25*

69

## METHYLMETHACRYLATE RECONSTRUCTION

Under special circumstances in patients with a limited life span who have tumorous involvement of vertebral bodies, polymethylmethacrylate (PMMA) may be used in spinal reconstructions. The dura and posterior longitudinal ligament are protected from thermal injury with several layers of Gelfoam. Small stabilizing K wires are placed in the vertebrae above and below the decompression (Fig. 4–26). The PMMA is mixed according to the manufacturer's instructions and used in the doughy state. It is gently packed within the interstices of the decompression trough as well as above and below the sculpted endplates of the vertebral bodies. It is continuously irrigated with cool saline to protect against thermal damage to the delicate neural structures posteriorly. Concomitant posterior stabilization should be considered if such a technique is employed. In patients with an uncertain prognosis, PMMA is best used in reconstructions requiring resistance to compression. Supplemental bone arthrodesis is needed in all cases for long-term stabilization (Fig. 4–27).

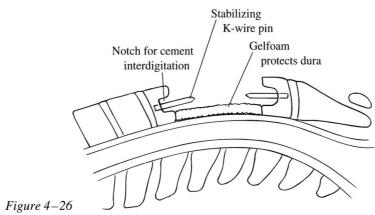

Figure 4–26

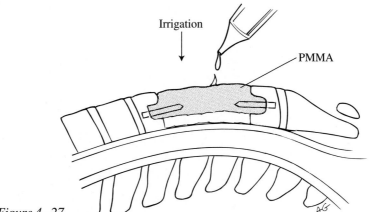

Figure 4–27

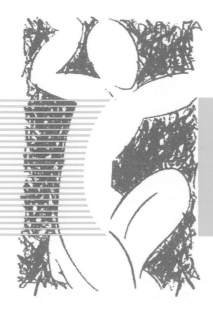

# 5

# POSTERIOR LOWER CERVICAL PROCEDURES

# Basic Exposure

The midline posterior exposure is the most common approach. Strong resilient retractors, such as Gelpe retractors, are used to maintain continuous retraction of the lateral soft tissue. This aids in identifying the meandering ligamentum nuchae and helps minimize blood loss. Do not advance into the paraspinal muscle because of the risks of denervation and the potential for kyphotic deformities (Fig. 5–1).

Once the tips of the spinous processes at the appropriate levels have been identified and confirmed radiographically, a subperiosteal dissection is carried out using medium-sized Cobb elevators. The muscles should be swept laterally, using the sharp edge of the elevator. In situations with incompetent posterior elements due to trauma, tumor, or infection, the spinous process should be stabilized with a grasping clamp and the dissection done sharply with a scalpel (Fig. 5–2).

Thorough hemostasis is essential. The dissection should not be excessively lateral, because of the potential to denervate the posterior erector spinal muscles. If an arthrodesis is to be done, dissection should be carried until the lateral aspect of the lateral masses is clearly visible bilaterally. Constant lateral retraction of the muscle by angled cerebellar retractors, or deep Gelpe retractors, aids in the dissection. The retractors should be adjusted often. At this point, bleeding should be minimal. The dissection should not expose facet joints or lamina or disrupt the interspinous ligaments adjacent to the proposed areas of decompression and fusion lest iatrogenic injury to those areas occurs. Taking extra time to develop a wide bilateral exposure and obtaining hemostasis ultimately speeds the operative procedure (Figs. 5–3 and 5–4).

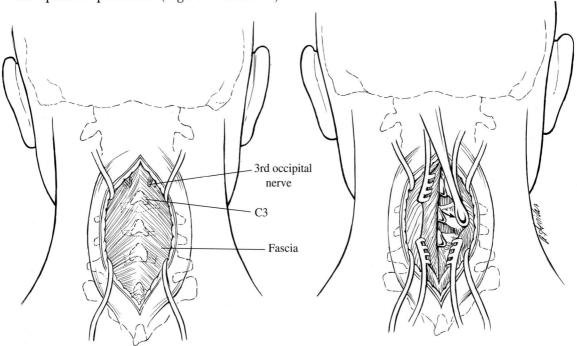

*Figure 5–1*                    *Figure 5–2*

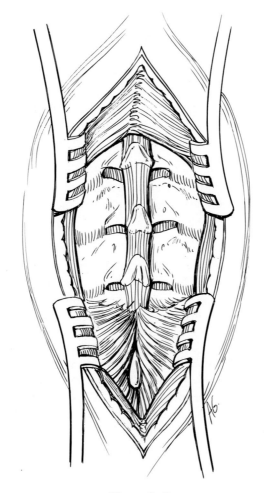

*Figure 5–3*

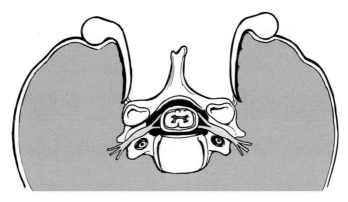

*Figure 5–4*

# *Hemilaminectomy*

## Soft Disk Excision with Foraminotomy

A unilateral exposure of the cervical spine at the level to be decompressed is carried out. A confirming lateral radiograph, with a metallic marker in place, is the only way to confidently assess the appropriate spinal level. Minimal resection of bone, ligamentum flavum, and facet joint is necessary in most soft disk herniations (Fig. 5–5).

A high-speed diamond burr, under continuous water irrigation, is used to thin and perforate the inner laminar cortex. A small portion of the upper and lower lamina and the medial facet joint are resected. Meticulous hemostasis of the epidural vessels is obtained by bipolar cautery and judicious use of Gelfoam packing (Fig. 5–6).

The takeoff of the cervical nerve root is clearly identified and additional interposing tissue, either the ligamentum flavum or facet capsule, is cautiously removed with a small curette. Operative trauma to the spinal nerve root should be avoided at all times, and this includes the insertion of a Kerrison punch into the nerve root foramen (Fig. 5–7).

Limited and judicious retraction of the nerve root is possible once thorough exposure of the nerve root above and below its takeoff has been carried out by sufficient resection of bone and facet joint capsule. A typical herniated cervical disk is present in the inferior portion of the axilla of the nerve root, and with gentle superior retraction of the nerve root, the fragment should be easily accessible. The fragment can be removed with small curettes or a pituitary-grasping forceps. At no time should instruments be inserted underneath the spinal cord lest iatrogenic damage occurs (Fig. 5–8).

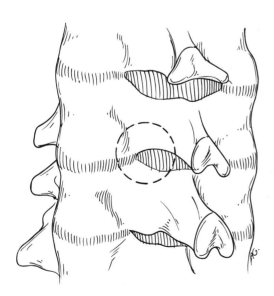

*Figure 5–5*

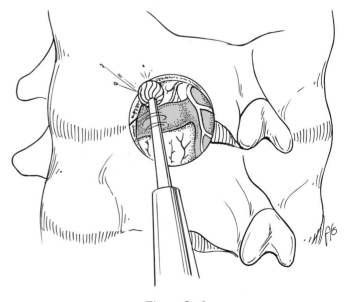

*Figure 5–6*

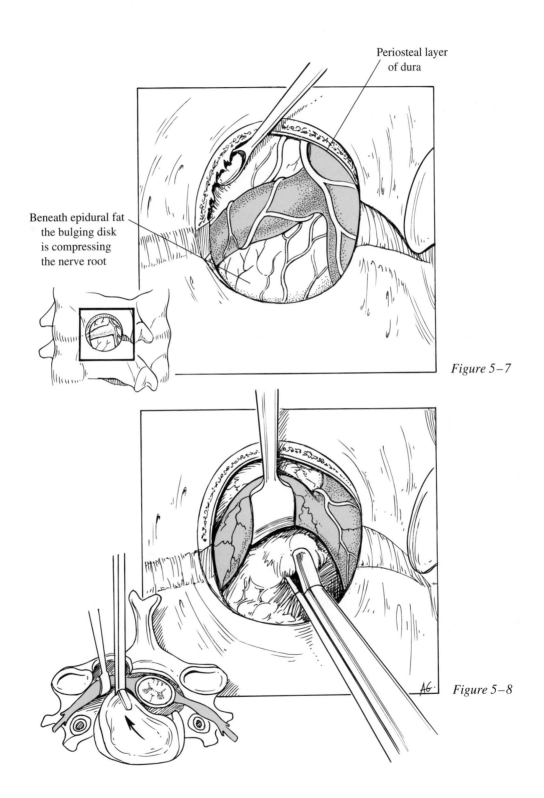

Periosteal layer
of dura

Beneath epidural fat
the bulging disk
is compressing
the nerve root

*Figure 5–7*

*Figure 5–8*

77

# BONE SPUR REMOVAL

A unilateral exposure of the posterior cervical spine, similar to that used for soft disk excision, is carried out. Routine removal of a spondolytic spur is controversial. Often sufficient foraminotomy, by resection of greater degrees of the lateral mass and facet joint, allows for suitable nerve root decompression with subsequent relief of radiculopathy. Spur removal is facilitated by the use of small-angled, reverse-directed currettes and working in a direction away from the spinal cord and exiting nerve roots, as described above for the foraminotomy for soft disk excision. Motorized burrs have a greater risk of iatrogenic injury to the root or cord. Surgical loupe magnification, or an operative microscope, facilitates dissection (Fig. 5-9).

Bone spur removal is controversial. Some authorities feel that an adequate foraminotomy by sufficient resection of the hypertrophic facet joint capsule and osteoarthritic spur is sufficient for relief of radiculopathy. The disk is degenerate and therefore stable. Others feel the bone spur provides an irritative focus for ongoing low levels of symptoms and, therefore, removal would provide an optimal environment for relief.

The sitting position facilitates dissection by less hydrostatic distention of the epidural veins and blood drainage away from the operative field. Surgical loupe magnification or an operative microscope facilitates dissection.

A unilateral exposure is achieved; placement of hemilaminectomy cervical retractors facilitates exposures with minimal skin and muscle dissection. A radiograph is obtained to confirm the operative level. The confluence of the lamina in the facet joint is thinned, utilizing a high-speed carbide burr. The inner table of the lamina is identified by a gradual exposure of the cortical bone; the cortical shell is removed from the spinal canal using fine, small-angled straight and reversed-directed curettes. The working direction is always away from the spinal canal and exiting nerve roots, as described for the keyhole foraminotomy for soft disk excision. Introduction of motorized burrs into the spinal canal and the nerve root region has a great risk of iatrogenic injury to the spinal cord and nerve root. With judicious use of small, reverse-angle curettes and suitable mobilization of the nerve root to allow gentle cephalad traction, the osteophytic spur can be removed. Placement of small pledgets of Gelfoam proximal and distal to the area of the dissection aids in hemostasis. Judicious use of bipolar cautery is recommended in order to avoid thermal injury to the nerve root. The end of a blunt tip probe should pass easily into the nerve root foramen to ensure an adequate lateral nerve root decompression.

Spur Removal

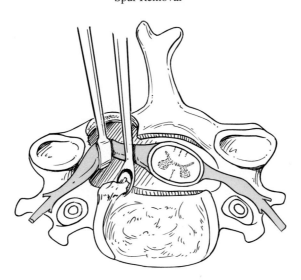

*Figure 5–9*

# *Laminectomy*

## CENTRAL CANAL STENOSIS

A wide bilateral exposure of the posterior elements from the inferior portion of C2 through the upper portion of T1 is carried out. Great care is used to preserve the integrity of the facet joint capsules bilaterally. The muscular attachments inserting on C2 and T1 are preserved to maintain an important insertion point for the erector spinal musculature. Bilateral subperiosteal exposure of the muscle, with limited use of unipolar cautery, helps preserve the innervation to the muscle and avoid mechanical derangement and an increased likelihood of postlaminectomy kyphosis. Periodically, the self-retaining retractors should be released to allow muscle reperfusion (Fig. 5–10).

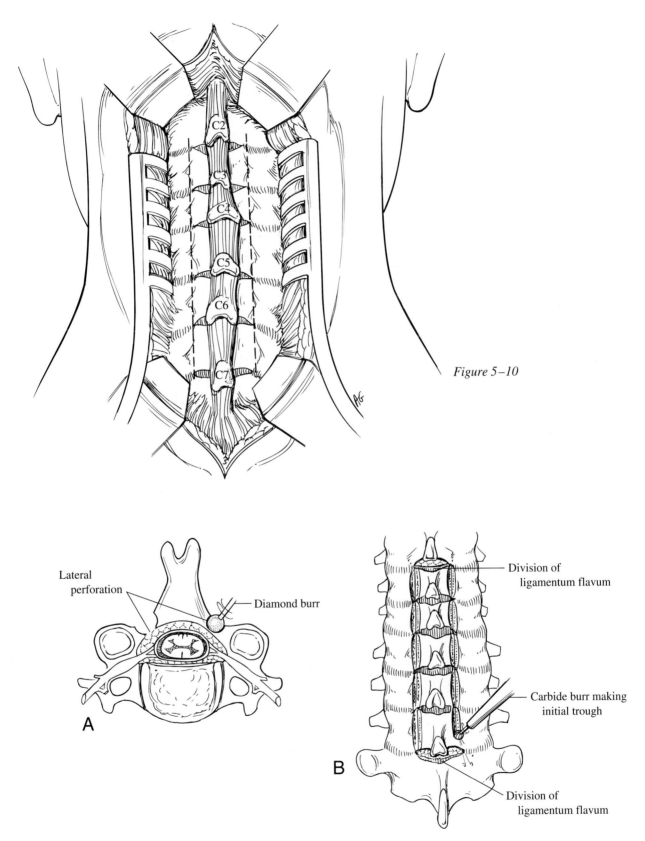

*Figure 5–10*

Lateral
perforation

Diamond burr

A

Division of
ligamentum flavum

Carbide burr making
initial trough

Division of
ligamentum flavum

B

*Figure 5–11*

The laminectomy is carried out by first developing the interval between the junction of the lamina and the facet joint with a high-speed carbide burr. This is done with loupe magnification and a headlight or a microscope visualization. The inner laminar cortex is cautiously approached. A slightly smaller radius high-speed diamond burr is used to perforate the inner laminar cortex. This frees the lamina from its osseous insertions laterally. The ligamentum flavum is then divided in its most proximal and distal insertions (Fig. 5–11).

Grasping the inferior spinous process, the lateral insertions of the ligamentum flavum are divided sequentially and the laminectomy is carried out en bloc. At no time is any instrument introduced into the spinal canal lest an iatrogenic spinal cord problem result. Hemostasis is obtained with gelatin sponge, tamponade, or bipolar cautery, as necessary. Limited use of bipolar cautery is recommended (Fig. 5–12).

When preoperative studies indicate facet hypertrophy and signs or symptoms of nerve root compression exist due to spondylosis or disk material, a foraminotomy, similar to the keyhole technique previously described (Fig. 5–13; see Figs. 5–5 and 5–6), may be carried out. This is done by medial facet resection with burrs or a sharp fine curette. A secure closure of the ligamentum nuchae is carried out over a small, flexible suction drainage system. Suction wound evaluation decreases the likelihood of a postoperative hematoma.

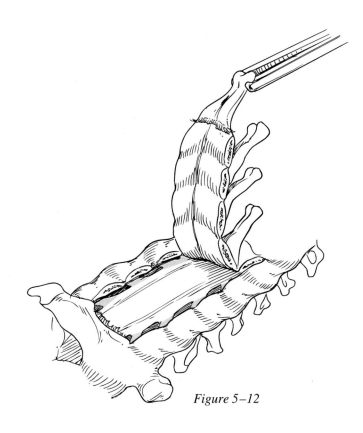

*Figure 5–12*

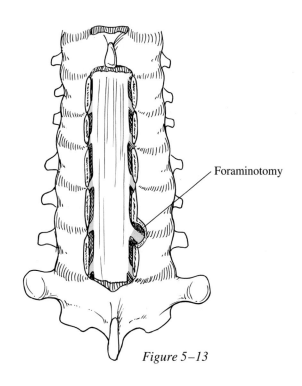

Foraminotomy

*Figure 5–13*

# LAMINAPLASTY

A standard laminectomy exposure is carried out, avoiding insult to the facet joints. Using a high-speed carbide burr, the outer cortex and the cancellous bone of the lamina are removed bilaterally at the junction of the lamina and the facet joint. Using a diamond burr, under continuous water irrigation, the inner laminar cortex is perforated on one side only (Fig. 5–14A).

There are a variety of techniques for laminaplasty. One technique is an alternating open door method in which a set of lamina, generally the upper three (C3, C4, and C5), are opened on one side and the inferior lamina, generally C6 and C7, are opened on the other side. The same side opening should be done in those who required a concomitant ipsilateral foraminotomy. For instance, if there is a left C7 radiculopathy due to herniated disk or spur and a left C6–C7 foraminotomy is necessary, the left side gutter is perforated with the smaller diamond burr at C6 and C7 and the remaining lamina are hinged upward on the right side (Fig. 5–14B).

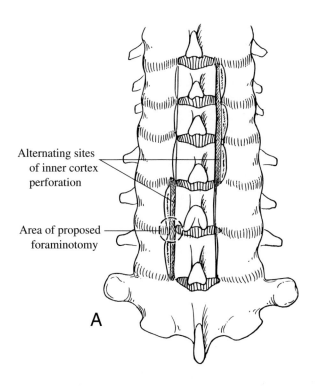

Alternating sites
of inner cortex
perforation

Area of proposed
foraminotomy

A

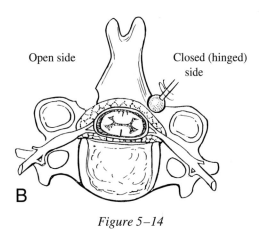

Open side

Closed (hinged)
side

B

*Figure 5–14*

# POSTERIOR LOWER CERVICAL PROCEDURES

Before the osteotomy is carried out, the spinous processes are removed. For sufficient opening, the ligamentum flavum is divided between the C2-C3, the C5-C6, and the C7-T1 lamina. Failure to do so will result in closure of the open door or difficulty in obtaining sufficient opening (Fig. 5-15).

The alternating door laminaplasty is held open by multiple stout sutures. For example, a suture would be placed through a tiny drill hole in the inferolateral corner of the left side of C5, and another hole is placed through the superolateral lamina of C6. A stout nonabsorbable suture is then passed through these drill holes twice to approximate respective edges of the lamina. This maneuver effectively maintains the hinges in an open position. Additional tethering sutures are placed through the spinous process of T1 and the inferolateral open side of the C7 and through the C2-C3 junction (Fig. 5-16A,B).

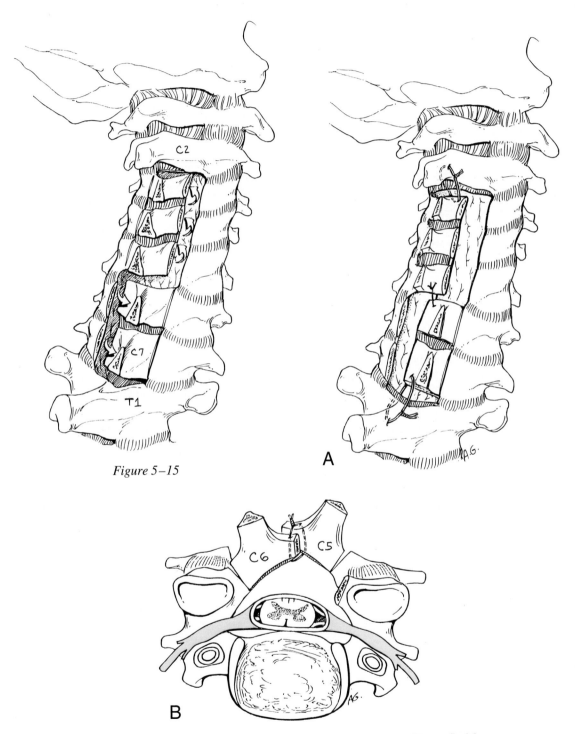

Figure 5–15

A

B

Figure 5–16

# *Arthrodesis*

## BASIC, NO INTERNAL FIXATION

There are numerous ways to provide a solid cervical spine arthrodesis. A wide bilateral exposure is carried out only in those areas to be fused. The facet joint capsules are opened, and the facet joint cartilage is removed with fine curettes and small motorized air drills. Cartilage removal should be restricted to the dorsal 1/3 of the joint to avoid iatrogenic injury to the exiting nerve root below (Fig. 5–17).

If an onlay fusion is performed, the posterior elements are then decorticated with a high-speed burr, and substantial grafting with autogenous bone is carried out. Careful placement of the bone graft is necessary to prevent migration of the grafts during wound closure at the inferior aspect of the fusion to avoid an undesirable iatrogenic extension of fusion (Fig. 5–18).

## KIRSCHNER WIRE TECHNIQUE

For additional fixation, a threaded Kirschner (K) wire is inserted percutaneously through the base of the spinous process. The wire is cut off and a malleable 18 or 20 gauge stainless steel monofilament wire is tied around the K wire in a figure 8 style to tether the posterior elements. Supplemental autogenous bone grafting is used. Occasionally, the threaded K wire can be used to pierce and transfix the cortical cancellous slab, and the bone is included in the overall mechanical construction (Fig. 5–19).

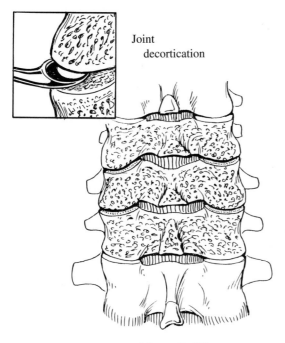

Joint decortication

*Figure 5–17*

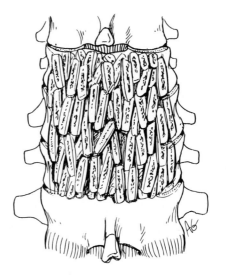

*Figure 5–18*

THREADED KIRSCHNER WIRES

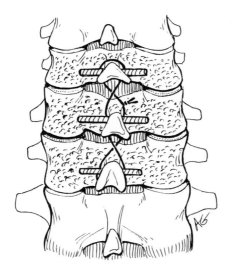

*Figure 5–19*

89

## SIMPLE MIDLINE WIRE TECHNIQUE

For the simple midline wire technique, holes are made at the junction of the base of the spinous process and lamina with a small right angle dental drill or large towel clip. This wire is then wrapped in a figure 8 around the spinous processes. It is important to pass the inferior and superior loops around the stronger cortical bone of the spinous processes, by a cerclage technique, at the ends of the fusion area. This technique helps improve the resistance of the wire to pull-through type of failure (Fig. 5–20).

## TRIPLE WIRE TECHNIQUE

In addition to the standard midline tethering wire, a triple wire technique can be used to incorporate corticocancellous strips over the area for arthrodesis (Fig. 5–21A). This increases the overall effectiveness of the fixation. A possible disadvantage of this technique is that a slightly larger drill hole is required at the base of the spinous process in the most cephalad and caudad vertebral body to be fused for multiple wide passage increasing the likelihood of fracture of the spinous process. Once the grafts are wired securely onto the opposing lamina, the interstices of the bone graft are grafted with morselized bone (Fig. 5–21B).

SIMPLE MIDLINE WIRE TECHNIQUE

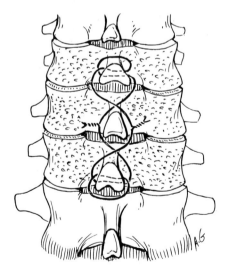

*Figure 5–20*

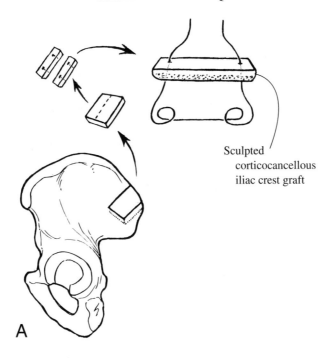

Sculpted
corticocancellous
iliac crest graft

A

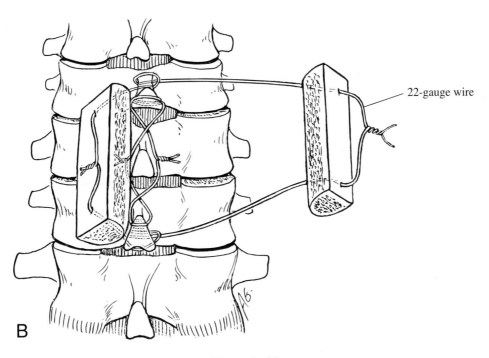

22-gauge wire

B

*Figure 5–21*

## SUBLAMINAR WIRE TECHNIQUE

Occasionally, deficiencies of the spinous processes do not allow for a spinous process wiring technique. The sublaminar wire technique has the neurologic risks associated with cord contusion during wire passage, and the canal dimensions must be kept in mind during its use. The passage of sublaminar wires in the cervical spine has greater risk than in the thoracic or upper lumbar regions. It is imperative that the wire be appropriately shaped. A slight upward deviation of the distal end of the double wire is recommended. Small amounts of ligamentum flavum are resected, and the wire is passed underneath the lamina keeping the tip of the wire in contact with the inferior surfaces of the lamina at all times. Once the wire is visible in the superior edge of the lamina, grasp the opening at the folded portion of the wire with a blunt nerve hook, or needle drivers, and pull through, again keeping the wire firmly in contact with the lamina. In most circumstances, the wires are most easily passed in a caudad to cephalad direction (Fig. 5–22).

Although rib grafts may be used because the curvature of the ribs conforms nicely to the cervical lordosis, contoured corticocancellous grafts from the posterior pelvis are equally effective (Fig. 5–23).

An appropriately sculpted graft is held in place by gently twisting the wires. Ideally, the grafts should be placed through the loop so when the loop is twisted, the tightening action of the wire will keep the graft in a slightly lateral position (Fig. 5–24).

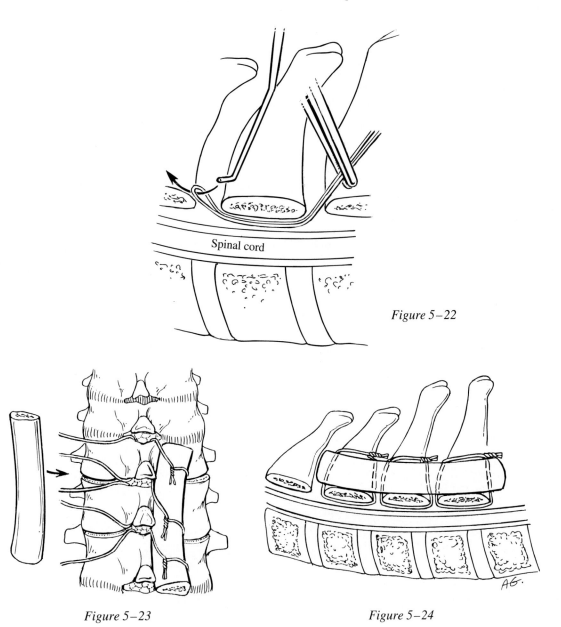

Figure 5–22

Spinal cord

Figure 5–23

Figure 5–24

93

## LUQUE CONSTRUCT

Occasionally, more substantial fixation is needed. In this case, sublaminar wires used with a luque rectangle, or an appropriately-sized and bent heavy Steinmann pin or Kirschner wire incorporated with sublaminar wires can provide additional stability. Again, caution must be followed during the passage of the sublaminar wires (Fig. 5–25).

Gentle contouring of the rod to accommodate the cervical lordosis and to keep the rod from impinging on the adjacent facet joints is essential. If at all possible, the ligamentum flavum between the fused and unfused spinal regions should be preserved, lest junctional kyphosis develops (Fig. 5–26).

## PLATE AND SCREW SYSTEMS

These systems provide strong fixation by rigid plate fixation of the lateral masses. The screws are inserted in the midportion of the lateral masses angled 10° laterally and 30–45° superiorly. The insertion point is slightly medial (1–2 mm) to the dome of the facet joint (Fig. 5–27).

The insertion point is drilled laterally with a calibrated depth guide. The initial drill hole is 14 mm deep, and rarely exceeding 18 mm; these depths were chosen to prevent perforation through the anterior cortex of the lateral mass with subsequent iatrogenic injury to the spinal nerve root. With fluoroscopy, the appropriate caudad–cephalad orientation of the screw can be checked. A small amount of autogenous graft is inserted into the intervening facet joints for arthrodesis. Supplemental laminar bone graft is placed if the remaining posterior elements are adequate (Fig. 5–28).

LUQUE CONSTRUCT

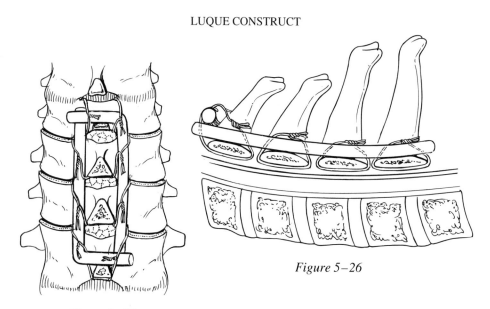

*Figure 5–26*

*Figure 5–25*

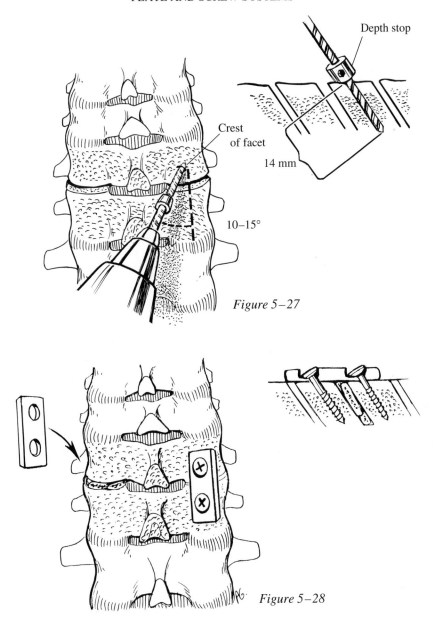

Crest
of facet

Depth stop

14 mm

10–15°

*Figure 5–27*

*Figure 5–28*

## LATERAL FACET WIRING

Lateral facet wiring is often used in patients with deficient posterior elements, and only the lateral mass and facet joints are available for arthrodesis. A wide bilateral exposure is necessary. The facet joints are individually opened and gently cleaned of soft tissue. A small dural elevator is placed beneath the facet joint. A small drill hole is made in the midportion of the facet joint and then into the protective periosteal elevator below (Fig. 5–29). Using a fine, strong clamp, a twisted 24-gauge wire, or a monofilament 20-gauge malleable stainless steel wire is inserted into the drill hole and pulled out inferiorly (Fig. 5–30). Multiple wires are passed at all levels to be fused. Because this technique injures the facet joint at the inferior portion of the laminectomy, the dissection is carried down to the next remaining anatomically normal level. A long strip of corticocancellous bone, either rib or the curved portion of the posterior ilium, is carefully harvested, sculpted, and inserted between these wire loops (Fig. 5–31). The graft must be kept in a lateral position. The portion of the wire entering the facet joint should be positioned against the medial aspect of the graft; the portion exiting the facet should be lateral. Deliberate and careful application of the wire twists keeps the graft situated over the decorticated remaining facet joints and lateral masses. An additional tethering spinous process wire in the inferior and superior junctions of the fusion completes the fixation of the grafts (Fig. 5–32). Although this technique does provide increased fixation, supplemental rigid, external immobilization, such as a halo vest or cast, is often necessary.

LATERAL FACET WIRING

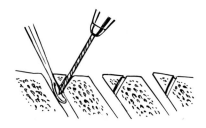

Figure 5-29

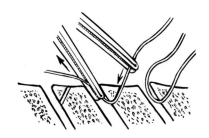

Figure 5-30

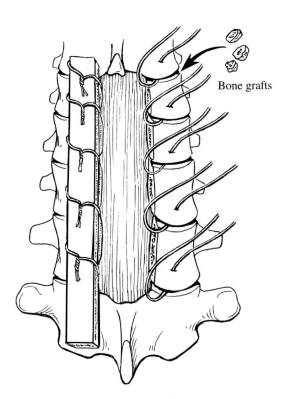

Bone grafts

Figure 5-31

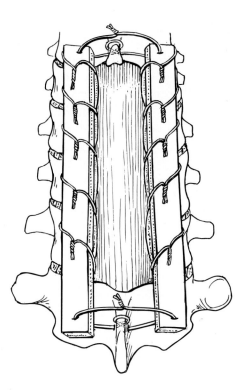

Figure 5-32

# Fracture Dislocations

Facet dislocations, or fracture dislocations, are commonly treated by posterior reduction and arthrodesis. The normal protective bony and ligamentous tissues commonly are not present. Extreme care should be used during exposure to prevent injury to the spinal cord or nerve roots. Often, concomitant laminar fractures are present and the dissection is carried out by sharply releasing the musculature with a scalpel, while simultaneously stabilizing the loose posterior elements with a Kocher clamp. A periosteal elevator is not used.

## UNILATERAL DISLOCATIONS

Cervical facet dislocations are a common occurrence. Fracture dislocations are typically unstable and care must be taken during exposure in a particularly unstable spine. Once a thorough bilateral exposure of the posterior elements over the areas requiring arthrodesis has been accomplished, reduction is performed as follows. First, the spinous processes spanning the dislocated segment is grasped firmly with Kocher clamps. The base of the spinous process near its junction with the lamina provides best mechanical grasping points. The reduction is carried out by first increasing the local amount of kyphosis to gently disengage the dislocated facets. This traction is applied in a superior and inferior direction. Second, once suitable facet distraction has been achieved, the rotation deformity is corrected by realigning the spinous processes to their normal sagittal position. Third, the widening of the interspinous distance is reduced, taking care to preserve a normal facet joint relationship. Fusion can then be carried out. Supplemental fixation is recommended (Figs. 5–33 to 5–36).

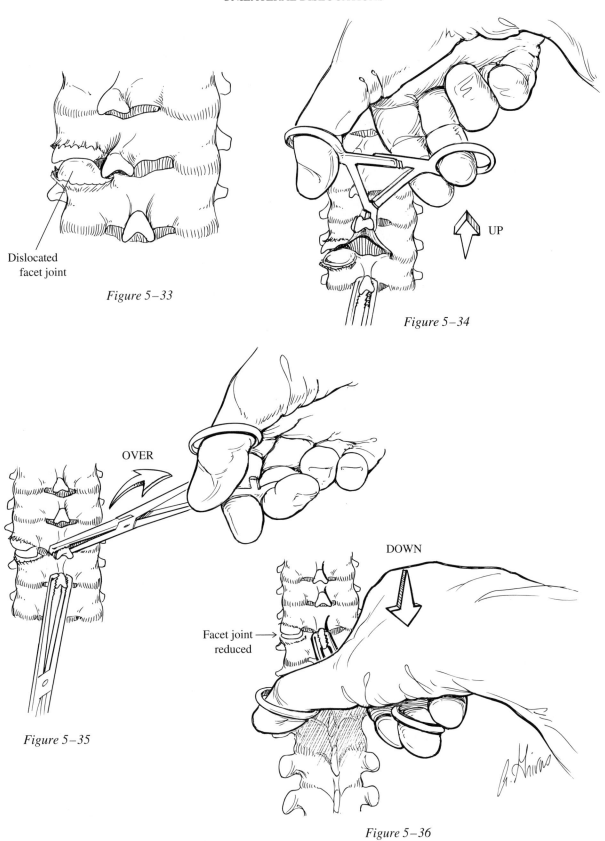

Dislocated
facet joint

*Figure 5-33*

UP

*Figure 5-34*

OVER

Facet joint
reduced

DOWN

*Figure 5-35*

*Figure 5-36*

## BILATERAL DISLOCATIONS

Bilateral facet dislocations have a higher incidence of spinal cord injury. These injuries are quite unstable because of the greater anterior translation and the extent of soft tissue, disk, and osseous injury. There is generally little rotatory deformity. There can be an associated herniated disk with this injury; this possibility should be considered preoperatively.

The reduction maneuver is similar to that of unilateral facet dislocations. There is generally no need to correct a rotational deformity. The facets are disengaged by axial distraction and by slightly increasing the local kyphosis. The interspinous space is reduced, keeping the facets in proper relationship. Subsequent posterior arthrodesis, with supplemental wire or plate fixation, should be carried out (Figs. 5–37 to 5–40).

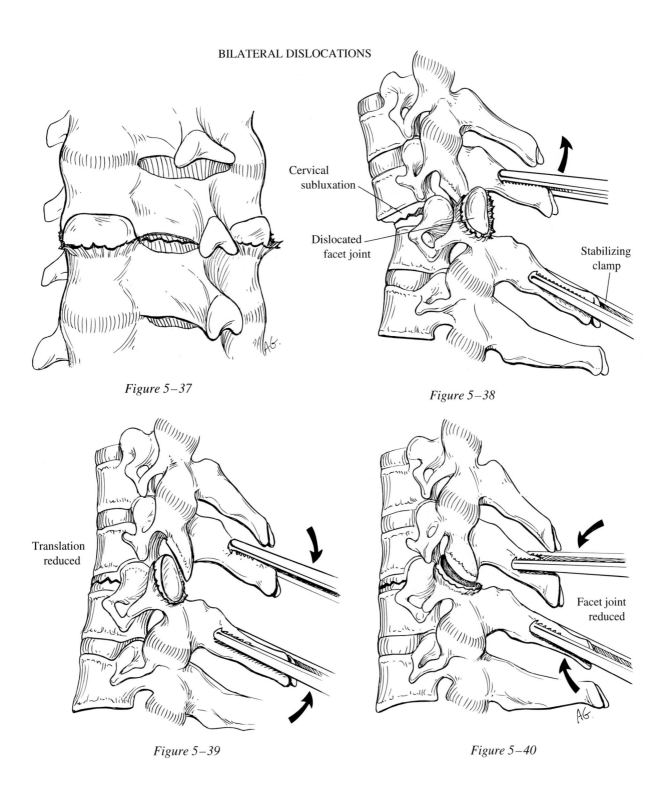

*Figure 5–37*

Cervical
subluxation

Dislocated
facet joint

Stabilizing
clamp

*Figure 5–38*

Translation
reduced

*Figure 5–39*

Facet joint
reduced

*Figure 5–40*

# Cervical Osteotomy

Wide bilateral exposure of the posterior elements of C6, C7, and T1 is performed. Typically, the operation is carried out with the patient in a sitting position under local anesthesia. A halo cast, for secure cervical spine immobilization, is applied prior to the operation (see Halo Application). The pathologic kyphosis is corrected by shortening of the posterior column, which requires considerable resection of the lamina and facet joints at the level of the proposed osteotomy. The osteotomy is carried out at the cervicothoracic junction because the vertebral arteries are less likely to be injured prior to their entrance into the fibro-osseous foramen transversarium of the C6 vertebral body (Fig. 5–41).

Laminectomy of C6, C7, and T1 is carried out, which allows for spinal cord movement during the osteotomy. An extensive foraminotomy and wide decompression of the C8 nerve root is carried out bilaterally. This often requires considerable resection of bone and a portion of the upper part of the transverse process of T1. The posterior aspect of the first rib may require partial resection, as well. It is imperative to carry the foraminotomy a suitable distance laterally to prevent any lateral residual bone from obstructing closure of the osteotomy (Fig. 5–42).

A small, high-speed diamond burr is used to partially undermine and remove the pedicles of C7 and T1. This undermining is done to provide room for the exiting C8 nerve root so the root is not compressed during osteotomy closure. The spinal nerve root and dura must be protected during the undermining process (Fig. 5–43).

With slow and deliberate care, the head is gently brought posteriorly. The osteoclasis/osteotomy is produced and a lead pipe-type rigidity is noted during an osteoclasis. The osteotomy is closed and additional bone grafting for arthrodesis is carried out using the resected posterior elements as a donor graft. The halo suprastructures are readjusted to accommodate the new posture, and a standard wound closure is carried out (Fig. 5–44).

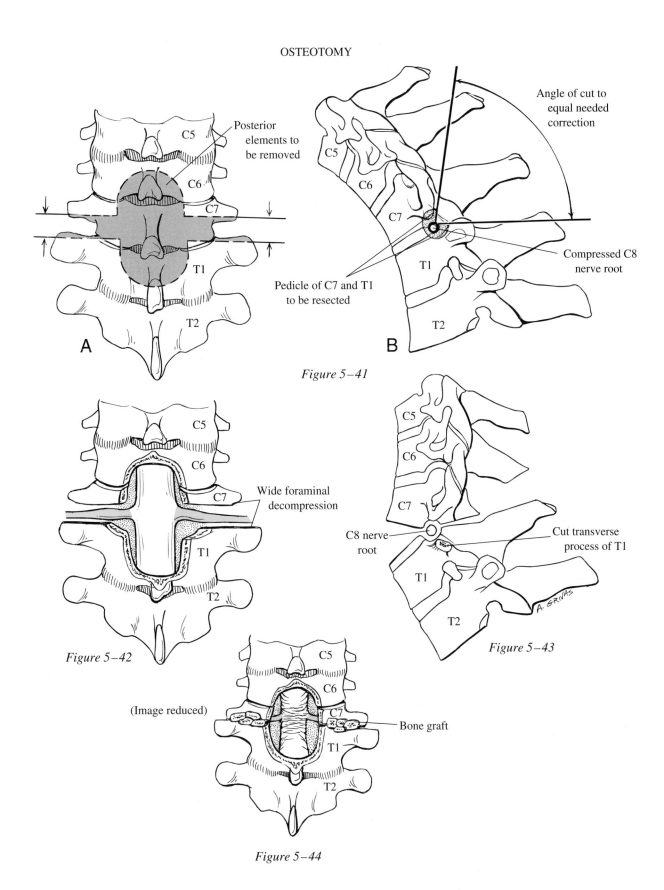

*Figure 5–41*

*Figure 5–42*

*Figure 5–43*

(Image reduced)

*Figure 5–44*

103

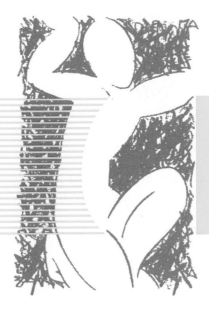

# 6

# ANTERIOR THORACIC AND THORACOLUMBAR PROCEDURES

# Anterior Surgical Approach of the Spine for Orthopedic Procedures

The anterior approach to the spine provides direct vision and extended access to the vertebral column. Through the anterior approach, the more severe and fixed deformities of the spine, whether due to congenital (hemivertebrae) or acquired (degenerative, infective, neoplastic, or traumatic) lesions, lend themselves for more complete removal and better correction by more solid fusion or fixation using bone and/or instrumentation.

The anterior approach alone or combined with posterior procedures reduces the chances of pseudoarthrosis, recurrent pain, and inadequate cord decompression, and often provides better functional and cosmetic results with quicker recovery and rehabilitation.

The details of anterior approaches to various segments of the spine are limited to the techniques of surgical exposure. Details of concomitant orthopedic procedures for fusion and fixation are discussed in Chapter 13. Anterior exposure of the spine may be carried out by the same orthopedic team, in collaboration with a general surgeon having thoracic and cardiovascular surgical experience, or with a thoracic and cardiovascular surgeon. The two-team approach preoperatively, perioperatively, and postoperatively reduces demands on the orthopedic surgeon, expedites surgery for the benefit of the patient, lessens chances of blood loss and complications, and hastens recovery.

## Preparation of the Patient

Patients are premedicated. Vascular lines are inserted and general endotracheal anesthesia is established. For special indications, a biluminal endotracheal tube is used. Monitoring electrodes for electrocardiogram and peripheral nerves are applied. An indwelling Foley catheter is inserted and inflatable pneumatic boots are applied to the lower extremities.

## Surgical Approach

Selection of the right- or left-sided approach depends upon the underlying spinal pathology such as scoliosis or abscess, reoperation, and personal preference. A right-sided abscess would dictate a right-sided approach—thoracic, thoracolumbar, or lumbar—and a left-sided abscess a corresponding left-sided approach. For patients with scoliosis, surgery is on the side of convexity. Patients undergoing reoperation may have surgery on the opposite side to avoid scar tissue, adhesions, and added blood loss, and to permit removal of another rib in thoracic or thoracolumbar cases for use in the fusion without leaving a wider interspace to close at the end of the procedure and thus promoting better healing. However, there is always concern for compromise of the spinal cord circulation if segmental arteries are divided on both sides. Consequently, some consider reoperation to be safer on the previously operated side. In thoracic and thoracolumbar cases, operating on the previously operated side avoids the additive loss of pulmonary function. From the left approach, one deals with the aorta and segmental vessels, which are more easily managed than dealing with the more fragile vena cava and azygos systems. In the lower thorax, the diaphragm elevated by the liver may provide less exposure on the right than the left. Although several of these variables are basically a matter of familiarity, experience, and personal preference, the left-sided approach generally is used for a straight, nonscoliotic spine.

## Position

Patients are placed in a right or left lateral decubitus position. The lower thigh is flexed. The kidney rest is elevated at the flank level, and the table is extended, dropping the leg position, allowing for better stretch and exposure of the spine. Pressure points and the lower axilla are padded. Pillows are placed between the legs and between the arms, which rest in the prayer position. The shoulder is free. A strap or broad tape across the upper hip stabilizes the patient. The operative area is shaved in the operating room after the aforementioned procedures are completed. The skin is prepared with a soap scrub followed by application of betadine and alcohol. The surgical field is draped. Sterile spray is applied to the skin followed by the application of an iodoform incise drape.

# SELECTION OF RIB RESECTION FOR GIVEN LEVEL

## Methods and Considerations

1. Choose the rib directly horizontal to the desired vertebral level at the mid-axillary line in the anteroposterior chest x-ray. The rib removed must be cephalad to the lesion or vertebral level sought to give adequate exposure *working down* on the lesion.

2. When direct access to the spinal canal is needed at one disk, as for thoracic disk excision, resect the rib that leads to the disk, that is, the ninth rib to the T8–T9 disk.

3. For scoliosis, select that rib cephalad to the highest disk to be resected.

4. A higher rib resection is needed for sloping ribs.

ANTERIOR THORACIC AND THORACOLUMBAR PROCEDURES

**Table 1. Thoracic, Thoracolumbar, and Lumbar Exposures**

| Level | Normal Spine | Focal Path | Scoliosis Convex L | R | Kyphosis | Kyphoscoliosis Convex L | R | Thoracolumbar L | R | Lumbar | Thoracotomy L | R | Rib Resection/Vortex |
|---|---|---|---|---|---|---|---|---|---|---|---|---|---|
| T1–4 | + | + | − | − | − | − | − | − | − | − | + | − | 3? |
|  | − | − | + | − | − | − | − | − | − | − | + | − | 3? |
|  | − | − | − | + | − | − | − | − | − | − | − | + | 3? |
|  | − | − | − | − | + | − | − | − | − | − | + | − | 3? |
|  | − | − | − | − | − | + | − | − | − | − | + | − | 3? |
|  | − | − | − | − | − | − | + | − | − | − | − | + | 3? |
| T5–12 | + | + | − | − | − | − | − | − | − | − | + | − | 7 |
|  | − | − | + | − | − | − | − | − | − | − | + | − | 7? |
|  | − | − | − | + | − | − | − | − | − | − | − | + | 7? |
|  | − | − | − | − | + | − | − | − | − | − | + | − | 7? |
|  | − | − | − | − | − | + | − | − | − | − | + | − | 7? |
|  | − | − | − | − | − | − | + | − | − | − | − | + | 7? |
| T8–L2 | + | + | − | − | − | − | − | + | − | − | − | − | 9 |
|  | − | − | + | − | − | − | − | − | − | − | − | − | 9? |
|  | − | − | − | + | − | − | − | − | + | − | − | − | 9? |
|  | − | − | − | − | + | − | − | + | − | − | − | − | 9? |
|  | − | − | − | − | − | + | − | − | − | − | − | − | 9? |
|  | − | − | − | − | − | − | + | − | + | − | − | − | 9? |
| T8–S1 | + | + | − | − | − | − | − | − | − | − | + | − | 9-10? |
|  | − | − | + | − | − | − | − | − | − | − | − | − | 9-10? |
|  | − | − | − | + | − | − | − | − | + | − | − | − | 9-10? |
|  | − | − | − | − | + | − | − | + | − | − | − | − | 9-10? |
|  | − | − | − | − | − | + | − | + | − | − | − | − | 9? |
|  | − | − | − | − | − | − | + | − | + | − | − | − | 9? |
| T10–L2 | + | + | − | − | − | − | − | − | − | − | + | − | 9 |
|  | − | − | + | − | − | − | − | + | − | − | − | − | 9? |
|  | − | − | − | + | − | − | − | − | + | − | − | − | 9? |
|  | − | − | − | − | + | − | − | + | − | − | − | − | 9? |
|  | − | − | − | − | − | + | − | + | − | − | − | − | 9? |
|  | − | − | − | − | − | − | + | − | − | − | − | − | 9? |
| L2–S1 | + | + | − | − | − | − | − | − | − | + | − | − | 9-10-11-12? |
| L3–L4 | + | + | − | − | − | − | − | − | − | + | − | − | − |
| L4–L5 | + | + | − | − | − | − | − | − | − | + | − | − | − |
| L5–S1 | + | + | − | − | − | − | − | − | − | + | − | − | − |

# SURGICAL EXPOSURE OF THE UPPER THORACIC SPINE T1–T4

## Position

If there is no scoliosis, the approach may be from either side. If scoliosis is present, the patient is placed in the lateral decubitus position with the convexity of the curve uppermost.

## Incision

A standard, posterolateral thoracotomy is made, commencing at a point midway between the vertebral border of the scapula and the spine and curved around the inferior angle of the scapula to the midaxillary line (Fig. 6–1). The lower portions of the trapezius and the latissimus dorsi muscles are divided. For higher rib resection, sixth and above, the trapezius and rhomboid muscles are divided, as necessary (Fig. 6–1).

## Rib Counting and Rib Selection

At this point, the scapula is retracted and the surgeon's hand is passed beneath the scapula to palpate the uppermost ribs. Generally, the highest rib palpated in this position is the second rib, since the first rib is essentially inside the second. Another guide is the wider interspace between the second and third ribs compared with those below. Once the rib counting is done, the thoracic incision is extended anteriorly to the costal arch dividing the serratus anterior muscle in line with the rib to be resected.

Rib counting for lower rib resection (8–12) is done from below upward, using the chest x-ray as a guide for short, long, or absent twelfth ribs.

For T1–T4 exposure, the scapula is elevated and the fourth rib is identified and removed in the following manner.

## Rib Resection

After the appropriate rib is selected and counted, the periosteum over the anterior surface is incised with electrocautery along the length of the rib and then scored transversely at intervals of 1 to 2 cm. The rib is then removed subperiosteally, using periosteal elevators to separate the rib from its surrounding periosteum. Removal is done anteriorly, inferiorly, superiorly, and, lastly, posteriorly to avoid injury to the intercostal neurovascular muscle bundle and intercostal muscles. When working on the inferior then superior rib margins, the periosteal elevators are directed upward anteriorly to posteriorly on the downward (inferior) margin of the rib, starting at the costochondral juncture to the posterior angle of the rib, then downward on the upside (superior) margin of the rib from the posterior angle back to the costochondral juncture. ("Up on the downside and down on the upside.") The paraspinal muscles are retracted to expose the posterior angle of the rib. A double-action cutter is used to cut the rib at the costochondral juncture and at the posterior angle (Fig. 6–2).

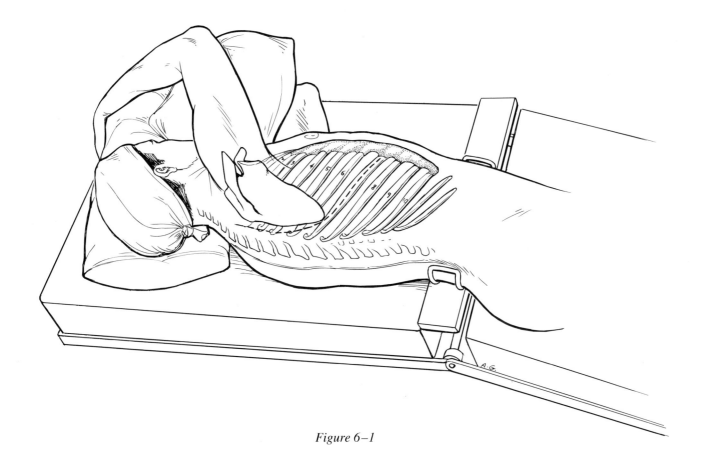

*Figure 6–1*

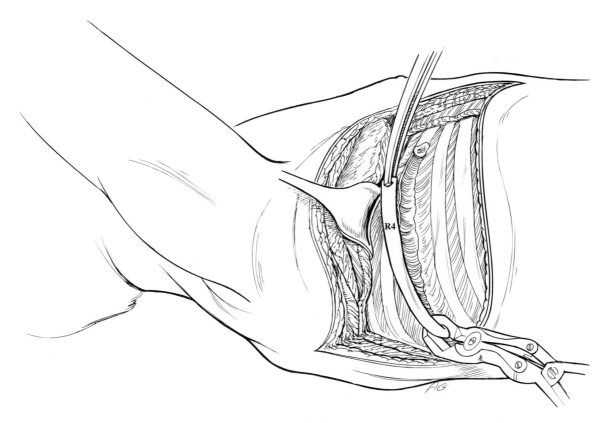

*Figure 6–2*

111

Removing the rib, the underlying parietal pleura is exposed and incised the length of the incision and the chest is entered. Any adhesions are lysed by blunt dissection or divided. The wound edges are protected with moist pads. A self-retaining rib spreader is inserted, which allows exposure of one disk space above and one below the rib removed. For more exposure, more rib resection may be needed posteriorly. For additional exposure, resection of 1 or 2 cm of rib at the posterior angle, above or below the resected rib, may be needed and cartilage resection anteriorly (Fig. 6–3A). In selected cases, confirmation of rib and vertebral level is made by radiography.

## Intrathoracic Procedures

The lung on the operated side is deflated, if a biluminal endotracheal tube is used, or packed with moist sponges and retracted after the lung and thorax are inspected.

## Anatomy of Chest

In the left thorax, above the aortic arch, which is at the level of the fourth vertebral body, the esophagus, thoracic duct, and subclavian artery are in proximity to the spine, with the esophagus being most posterior (Fig. 6–3B). Lower in the chest, the aorta lies to the left of the midline, anterior to the vertebral bodies, and exits the thorax at the level of the twelfth thoracic vertebra, while the splanchnic nerves and thoracic duct are to the right of the midline. In the right thorax are the brachiocephalic vein, superior vena cava, and azygos vein (Fig. 6–3C).

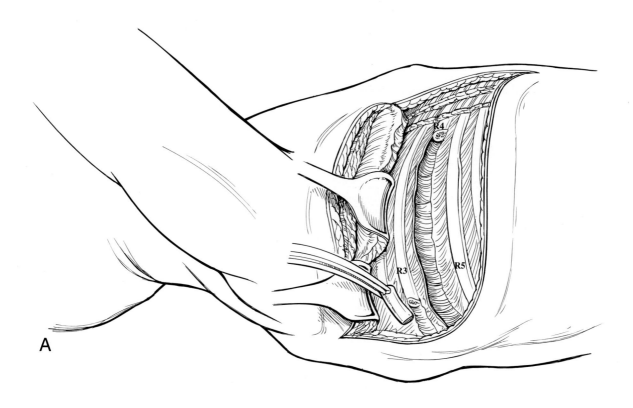

*Figure 6–3*

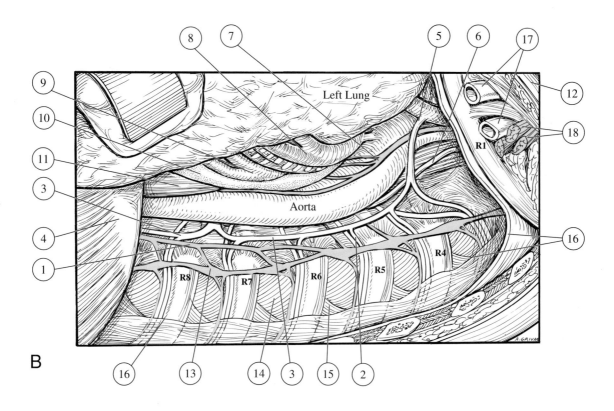

B

1. Greater thoracic splanchnic nerve
2. Intercostal artery and vein
3. Hemiazygos accessory veins
4. Diaphragm
5. Left brachiocephalic vein
6. Thoracic duct
7. Vagus nerve
8. Left pulmonary artery
9. Left pulmonary veins
10. Pericardium
11. Esophagus
12. Clavicle
13. Sympathetic trunk
14. External intercostal muscle
15. Internal intercostal muscle
16. Cut edge of costal pleura
17. Left subclavian artery and vein
18. Brachioplexus

*Figure 6–3 Continued*

114

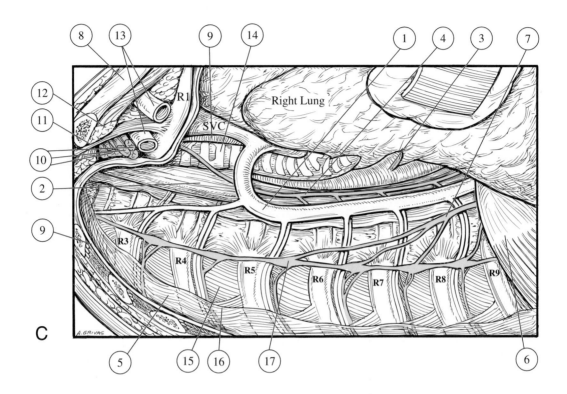

C

1. Azygos vein
2. Esophagus
3. Pulmonary vein
4. Vagus nerve
5. Cut edge of costal pleura
6. Diaphragm
7. Greater splanchnic nerve
8. Clavicle
9. Cut edge of costal pleura
10. Brachioplexus
11. Sternocleidomastoid muscle
12. Subclavius muscle
13. Subclavian artery and vein
14. Trachea
15. External intercostal muscle
16. Internal intercostal muscle
17. Sympathetic trunk
SVC. Superior vena cava

*Figure 6–3 Continued*

115

The mediastinal pleura over the anterolateral aspect of the spine is incised with electrocautery and peeled medially and laterally using a Küttner dissector, exposing the segmental arteries and veins (Fig. 6–4).

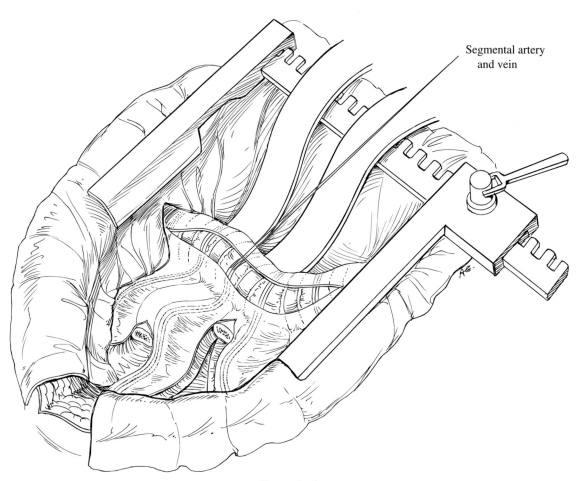

Segmental artery
and vein

*Figure 6–4*

## Anatomy of Thoracic Intercostal and Lumbar Arteries

Variations of the thoracic and lumbar arterial branches of the aorta are of surgical importance. The arterial topography varies according to the spinal sectors. At *T1–T3,* the anterior surfaces of the vertebral bodies are generally free of overlying intercostal arteries. The most frequent variation is the presence of vertically descending small arteries from the inferior thyroid and vertebral arteries, with anastomosis sometimes occurring with the second or third intercostal artery.

This first pair of intercostal arteries does not usually run over the vertebral bodies since they ascend directly from the costocervical trunk, which arises from the subclavian artery (95% on the right and 90% on the left), or from a common trunk with the second intercostal artery.

In 62% of cases, the second intercostal artery arises from the aorta and runs vertically over the vertebra; in the remaining cases, it arises from the costocervical trunk, the inferior thyroid artery, or a common trunk with a third intercostal artery.

The segmental arteries arising from the aorta can run in varying directions. An ascending recurrent course, especially involving the upper intercostals, decreases in frequency from the third intercostal (100%) to the fourth lumbar (7%). Similarly, a descending course of the segmental arteries increases in frequency from the sixth intercostal (1%) to the first lumbar (53%) and, finally, to the fifth lumbar (100%).

The frequency of a strictly horizontal direction resembles a *parabolic curve* from the fourth intercostal to the fourth lumbar artery with a maximum occurrence (42%) at T12.

The fact that the segmental arteries arising from the aorta can run in an ascending, recurrent, horizontal, or descending direction probably results from the differential rate of growth of the aorta and spine.

From *T3–T5,* the third through sixth intercostal arteries run almost vertically over the vertebral bodies. They arise as a group from the posterior origin of the thoracic aorta at the level of T4–T5 and ascend almost vertically with a very slight lateral slant, running over several disks and vertebrae before reaching the lower margin of their corresponding ribs.

From *T6–T10,* the intercostal arteries are generally in a segmental, recurrent distribution. Their origin is on each side of the posterior aortic midline followed by a short, vertically ascending segment. They then run horizontally from the flank of the aorta below the middle of their corresponding vertebral body to reach the intervertebral foramen. *The disks are free of overlying arteries in this spinal region.* Identification of the intercostal artery is achieved on the aortic flank at a point half-way between two neighboring disks.

From *T10–L2,* the intercostal and lumbar arteries display essentially a horizontal segmental distribution. Arising on each side of the posterior aortic midline, they run horizontally across the middle of the corresponding vertebral bodies.

From *L2–L4,* the lumbar arteries run in a descending direction, ascending on each side of the posterior aortic midline at the level of the disk just above their numerically corresponding vertebrae, then run vertically downward behind the

117

aorta, and, finally horizontally toward the middle of the vertebral bodies before entering the intervertebral foramen.

Variations in the origins, common origins, and distribution occur. In cases where the aortic bifurcation is cranial to its typical position, the lumbar arteries may rise from the middle sacral artery rather than from the aorta.

The aorta gives rise to 10 intercostal arteries in 51% of subjects and 11 in 44%. The presence of 12 intercostal arteries is relatively rare (2.1% on the right and 4% on the left). In 1% of subjects, only six or seven right and left intercostal arteries are found. The number of lumbar arteries may vary, four in 70–74%, three in 20–22%, and five in 5–7%. The caliber of the segmental arteries increases in cranial caudal fashion, the upper intercostals being 1.1 mm and the lower lumbar 1.5 mm.

The fatty areolar and lymphatic tissue is cleared away from the segmental vessels by sharp and blunt dissection, cauterizing small bleeding points as encountered. A fine, right-angled forceps is then passed around the segmental vessels, artery, and vein separately, or combined, depending on their size and local anatomy. These are quadruplicately occluded with Ligaclips or doubly ligated, stitched tied, if necessary, and divided. Often at this point, hemostasis is secured by cautery, and the vertebral bodies, the disks, and anterior longitudinal ligament are exposed for the orthopedic surgeon to proceed with the appropriate reparative procedures.

Following the corrective procedure on the spine, the mediastinal pleura is approximated with a continuous 3–0 catgut suture, loosely closed to allow any continued oozing of blood from the vertebral raw surfaces to find its way into the chest cavity where it will be drained, rather than dissect under a tightly closed pleura to form a hematoma. One or two siliconized chest tubes are inserted, one in the posterior gutter and one anteriorly, if there is concern of pneumothorax through stab wounds below the thoracotomy incision (Fig. 6–5). The chest wall is then closed anatomically. Five or six pericostal sutures of 0 braided dacron are placed, followed by a running suture of 0 monofilament polydioxanone to approximate the intercostal muscle bundles above and below the resected rib. This suture is not pulled taut until the tension on the suture lines is removed by a rib approximator. Next, the pericostal sutures are tied. The divided chest wall muscles are approximated with a continuous 0 monofilament suture. If the chest wall muscles are unduly large, closure is done by separately approximating the inner and outer fascial layers in order to obliterate dead space and avoid seromas. An alternative method of muscle approximation consists of a "pulley stitch," essentially a modified continuous mattress suture with a deep bite of tissue passing through the full thickness of muscle and a superficial bite, not reversed, passing through the outer fascial layer. The subcutaneous fat layer is approximated with a 2–0 Vicryl, and a 3–0 Vicryl suture is used for subcuticular approximation of the skin. Underwater-seal chest suction is maintained at minus 15 cm of water. The chest tubes are removed when the drainage is serous and is 30 to 50 cc or less for two or more consecutive 8 hour periods. If the lung has been injured during the surgery and an air leak is present, the chest tubes are not removed until the air leak has sealed and the lung remains fully expanded.

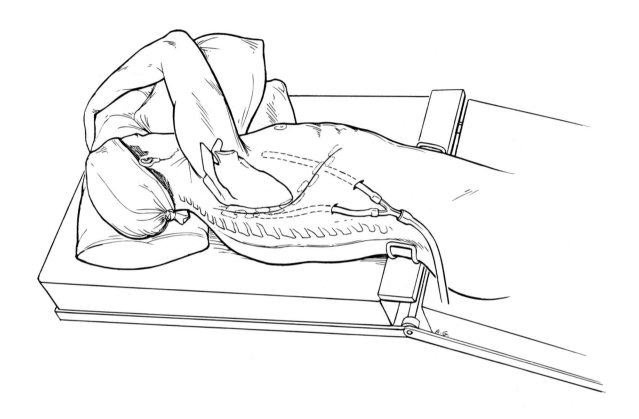

*Figure 6–5*

# SURGICAL EXPOSURE OF MID AND LOWER THORACIC SPINE T5–T12

Preparation of the patient and selection of the surgical approach are the same as described for the exposure of T1–T4 (see pp 110–119).

## Position

The patient is placed in the lateral decubitus position with the flank over the kidney rest and the lower thigh flexed. The kidney rest is elevated and table extended (Fig. 6–6). Pressure points and the lower axilla are padded. Pillows are placed between the legs and the arms, which rest in a prayer position. A strap or broad tape across the hip stabilizes the patient.

## Incision

A standard posterolateral thoracotomy incision is made for resection of the fifth or sixth, or sometimes seventh, rib dividing the trapezius and rhomboids, as necessary, then the latissimus dorsi and serratus anterior muscles (Fig. 6–6).

Follow the same methods of rib selection and rib counting as previously described. For the lower rib resections (7–10), the skin incision is made over the rib to be resected from the costochondral juncture, posteriorly, to a site corresponding to the posterior angle of the rib, dividing the latissimus dorsi and serratus anterior muscles.

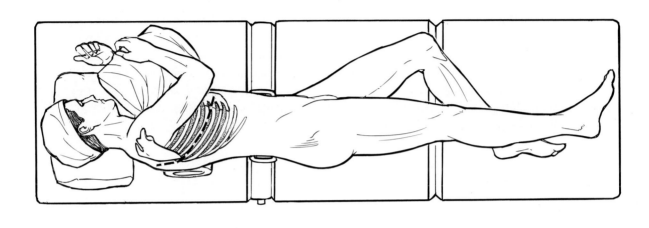

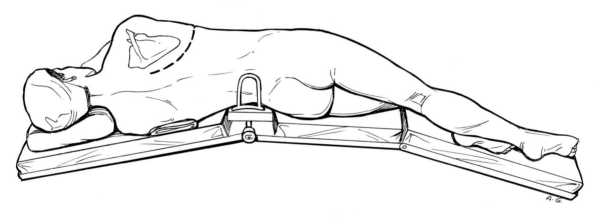

*Figure 6–6*

In severely kyphotic patients in whom the ribs run parallel and interspaces are very narrow, subperiosteal removal of 2 cm of adjacent ribs above and/or below, posteriorly, near the angles of the rib and, if necessary, additional division of the costal cartilage of the same ribs anteriorly, allows wider exposure and usually causes no problem during closure (Fig. 6–7).

The posterior periosteal layer of the rib bed is incised and the chest entered. The wound margins are padded with moist gauze, and a self-retaining rib spreader is inserted. The lung is packed with moist compresses. The mediastinal pleura over the anterolateral spine is incised with electrocautery in a vertical direction and peeled medially and laterally with gauze dissection. This exposes the vertebral bodies, disks, and segmental vessels. The segmental vessels are dissected free, encircled with a right angle forceps, doubly occluded with Liga-clips, or doubly ligated and divided, and peeled medially and laterally. The anterior longitudinal ligament is exposed and the orthopedic surgeon can proceed with the corrective procedure.

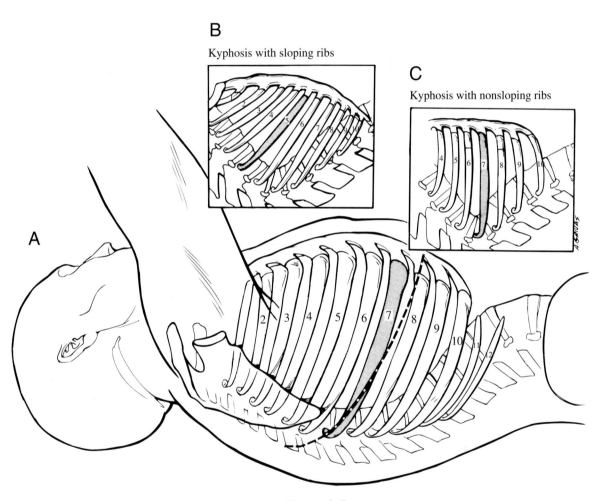

B

Kyphosis with sloping ribs

C

Kyphosis with nonsloping ribs

A

*Figure 6–7*

123

# ANTERIOR THORACIC AND THORACOLUMBAR PROCEDURES

The exposure of the mid to lower thoracic spine, T5–T12, may be obtained without need to divide the costal arch anteriorly (Fig. 6–8). It may be necessary, however, to detach the crus of the diaphragm from the prevertebral tissues to expose T12–L1 (Fig. 6–9). If the approach is the right thoracotomy with exposure down to the T12–L1 level, it is advisable, after dividing the prevertebral tissues and the crus of the diaphragm, to peel the tissues away from the spine as close to the spine as possible using blunt gauze or finger dissection to avoid injury to the cisterna chyle and thoracic duct. If the duct is injured, which will be evident by clear or milky lymph fluid, the thoracic duct or major lymphatic vessel should be tied or stitch-tied as with any major blood vessel.

Following the orthopedic correction, the mediastinal pleura is loosely approximated over the spine using 3–0 chromic catgut. One or two #24 siliconized chest tubes are inserted, one in the posterior gutter and one anteriorly. The surgeon follows the method previously described for chest closure (see p 118).

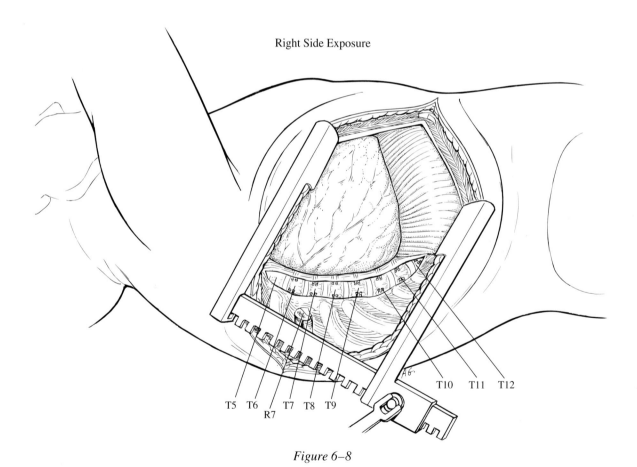

*Figure 6–8*

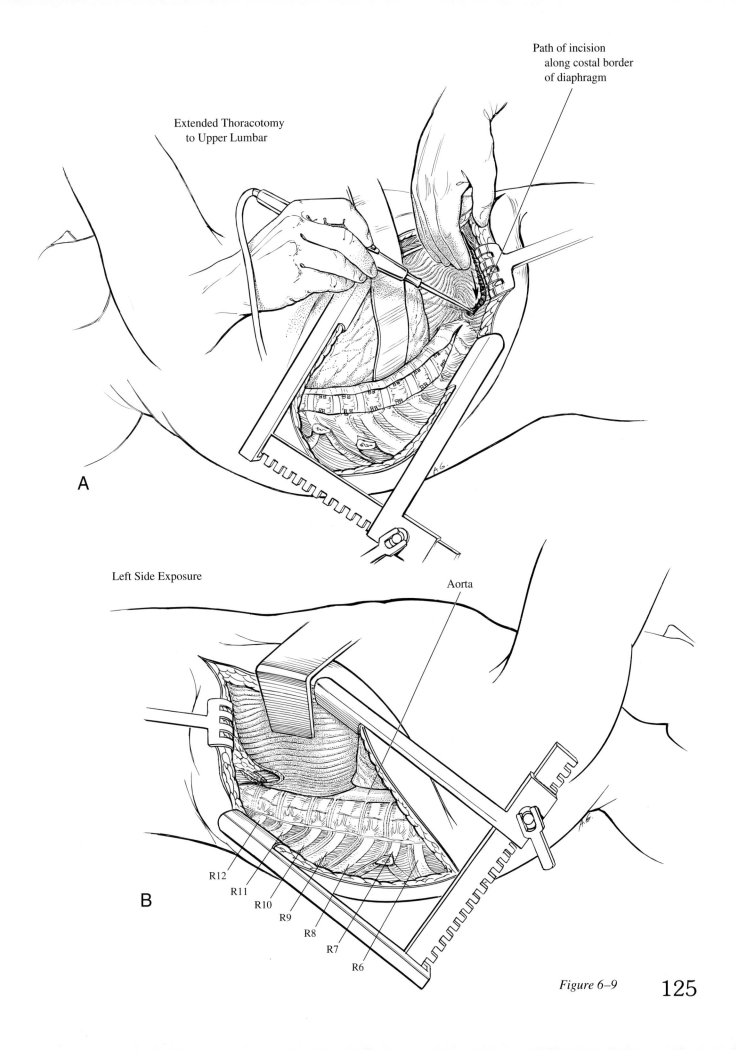

Extended Thoracotomy
to Upper Lumbar

Path of incision
along costal border
of diaphragm

A

Left Side Exposure

Aorta

R12
R11
R10
R9
R8
R7
R6

B

*Figure 6–9*    125

# Surgical Exposure of the Thoracolumbar Spine T8–S1

For the anterior exposure of the thoracolumbar spine in patients without scoliosis, the approach can be made from either side. Because of scar tissue and its associated problems, it may be preferable to avoid the previously operated side. The lateral surgical approach and the spinal circulation have been previously discussed (see pp 110–119). Patients with scoliosis are positioned with the major convexity of the curve uppermost. The kidney rest is elevated at the flank level and the feet dropped to extend and stretch the spine for better exposure.

## Incision

Exposure of the vertebral bodies and disk spaces from T8–S1 is through a thoracolumbar incision starting from the lower angle of the scapula, curving and continuing over the ninth rib, and crossing the costal arch (Figs. 6–10A–D). The incision is then directed toward the midinguinal ligament obliquely, staying lateral to the rectus sheath (Fig. 6–11). The latissimus dorsi and serratus anterior muscles are divided with electrocautery (Fig. 6–12). The ninth rib is removed subperiosteally (Figs. 6–13 and 6–14).

Before the abdominal muscles are divided, attention is directed to entering the chest. The periosteal layer of the removed rib bed is incised longitudinally. The chest cavity is opened. The margins of the wound are padded with moist sponges, and a rib spreader is inserted. The costal arch at the level of rib resection is divided or the costal cartilage of the resected rib is split. Intercostal vessels are ligated as encountered.

A

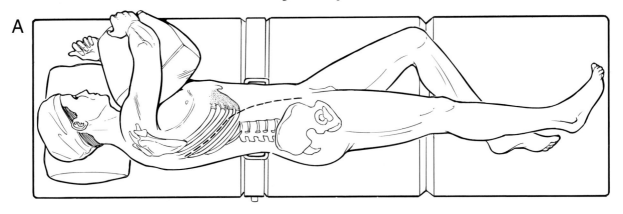

B

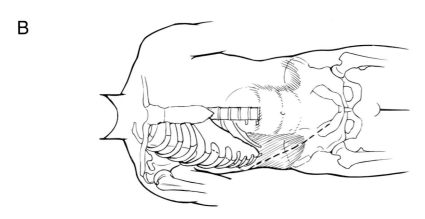

C

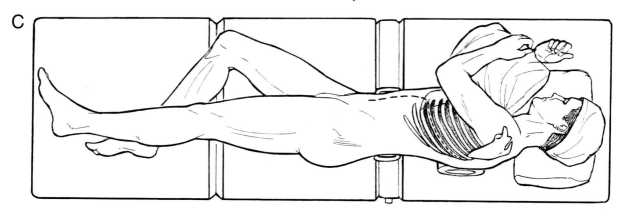

D

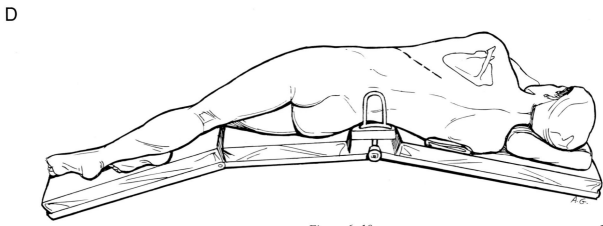

*Figure 6–10*

127

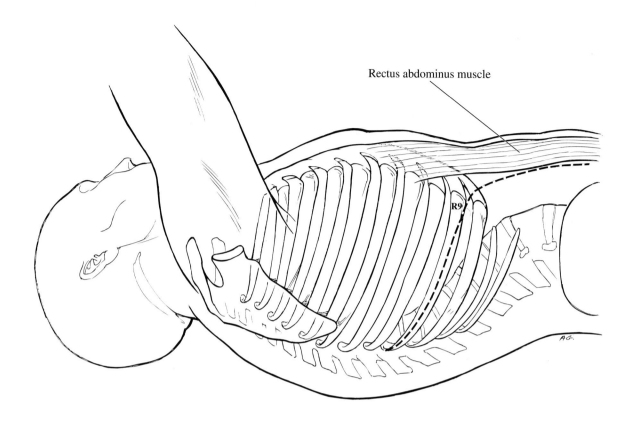

Rectus abdominus muscle

R9

*Figure 6–11*

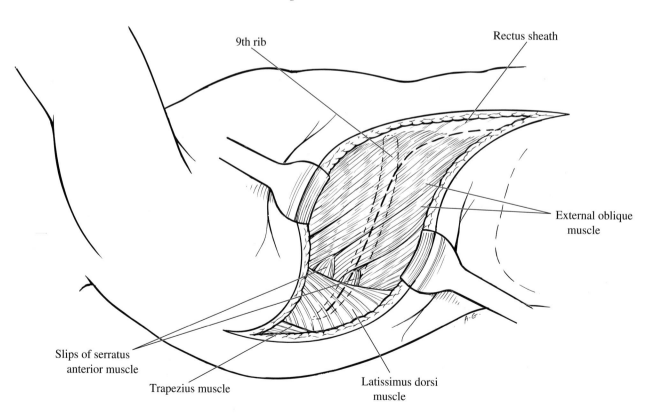

9th rib

Rectus sheath

External oblique muscle

Slips of serratus anterior muscle

Trapezius muscle

Latissimus dorsi muscle

*Figure 6–12*

128

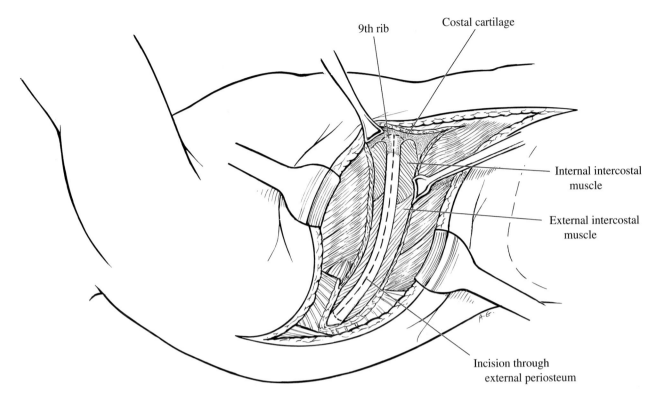

9th rib

Costal cartilage

Internal intercostal muscle

External intercostal muscle

Incision through external periosteum

*Figure 6–13*

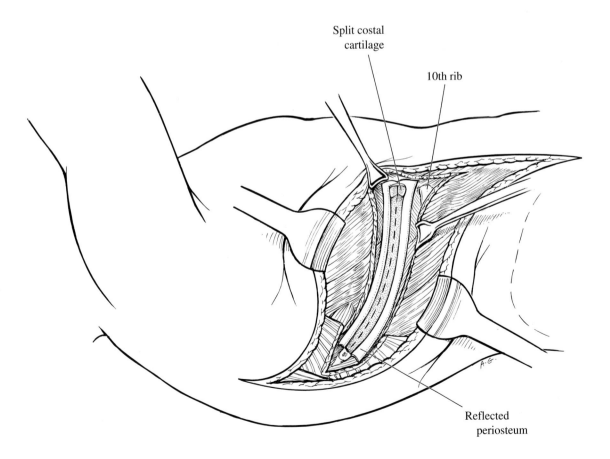

Split costal cartilage

10th rib

Reflected periosteum

*Figure 6–14*

## Separation of the Diaphragm

The diaphragm is separated peripherally (Figs. 6–15A, B and 6–16).

The attachments of the diaphragm anterolaterally are the xyphoid process and the cartilagenous ends of the lower six ribs. Posteriorly, the diaphragm arises from the lumbar vertebrae by way of the crura, the aponeurotic ligaments, and the twelfth ribs. The crura are fibromuscular structures that arise from the anterior longitudinal ligaments of the lumbar vertebrae and extend superiorly to surround the aorta and esophageal hiatus. The median arcuate ligaments arise from the crura on the respective sides, cross the psoas muscle as a bridge, and insert on the transverse processes of the first lumbar vertebrae. The lateral arcuate ligaments arise from the transverse process from the first lumbar vertebrae extending over the quadratus lumborum muscle to the tips of the twelfth ribs.

A Duval forceps, or hand pressure, may be used on the central tendon of the diaphragm to tent it, putting the peripheral diaphragm under tension.

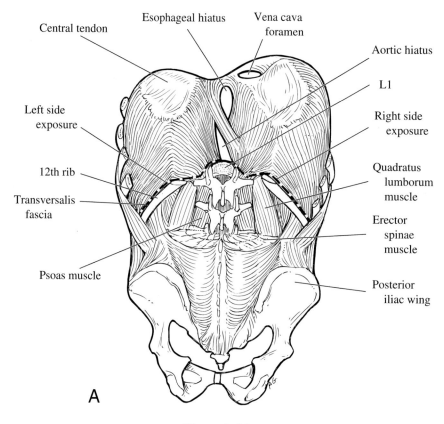

*Figure 6–15*

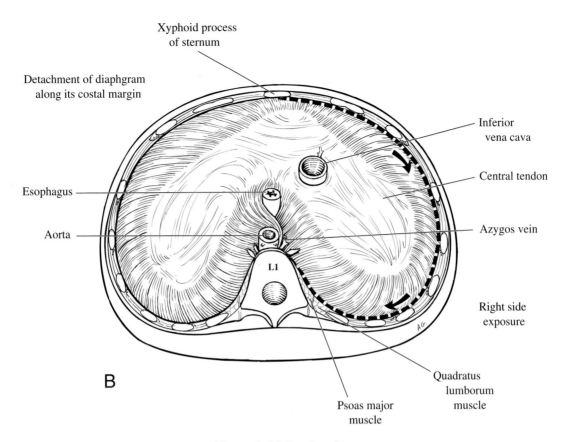

Xyphoid process
of sternum

Detachment of diaphgram
along its costal margin

Inferior
vena cava

Central tendon

Esophagus

Aorta

Azygos vein

L1

Right side
exposure

B

Quadratus
lumborum
muscle

Psoas major
muscle

*Figure 6–15 Continued*

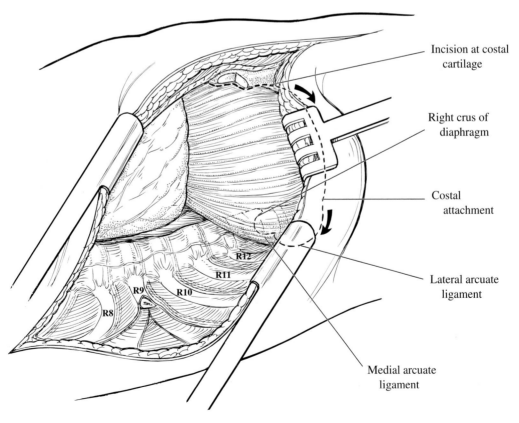

Incision at costal
cartilage

Right crus of
diaphragm

Costal
attachment

R12

R11

R9    R10

R8

Lateral arcuate
ligament

Medial arcuate
ligament

*Figure 6–16*

131

Using electrocautery (Fig. 6–17), the parietal pleura at the very subcostal diaphragmatic angle (where the costal arch has been transected or the cartilage split) is incised, followed by the division of the subjacent insertion fibers of the diaphragm. When the insertion fibers are divided close to the chest wall, the extraperitoneal fat layer is entered. *This is the key to separation of the diaphragm.* Incising outside the margin of the diaphragm peripherally, more than 5 to 10 mm, the peritoneum may be directly entered, causing injury to the stomach and spleen or bowel on the left or liver on the right. Even when the insertion fibers are literally shaved off the chest wall, enough of the fibers remain with the parietal pleura to approximate the diaphragm to the chest wall on closure without difficulty.

Once the properitoneal fat is visualized, finger or manual dissection with or without gauze is carried out, separating the properitoneal fat and peritoneal contents from the anterior abdominal muscles.

In some instances, temporarily removing the rib spreader and using a rake retractor, the pleurodiaphragmatic angle can be further exposed and the diaphragm can be separated to the lateral arcuate ligament. The rib spreader can be replaced. Having dissected the peritoneum from the abdominal muscles to the lateral margin of the rectus, the ligaments can be divided with electrocautery. With added exposure, the separation of the diaphragm can be completed by further dividing the lateral and medial arcuate ligaments over the quadratus lumborum and psoas muscles. Lastly, the crus is divided or detached from the lumbar vertebrae (Fig. 6–18).

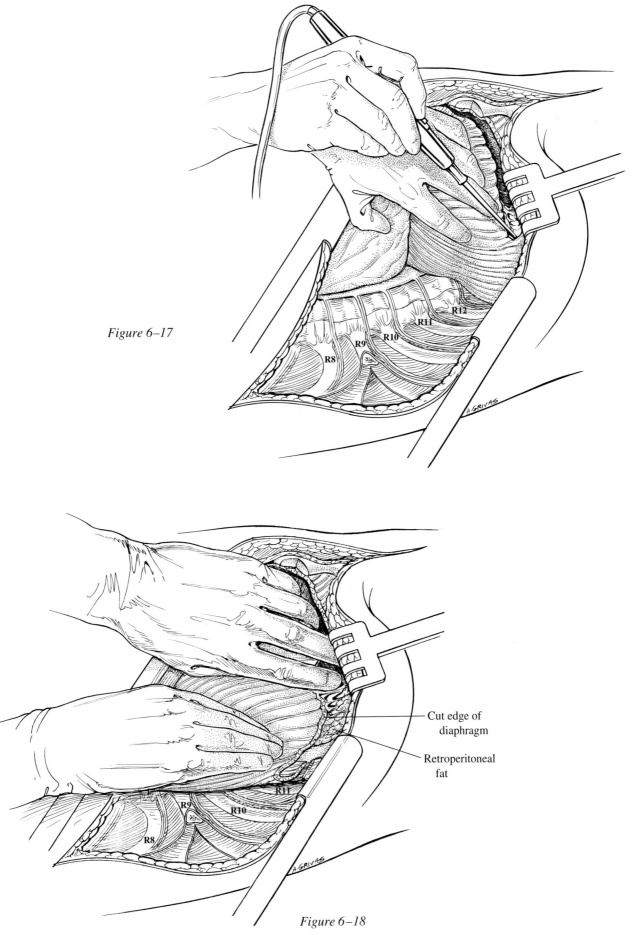

*Figure 6–17*

R12
R11
R10
R9
R8

A. GRIVAS

Cut edge of
diaphragm

Retroperitoneal
fat

R11
R10
R9
R8

A. GRIVAS

*Figure 6–18*

133

SUMMARY OF STEPS FOR THORACOLUMBAR EXPOSURE
AND DETACHMENT OF DIAPHRAGM

1. Patient in lateral decubitus position.
2. Thoracolumbar incision overlying rib selected for resection.
3. Subperiosteal resection of rib.
4. Insertion of rib spreader.
5. Division of costal arch in line with rib resection or splitting costal cartilage of resected rib.
6. Division of pleurodiaphragmatic reflection subjacent to divided costal arch exposing properitoneal fat and gaining access to extraperitoneal space.
7. Division of costal attachments of diaphragm to lateral arcuate ligament.
8. Blunt dissection in extraperitoneal and properitoneal space, separating the anterior abdominal muscles from peritoneum, staying lateral to rectus sheath.
9. Division of the anterior abdominal muscles in line with the incision. In some instances, 9 and 10 may precede or digitate with 8.
10. Complete detachment of diaphragm, dividing lateral and medial arcuate ligaments and the crus.
11. Division or detachment of the diaphragmatic crus.

The peritoneum is then freed laterally and posteriorly, entering the retroperitoneal space (plane) between the renal or Gerota's fascia and the quadratus lumborum and psoas muscles. Gerota's fascia is continuous with the peritoneum, surrounds the kidney, ureter, adrenal gland, and peritoneal fat and is loosely applied to the quadratus lumborum and psoas muscles. The layer blends loosely with the psoas fascia and is attached to the vertebral column anterior to the medial margin of the psoas.

In this plane, by manual and blunt dissection in a sweeping motion, the peritoneum, peritoneal contents, Gerota's fascia, and contents are pushed forward and medially across the quadratus lumborum and psoas muscles (Fig. 6–19), exposing the lumbar spine posteriorly and medially and the pelvic brim and iliac vessels inferiorly (Fig. 6–20). Exposure from the left side is shown in Figure 6–21. If the peritoneum is inadvertently opened, it is simply repaired with a 3–0 chromic catgut suture.

The aorta is exposed from the left approach and the inferior vena cava from the right approach. The mediastinal pleura over the lower thoracic spine is divided longitudinally from the desired level to the aortic hiatus and peeled medially and laterally. The diaphragmatic crus is then divided and the ligamentous origins of the psoas muscle are detached from the spine with electrocautery and reflected laterally. The wound margins of the lumbar incision are padded with moist sponges, packing the peritoneum and peritoneal contents. A self-retaining retractor is inserted to provide adequate exposure.

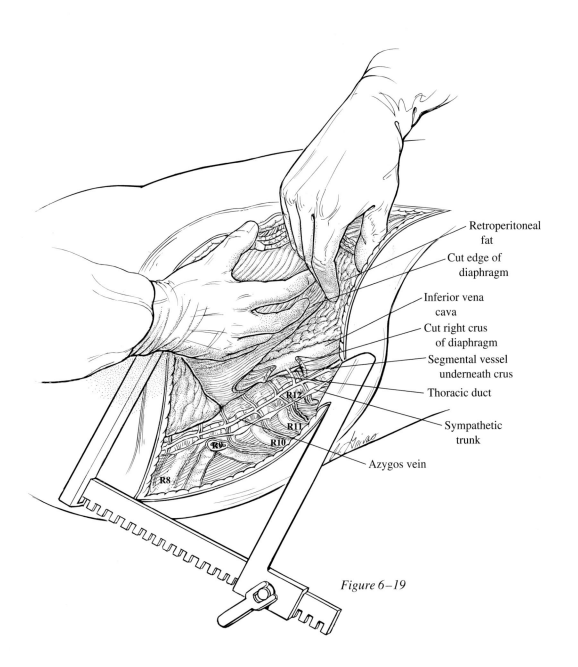

Retroperitoneal
fat

Cut edge of
diaphragm

Inferior vena
cava

Cut right crus
of diaphragm

Segmental vessel
underneath crus

Thoracic duct

Sympathetic
trunk

Azygos vein

R12

R11

R10

R9

R8

*Figure 6–19*

135

Right Side Exposure

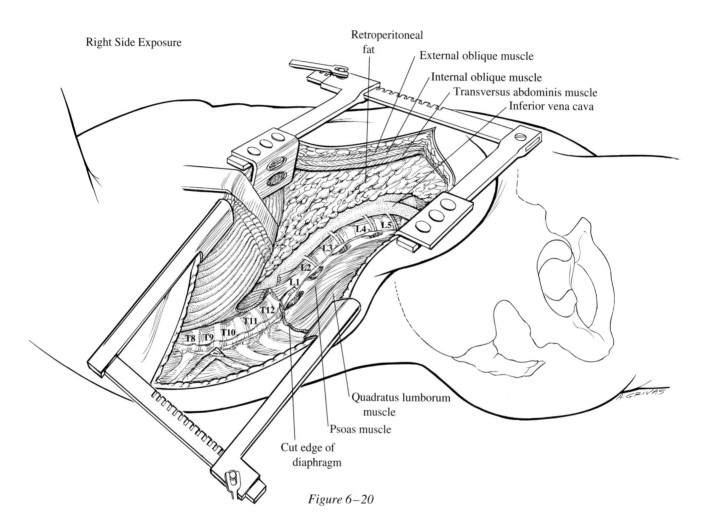

Retroperitoneal
fat

External oblique muscle

Internal oblique muscle

Transversus abdominis muscle

Inferior vena cava

L5

L4

L3

L2

L1

T12

T11

T10

T9

T8

Quadratus lumborum
muscle

Psoas muscle

Cut edge of
diaphragm

A.GRIVAS

*Figure 6–20*

136

Left Side Exposure

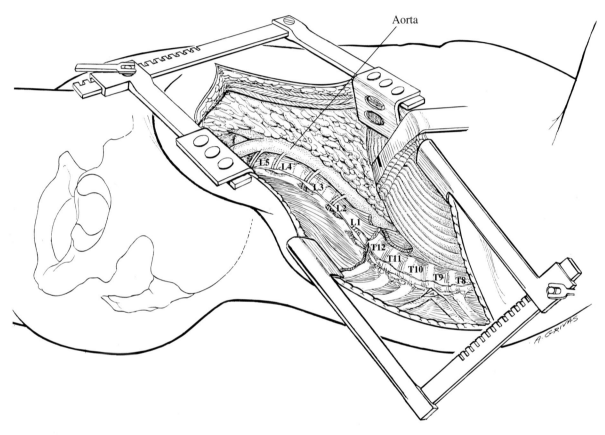

Figure 6–21

The segmental arteries and veins are then exposed. These arteries run in the depressions of the vertebral bodies, bordered by the avascular elevations of the intervertebral disks. Blunt Küttner dissection is used to move away the fatty areolar tissue overlying the vessels. A fine hemostat or right-angled forceps is used to free and encircle the vessels to allow quadruple occlusion with Ligaclips or double ligation and division. In some instances, ligation and application of Ligaclips may be suitable. Occasionally, a stitch-tie may be necessary.

When exposing L4–L5 cephalad to the iliac vein, a sizable *iliolumbar* vein may be encountered, which will require double ligation, division, or, if unduly large, vascular clamping, division, and oversewing (Figs. 6–22, 6–23, 6–24). Otherwise, if this vein is stretched, it tears readily and may cause undesirable bleeding before control is achieved. Since the vein also may be short, it retracts when divided. It is wise to doubly clip, stitch-tie, or oversew the cut ends after division. The L4–L5 disk space is then easily exposed cephalad to the iliac vessels, again using blunt dissection and pushing the loose areolar and fatty tissues anteriorly and medially, retracting the left common iliac artery and underlying vein as necessary. Variations in the venous anatomy are to be expected and need to be managed accordingly.

Exposure of the L5–S1 level also is achieved retroperitoneally, but usually caudad to the iliac vessels by bluntly pushing the loose areolar tissues and peritoneal contents anteriorly toward the dependent side. In this way, the promontory is first felt and exposed by gauze Küttner dissection. A malleable or Deaver retractor serves to hold the peritoneum and contents out of the field to expose the L5–S1 disk. The presacral artery, veins, and nerves are visualized. The artery and veins are double-clipped and divided. If nerve fibers are encountered, they may be pushed medially or laterally and preserved if exposure is not compromised.

When exposing the L5–S1 disk, special care must be taken to avoid injury to the iliac vessels. Undue continuous pressure on the iliac arteries is to be avoided. In older patients, these vessels are often atherosclerotic and may be predisposed to injury. The left iliac vein is mobilized laterally and cephalad for L5–S1 disk exposure, most often with blunt dissection alone. Vein retractors or Küttner dissectors may be used to sustain retraction during the diskectomy. Occasionally, one or two tethering tributaries on the medial side of the iliac vein are encountered and require division.

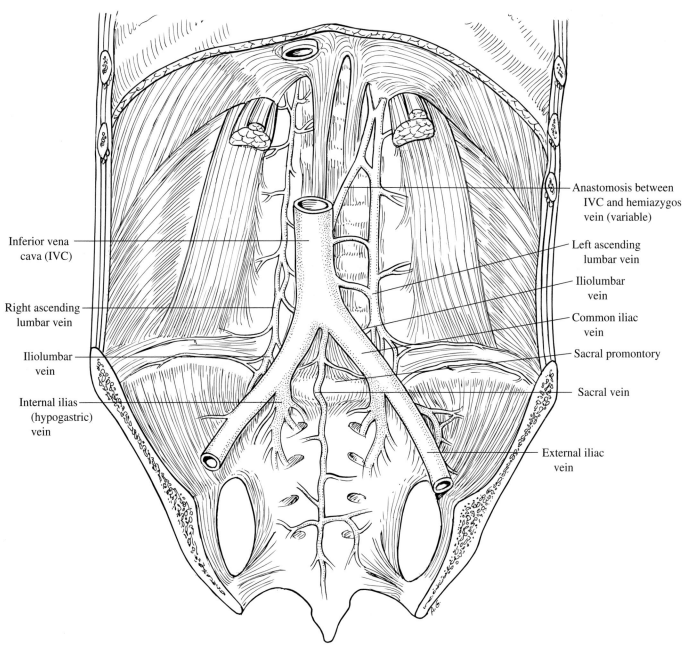

Inferior vena cava (IVC)

Right ascending lumbar vein

Iliolumbar vein

Internal ilias (hypogastric) vein

Anastomosis between IVC and hemiazygos vein (variable)

Left ascending lumbar vein

Iliolumbar vein

Common iliac vein

Sacral promontory

Sacral vein

External iliac vein

*Figure 6–22*

139

Most common bifurcation
(left side)

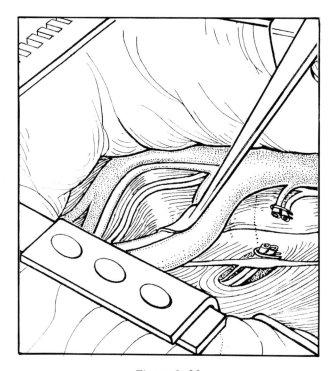

*Figure 6–23*

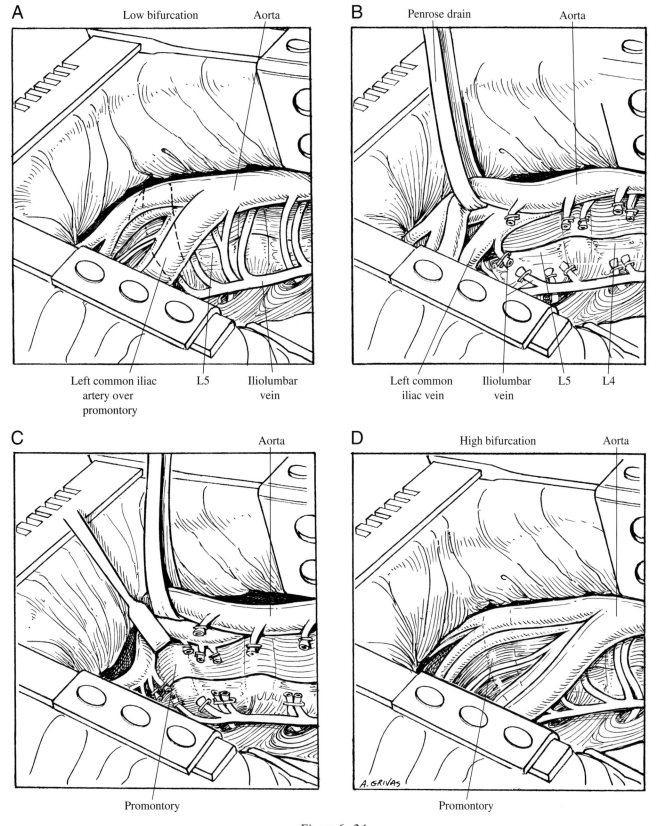

A **Low bifurcation**  **Aorta**

**Left common iliac artery over promontory**  **L5**  **Iliolumbar vein**

B **Penrose drain**  **Aorta**

**Left common iliac vein**  **Iliolumbar vein**  **L5**  **L4**

C **Aorta**

**Promontory**

D **High bifurcation**  **Aorta**

A. GRIVAS

**Promontory**

*Figure 6–24*

141

After completion of the orthopedic procedure, hemostasis is secured. There may be some oozing from the denuded vertebrae, but this usually ceases as the peritoneal contents fall back in place and serve as tamponade. No retroperitoneal drains are used. The kidney rest is lowered and the operating table leveled. The mediastinal pleura over the lower thoracic spine is loosely approximated with a 3–0 running chromic catgut down to the hiatus. The diaphragm is reattached starting with approximation of the divided crus using a polydioxanone 0 monofilament suture and then as a continuous suture following the line of the arcuate ligaments and subcostal insertions. This is carried around the periphery and anteriorly to the site of the division of the costal arch. The divided costal arch is approximated with two #0 or #1 braided dacron sutures in a figure eight. Once the divided costal arch is approximated, attachment of the subjacent portion of the diaphragm is completed with the running suture. The abdominal muscles are approximated anatomically with a continuous 0 suture, starting caudally and running toward the costal arch. The abdominal muscles usually require two layers of closure: one for the transverse and internal oblique muscles and one layer for the external oblique muscles. If the transverse muscle is well developed, it may be closed separately, or the medial part of the incision may combine the transverse and internal oblique muscles with the lateral segment closed separately. Polydioxanone suture or chromic catgut are preferred over Vicryl for muscle closure, as these have a "give" and are first placed without tension. The abdominal wall is pushed laterally to medially on each side of the incision as each loop of the running suture is tightened, thus avoiding tearing and allowing better distribution of the tension along the closing suture line. One or two chest tubes are placed. The chest wall is closed anatomically, as previously described, with pericostal sutures and 0 suture to the intercostal muscle bundles, the divided latissimus dorsi, and serratus anterior. Vicryl 2–0 is used as subcutaneous closure and 3–0 Vicryl as a subcuticular suture for the skin approximation.

## Surgical Exposure of the Thoracolumbar Spine T10–L3

The anterior exposure of the thoracolumbar spine from T10–L3 is a commonly used exposure as for "burst" fractures of T12, L1, L2, as well as spinal deformities, infections, and neoplastic lesions. It is similar to the exposure previously described to the T8–S1, although less extensive. A lateral approach, as previously described, applies to this exposure. The patient with scoliosis is placed in a lateral decubitus position with the major convexity of the curve uppermost. The flank overrides the kidney rest. The legs are dropped to extend and stretch the spine for better exposure.

A thoracolumbar incision is made overlying the tenth rib, crossing the costal arch, and extending about midway to the inguinal ligament and lateral to the rectus muscle. The tenth rib is subperiosteally resected. The pleura is incised and the chest cavity is entered. The measures previously described for T8–S1 for separations of the diaphragm apply to the T10–L3 exposure.

As shown in Figure 6–18, the diaphragm is incised peripherally at the level of the costal arch in line with the resected tenth rib, and the extraperitoneal fat layer is entered. With electrocautery, the diaphragm is divided along the costal margins and the lateral and medial arcuate ligaments, crossing the quadratus

142

lumborum and the psoas muscle, and then dividing the crus of the diaphragm, leaving about 5–10 mm of diaphragmatic muscle in the line of attachment.

With the properitoneal fat visualized, the anterior abdominal muscles are separated from this fat layer, peritoneum, and peritoneal contents by blunt finger dissection allowing the abdominal segment of the incision to be extended toward the inguinal ligament or pubic tubercle.

As shown in Figure 6–19, the retroperitoneal space is opened and in a sweeping motion, the peritoneum, peritoneal contents, and fascia are pushed forward and medially across the quadratus lumborum and psoas muscles exposing the lumbar spine.

Segmental vessels are exposed by cleaning away the overlying fatty areolar tissue and lymphatic vessels. Tethering attachments of the psoas muscles to L1, L2, and L3 may need to be separated for exposure. The vessels, singly or combined, are encircled with a right-angle forceps and occluded with Ligaclips or tied and then divided. Now the vertebral bodies disks and anterior longitudinal ligament are exposed for the orthopedic surgeon to proceed with the procedures of fusion and/or instrumentation.

# Transthoracic Diskectomy

A transthoracic spinal canal decompression for a herniated thoracic disk requires a limited thoracotomy. In general, the side of exposure is the side on which the disk is most prominent. If the disk is predominantly central in nature and results in a central canal stenosis, the right side is preferred because the intercostal vessels coming off the aorta are longer, generally easier to control, and the aorta is further away from the surgical field. A double lumen endotracheal tube allows for sequential deflation of the lung, and eliminates the need for excessive packing of the lung, manual retraction of the lung, or excessive manipulation of the lung parenchyma. In general, the rib corresponding to the disk requiring surgery is removed. For example, a T8–9 disk would require removal of the ninth rib. Positioning, preparing, and draping for a thoracotomy is similar to those for more extensive anterior releases and fusions (Fig. 6–25).

Once the chest has been opened, the parietal pleura is incised longitudinally along its anteromedial exposure. The segmental vessels are exposed and divided. The head of the rib is subperiosteally dissected and removed. A suitable section of rib should be removed so that the costotransverse joint is disarticulated, as well. This allows for a very suitable lateral and anterolateral exposure of the vertebral bodies (Fig. 6–26).

It is imperative to ensure correct intraoperative localization. This is done by carefully counting the ribs on the preoperative studies to ensure that there are indeed 12 ribs, and when the chest is opened, the proper rib will be resected. The surgeon and the assistant count separately and independently assess the level before coming to a decision. An intraoperative radiograph with a marker in the disk space also is taken. These precautions are necessary because of the monotonous and uniform intraoperative appearance of the midthoracic spine and the lack of specific discrete anatomic landmarks (Fig. 6–27).

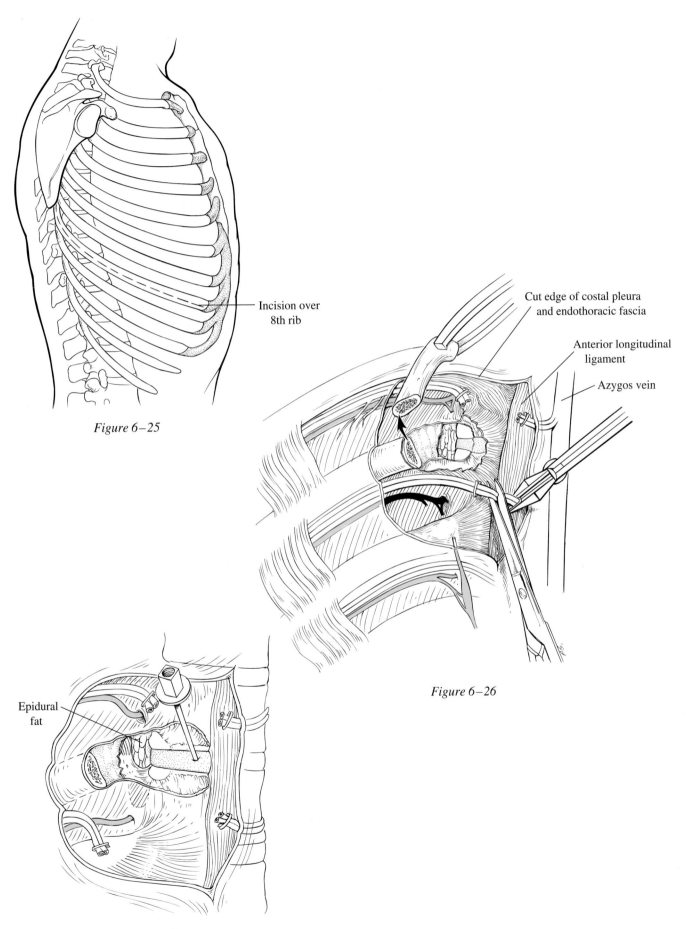

Incision over
8th rib

*Figure 6–25*

Cut edge of costal pleura
and endothoracic fascia

Anterior longitudinal
ligament

Azygos vein

*Figure 6–26*

Epidural
fat

*Figure 6–27*

145

Once the appropriate level has been clinically and radiographically confirmed, the confluence of the transverse process, lateral aspect of the pedicle, and the anterolateral aspect of the vertebral body are cleared of soft tissue. The pedicle is further resected using a small Kerrison punch to provide adequate access to the lateral aspect of the spinal canal. The longer (9 inch) thoracic-type Kerrison punch facilitates pedicle resection in the depths of the chest (Fig. 6–28).

If considerable central canal stenosis exists, and the insertion of the small foot plate about the medial aspect of the pedicle is a concern, a high-speed diamond burr, under continuous water irrigation, is used to cut away the upper and medial one third of the pedicle. This provides a very safe and atraumatic lateral exposure of the spinal canal (Fig. 6–29).

In a similar fashion, the costovertebral joints above and below the disk herniation are removed. This allows for definitive identification of the lateral and anterolateral aspects of the spinal canal. Generally, it is not necessary to dissect and trace the intercostal nerves. If the anatomy is markedly distorted, locating the intercostal nerve within its neurovascular bundle laterally, tracing it down around the pedicle, and performing a formal pedicle excision often allows the surgeon to develop similar appreciation of a lateral spinal canal anatomy (Fig. 6–30).

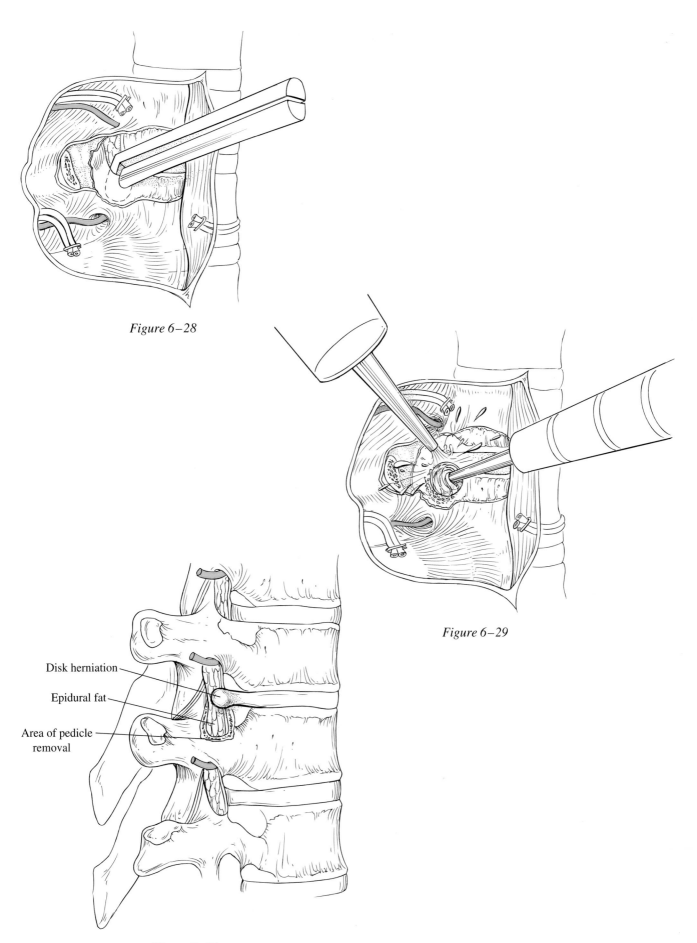

*Figure 6–28*

*Figure 6–29*

Disk herniation

Epidural fat

Area of pedicle
removal

*Figure 6–30*

147

The proposed hemivertebral body resection encompasses a portion of the disk material as well to a suitable proximal and distal extent. This would permit formal spinal canal decompression to be carried out in a region where relatively less canal stenosis exists. The decompression is carried out keeping the previously identified limits of the anterior and anterolateral aspects of the spinal canal in mind (Fig. 6–31).

The dissection is carried out with minimal disk manipulation. At no time is any instrument introduced into the spinal canal. A high-speed carbide burr is used to quickly remove the bone and most of disk material. The posterior vertebral cortex is cautiously approached but is not perforated with the carbide burr. Utilizing a high-speed diamond burr, under continuous water irrigation, the remaining cortex is divided. A transverse cut on the far lateral aspect of the spinal canal is then used to remove the bridging bone and osteophyte (Fig. 6–32).

This frees up an island of disk and bone material, which allows the disk and offending osteophyte to be pulled into the previously created surgical trough. If done properly, a fragment consisting of herniated disk and adjacent adherent osteophyte can be removed in one piece. This rapidly decompresses the spinal canal without any undue mechanical manipulation of the spinal cord itself (Fig. 6–33).

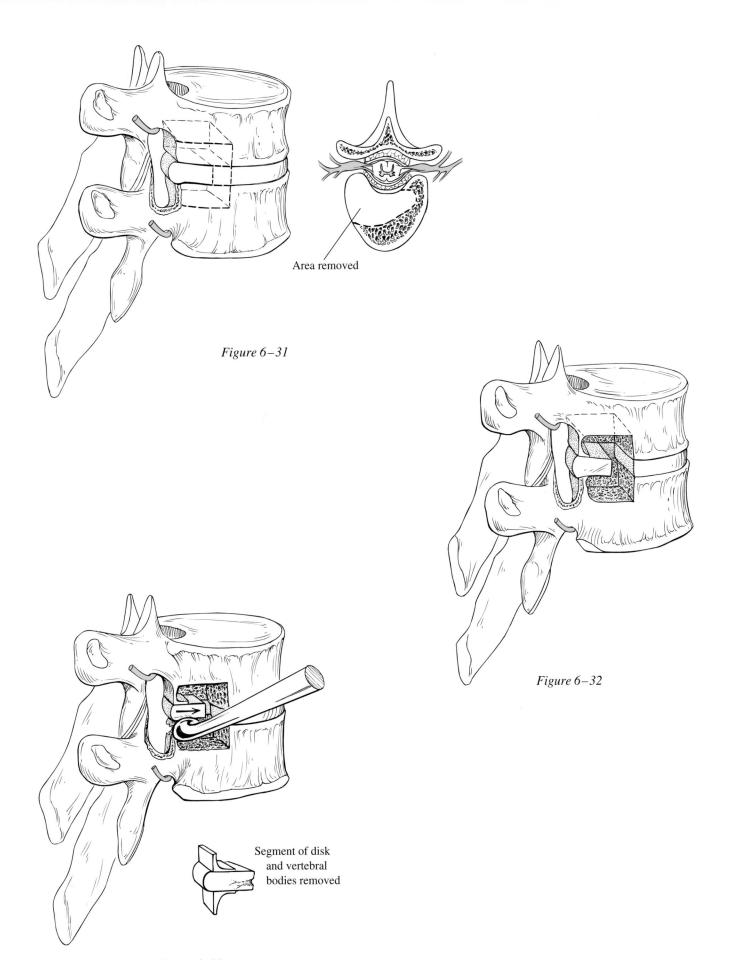

Area removed

Figure 6–31

Figure 6–32

Segment of disk
and vertebral
bodies removed

Figure 6–33

149

Once the formal hemicorporectomy and disk removal have been completed, deliberate hemostasis with a gelatine sponge and bone wax is carried out.

It is not necessary to take down the posterior longitudinal ligament in all cases. If there is any suggestion of a transligamentous process or if the adequacy of the decompression is in doubt, the ligament can be stretched by placing a thin, narrow elevator between the ligament and dura once the disk and osteophyte have been removed and dividing the ligament with a sharp knife using the elevator as protection. The ligament can be removed to allow for spinal canal inspection. Occasionally, epidural bleeding can be severe and precautions must be made for immediate tamponade and bipolar cautery (Fig. 6–34).

Once the decompression is completed, slots are cut in the upper and lower vertebral bodies using osteotomes. Care is used to preserve a posterior ledge to prevent posterior graft displacement. Multiple rib grafts are placed in a longitudinal fashion. These grafts are cut slightly longer than the measured length of the mortise and impacted.

Generally, three intact rib grafts can be impacted. Additionally, morsels of bone are placed around the grafts and into the resected disk space anteriorly. No graft is placed between the rib struts and the dura and posterior longitudinal ligament, posteriorly. It is important that all of the disk be removed, and bone grafting is done in the entire disk area, not just a small area on the side of surgical exposure (Fig. 6–35).

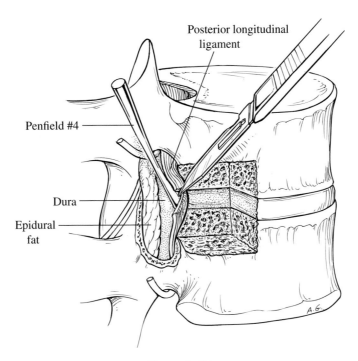

*Figure 6–34*

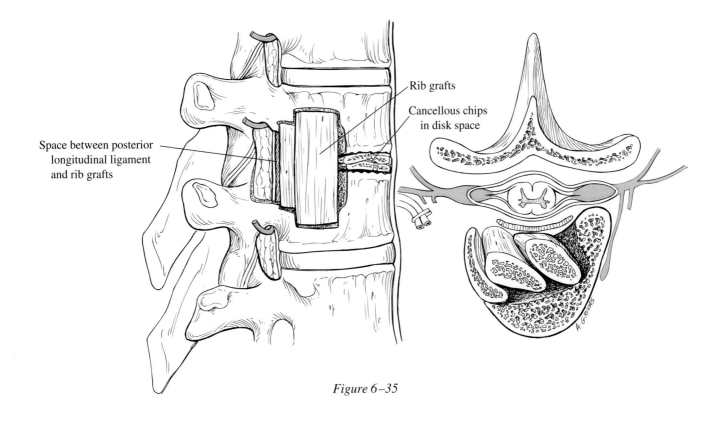

*Figure 6–35*

151

# Anterior Multilevel Ligament and Disk Release

This procedure is used both for frontal plane (scoliosis) and sagittal plane deformities (lordosis and kyphosis). The purpose of the procedure is to excise the disk and the annulus to provide a greater degree of mobility at each motion segment and to graft the disk space with chips of bone in order to enhance the rate of arthrodesis.

After exposure of the desired area by one of the anterior procedures previously described, the areolar soft tissue anterior to the disk space is dissected around to the side opposite the surgeon. This is usually a bloodless, avascular plane, especially in the thoracic region, but may be slightly more difficult in the lumbar spine. With a hot cautery knife, the annulus is outlined in a rectangular fashion and excised with a sharp knife and rongeurs.

For the correction of a kyphosis, it is highly desirable to remove the anterior longitudinal ligament and the annulus on both the near and far side. The near side is easy, but the far side is more difficult requiring a careful exposure and excision of the annulus with rongeurs under direct vision. Blunt retractors should be placed in the sulcus prior to excision of the annulus on the far side. This prevents inadvertent vascular injury.

For scoliosis correction, the far side annulus is a stabilizing hinge that the surgeon may wish to preserve, and, therefore, only the anterior longitudinal ligament, anterior annulus, and near side annulus are removed.

Once the annulus has been excised, the soft disk material is removed with rongeurs. The cartilaginous end plate is then incised at its junction with the vertebral body laterally, and a flat periosteal elevator is slipped into the interspace peeling the cartilaginous vertebral end plate off the bony end plate in this plane. If done carefully, an avascular plane can be found allowing a thorough but quick removal of the cartilage plate. Once this plate is peeled back, it can be quickly removed with rongeurs providing a bloodless view inside the disk space. Finally, the remaining fragments of cartilage and disk material are removed using curettes and rongeurs until only the posterior annulus remains. It is not necessary to enter the spinal canal, and it is usually desirable to leave the posterior annulus as a protective barrier between the bone fragments of the disk space and the spinal canal. If this procedure has been done carefully, there will be virtually no bleeding from the bony end plates, since there was no penetration into the cancellous bone. Each disk space is done in sequence over the area desired, packing each disk space with thrombin-soaked Gelfoam after removal of the disk material. At this point, penetration into the cancellous bone is to be avoided (Figs. 6-36 and 6-37).

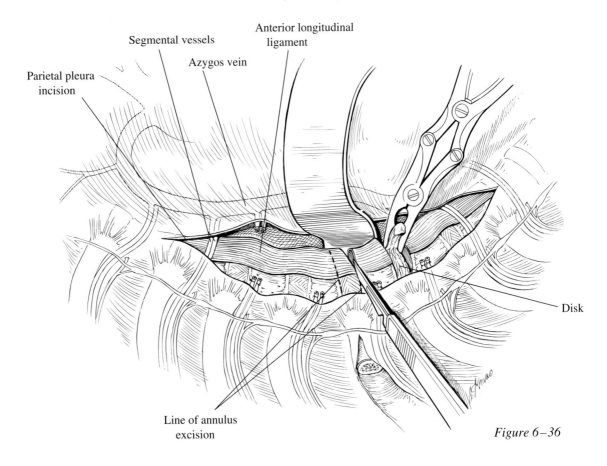

Parietal pleura incision

Segmental vessels

Azygos vein

Anterior longitudinal ligament

Disk

Line of annulus excision

*Figure 6–36*

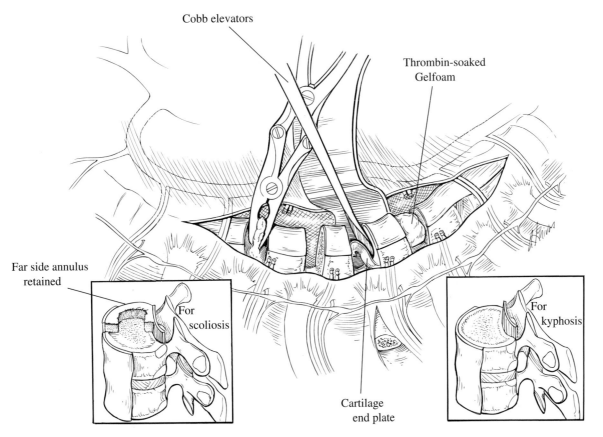

Cobb elevators

Thrombin-soaked Gelfoam

Far side annulus retained

For scoliosis

Cartilage end plate

For kyphosis

*Figure 6–37*

153

After all of the disks have been removed, one then proceeds with bone grafting each disk space in sequence. The thrombin-soaked Gelfoam pledget is removed at one level and, using a sharp curette or osteotome, the bony end plate is penetrated. The bone fragments are simply left in the disk space and additional autogenous bone fragments from the rib are packed into the disk space. These fragments are tamped into place using a drift, driving the fragments toward the opposite side and not toward the canal. At this point, the disk space will show some bleeding, but the packing of the space will usually slow down the oozing. It is then covered with a thrombin-soaked Gelfoam pledget. The surgeon proceeds to the next disk space, repeating this procedure until all levels are done (Fig. 6–38).

After completing the diskectomy, ligament release, and bone grafting of each disk space individually, the parietal pleura is resutured over this area, which reduces the amount of bleeding into the chest. In the lumbar spine, no tissue is available to sew over this space unless the psoas has been reflected and it can be brought forward to help control oozing. A chest tube is then inserted if the thorax has been opened and appropriate closure completed. This procedure is virtually always supplemented by a posterior procedure performed at the same time or at a later date.

Because there is no longitudinal strut graft used in this procedure, it is technically feasible to do the procedure without ligation of all or any of the segmental vessels. This may be advantageous in highly specialized cases in which there might be a compromise of the blood supply of the spinal cord.

This procedure can be used at any level of the spine from C1–S1. As stated earlier, it is a procedure designed to improve the mobility and correctability of the spine and to enhance the rate of arthrodesis.

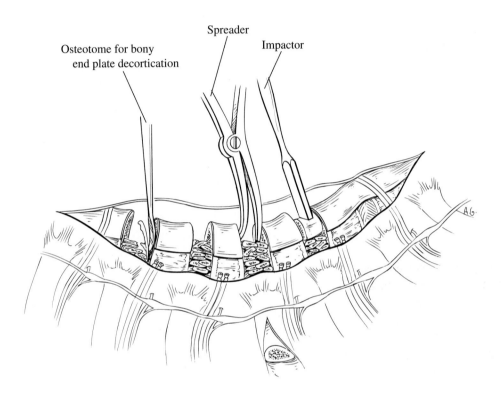

Osteotome for bony
end plate decortication

Spreader

Impactor

*Figure 6–38*

# Anterior Multilevel Diskectomy and Wedge Vertebrectomy for Scoliosis

This procedure is similar to Anterior Multilevel Ligament and Disk Release with the exception that additional bone wedges are taken at the disk levels in order to improve the amount of potential correction.

After exposure and excision of the disk as previously described, the annulus is removed and the disk excised, avoiding penetration into the cancellous bone and vertebral bodies. After all the disks have been exposed and excised, attention is then directed to the apical vertebra of the scoliosis, at which time the periosteum of the lateral vertebral body at the convexity, the side toward the surgeon, is peeled back off of the vertebral bodies using a periosteal elevator. The periosteum may be cut with a hot knife, and the surgeon can then peel back the lateral vertebral body.

There may be significant bleeders from the lateral wall of the vertebra and these should be stopped with bone wax. After the desired number of vertebrae have been exposed, an osteotome is used to outline a wedge of bone adjacent to the disk space. The osteotome is used to cut the vertebral body, taking care not to penetrate the posterior cortex or the spinal canal. The transected bone is removed with rongeurs, which will leave posterior bone that is removed back to the posterior cortex with a curette.

Since the outcome of this procedure is to have a greater degree of "closing wedge osteotomy effect," the wedge will not close if the posterior cortex is left in place. This, therefore, requires entering the spinal canal, which can be done through the disk space or through the posterior cortex of the vertebral body. The problem is usually bleeding from epidural veins, which should be controlled with thrombin-soaked Gelfoam pledgets or bipolar cautery.

Since the purpose of the procedure is to close wedges, do not place a large amount of grafting bone in these excised wedges. There is considerably more bleeding with this procedure (Figs. 6–39 and 6–40).

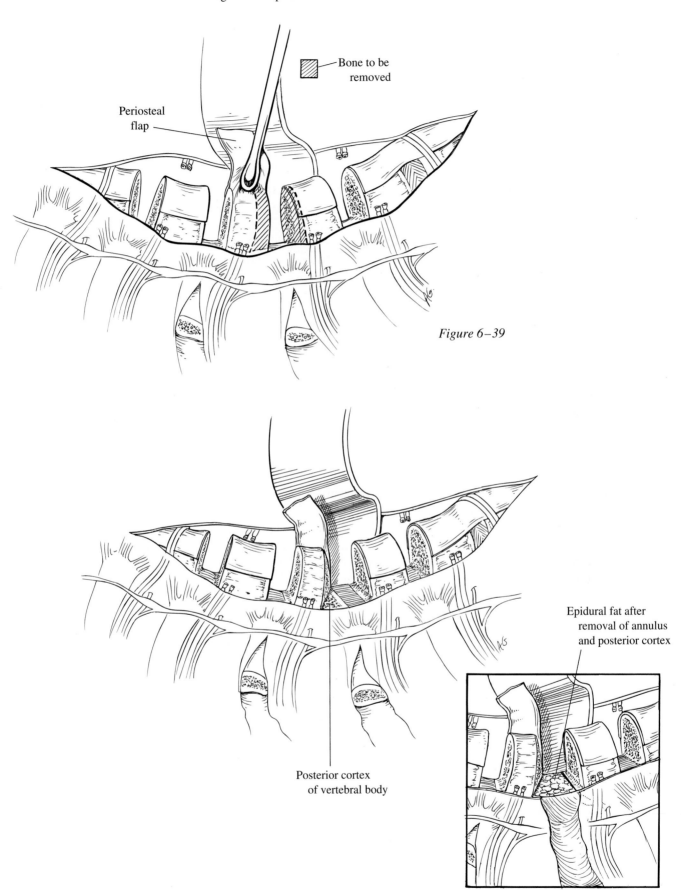

Bone to be
removed

Periosteal
flap

*Figure 6–39*

Epidural fat after
removal of annulus
and posterior cortex

Posterior cortex
of vertebral body

*Figure 6–40*

157

# Anterior Diskectomy and Vertebrectomy for Scoliosis

This relatively radical operation is for major spinal curvature where a great deal of angulation is taking place at the apical vertebra. To obtain significant correction of the curvature, the convexity is shortened by taking out a vertebra so that the upper and lower limbs of the curvature can be brought into better alignment. This is a more radical operation than a hemivertebra excision, which is designed to maintain the concave annulus as a stabilizing ligament hinge allowing shortening and correction of the curvature, but providing three-dimensional stability. That is, there is no anterior-posterior shear instability or lateral shear instability if the concave ligament complex is kept intact. However, in vertebrectomy surgery, the intent of the operation (as originally described by Luque) is to create a totally mobile segment of the spine allowing major correction to take place. Thus, major instability is deliberately created to obtain major correctability.

The spine is exposed along the convexity of the curvature by a transthoracic or transthoracic–retroperitoneal approach. Often the ribs of the convexity are lying on the vertebral body and it may be necessary to osteotomize or resect more than one rib to obtain adequate exposure. With the chest opened and the ribs excised, the periosteum is incised and reflected carefully as a periosteal flap, the outer layers of the annulus being in continuity with the periosteum. This dissection usually extends about three vertebrae above and three below the apical vertebra. The disks throughout the curvature are resected as previously described (Figs. 6–41, 6–42, and 6–43). Since the disks above and below the vertebra have already been dissected, the remainder of the vertebral body can be removed with a rongeur. The posterior cortex of the vertebral body and the posterior annulus at the two disks are the most difficult to remove.

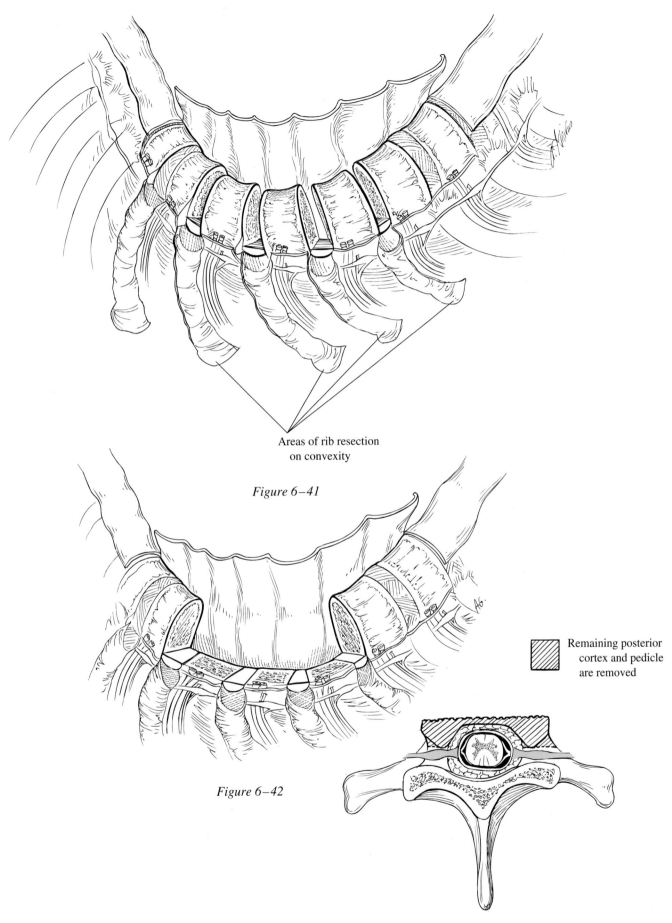

Areas of rib resection
on convexity

*Figure 6–41*

*Figure 6–42*

Remaining posterior
cortex and pedicle
are removed

*Figure 6–43*

159

Curettement of the bone using transversely oriented maneuvers is carried down to the posterior hard cortical bone, and bone holes are plugged with bone wax (Fig. 6–44). When the entire posterior cortex has been exposed, the spinal canal is entered centrally and the hole gradually enlarged in all directions, resecting the posterior annulus of the two disks (Figs. 6–45 and 6–46). The dissection is carried out first to the near side nerve root foramina and then the far side above and below the pedicle so only the two pedicles of the vertebra to be removed are in view. A fat graft or Gelfoam followed by mushed bone chips from the vertebral body are inserted into the tube of periosteum so that no matter what correction is obtained during the posterior procedure the bone chips will align themselves in the zone of the vertebral column (Fig. 6–47).

Because of the fairly extensive dissection in the spinal canal, bleeding from epidural veins can be significant. These veins should be managed with thrombin-soaked Gelfoam and/or bipolar cautery.

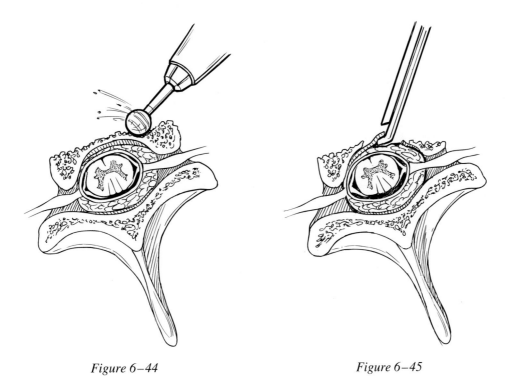

Figure 6–44

Figure 6–45

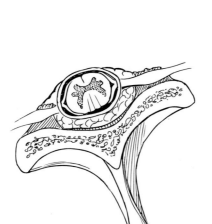

Figure 6–46

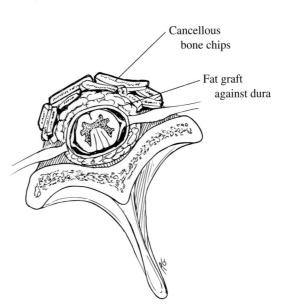

Cancellous
bone chips

Fat graft
against dura

Figure 6–47

# Anterior Inlay Graft for Round Kyphosis

This procedure is for a flexible round kyphosis such as Scheuermann's disease, where the anterior longitudinal ligament is left intact, and in a postlaminectomy kyphosis, where a severe deformity has not yet developed but the need for anterior fusion is obvious.

After opening the chest and ligating the segmental vessels over the desired area, the periosteum is incised just anterior to the rib heads with a T-shaped incision at each end so that the periosteum can be deflected forward to the anterior longitudinal ligament. The disk is resected from the anterior longitudinal ligament back to the rib head area. With a rongeur and/or gouge, a trough is created in the lateral aspect of the vertebral bodies to the opposite side, which can be done fairly rapidly. Large venous bleeders should be bone waxed, but smaller ones are ignored (Figs. 6–48 and 6–49). With manual correction of the kyphosis, the correct length of rib inlay graft is tapped into place (Fig. 6–50). It is beneficial to countersink each end of the rib graft to prevent dislodgement, which is highly unusual. The remaining disk spaces are packed with autogenous cancellous bone (Fig. 6–51). The periosteum and parietal pleura are sutured for hemostasis.

For more significant deformities, the periosteum is reflected past the anterior longitudinal ligament, which is divided into multiple levels anterior to the disk. This provides more flexibility to the curvature. The same type of trough is created and manual correction is utilized to gain the maximum improvement on the table. This approach permits more correction of the curvature if necessary by creating more flexibility but does involve a greater amount of anterior dissection.

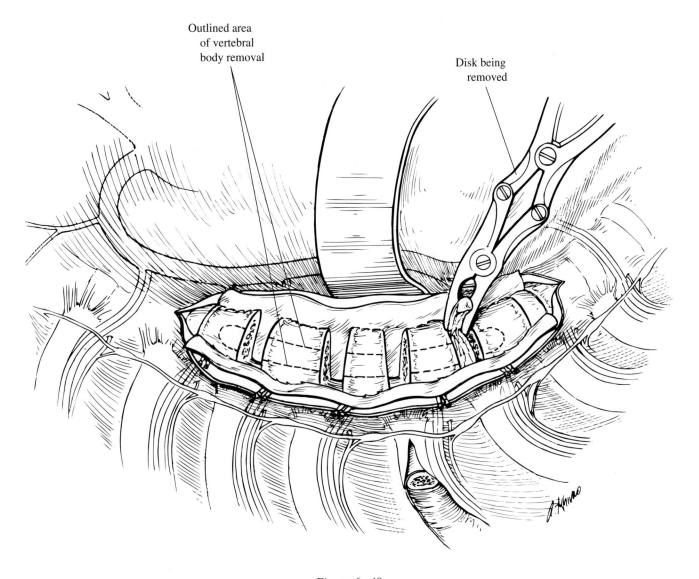

Outlined area of vertebral body removal

Disk being removed

Figure 6–48

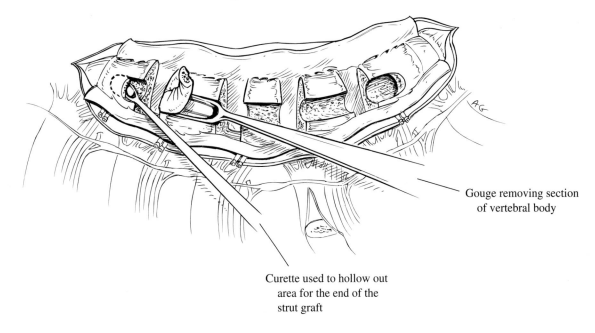

Gouge removing section of vertebral body

Curette used to hollow out area for the end of the strut graft

Figure 6–49

163

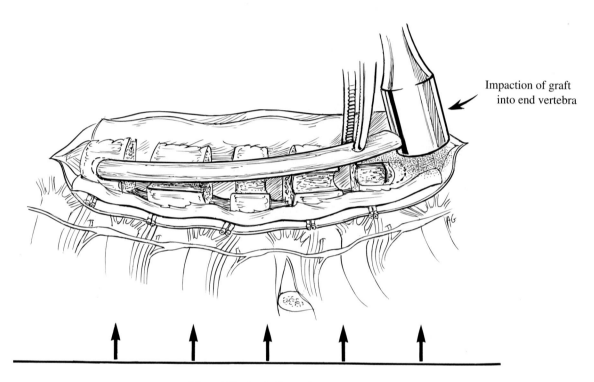

Impaction of graft
into end vertebra

Manual Kyphosis Correction

*Figure 6–50*

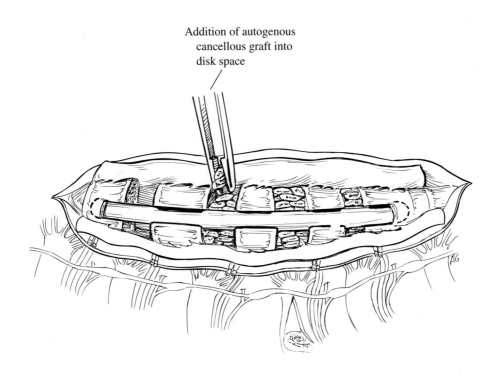

Addition of autogenous
cancellous graft into
disk space

*Figure 6–51*

# *Anterior Strut Graft for Angular Kyphosis*

For angular kyphosis the spine is exposed through the convex side if the kyphosis occurs in combination with a scoliotic deformity. If it is a pure kyphosis, it can be exposed from either the right or left. After ligation of the segmental vessels throughout the length of the planned surgical area, the spine is exposed by subperiosteal dissection. The periosteal flap begins at the head of the ribs posteriorly, and the flap is cut at the top and bottom in a "T" shape so it can be fully reflected. The subperiosteal dissection is carried past the anterior longitudinal ligament and around as far as possible to the convexity of the scoliosis or the far side of the kyphotic deformity. The periosteal flap can be used as a protective barrier against the soft tissues and the retractors can be placed within this flap.

The disks throughout the kyphotic area are fully excised to the posterior longitudinal ligament. It is not necessary to enter the spinal canal. In a congenital kyphotic patient, there is usually a large amount of cartilaginous material at the apex of the curve that should be liberally excised to good bleeding bone (Fig. 6–52).

General Principles of Anterior Release and Strut Grafting for Severe Angular Kyphosis of any Etiology

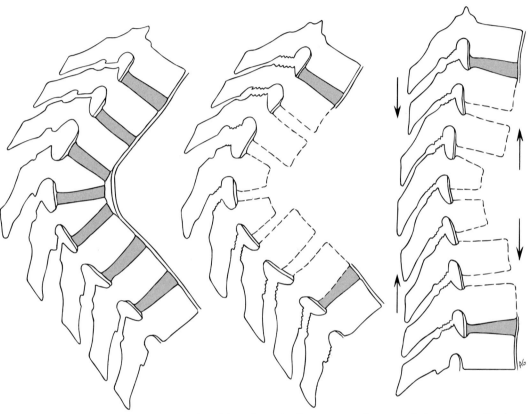

Radical excision of anterior ligament, annulus, cartilage, and disk material. The posterior longitudinal ligament is left intact.

Anterior elongation is followed by posterior shortening.

*Figure 6–52*

At this point an anterior distractor is placed at the furthest anterior position and gradually elongated. There are two types of distractor: the Santa Casa distractor (DePuy Company) and the Slot distractor (Ullrich Company). This should be done patiently, allowing for soft tissue "creep." Spinal cord monitoring and/or wake-up test can be done during or following the distraction. For the best results, this procedure is done with the patient's neck in extension, which relaxes the neural axis. Manual pressure over the apex of the gibbus can facilitate the corrective maneuver (Figs. 6–53 and 6–54).

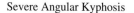

Severe Angular Kyphosis

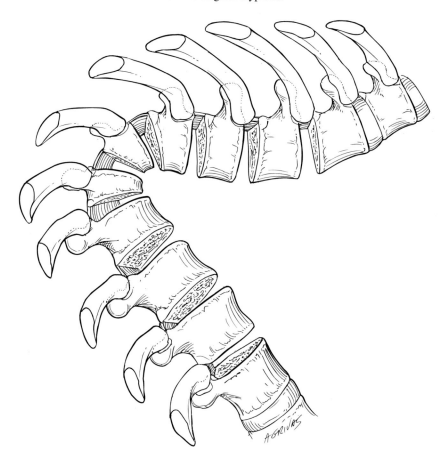

*Figure 6–53*

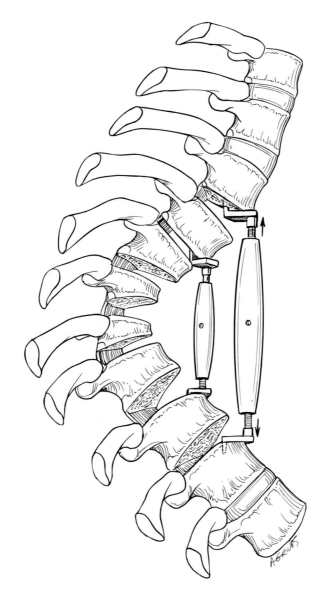

*Figure 6–54*

When the maximal amount of distraction is achieved, a solid strut graft (usually fibula) is prepared. A hole is made in the vertebral body just behind the distractor, the strut graft tucked into the superior vertebra and then into the inferior vertebra. Once this solid strut graft is firmly embedded, the anterior metallic distracting devices are removed (it is not an implant) and a larger strut graft is inserted in their place. Any space remaining behind and in between these grafts must be filled with autogenous bone from the rib, iliac crest, or any other possible source. Anterior strut grafts should never be free, that is, separated from the vertebral body tissue without interspersed grafts (Figs. 6–55 and 6–56).

An anterior fibular strut graft can be augmented by a vascularized rib graft (see pp 190–192). This aids in the revascularization of the fibular graft.

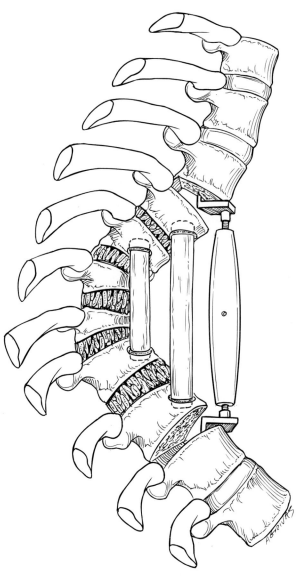

Figure 6–55

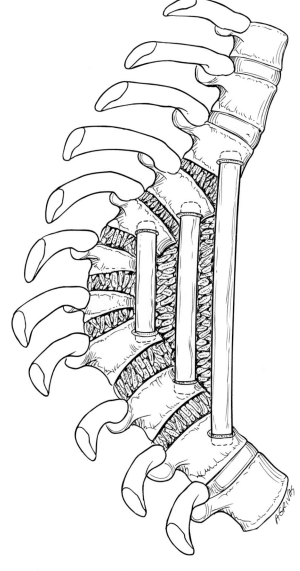

Figure 6–56

171

# Anterior Cord Decompression for Angular Gibbus

The purpose of this procedure is to anteriorly decompress the spinal cord because of an angular kyphosis or gibbus. The patient should have a significant neurologic deficit to justify this procedure. The thorax is opened either with a transthoracic or a thoracolumbar approach depending on the level involved. Usually the rib proximal to the apex of the deformity is removed so that the midaxillary point of that rib is directly opposite the apex of the gibbus (Fig. 6–57). The segmental vessels are ligated throughout the entire kyphosis and the

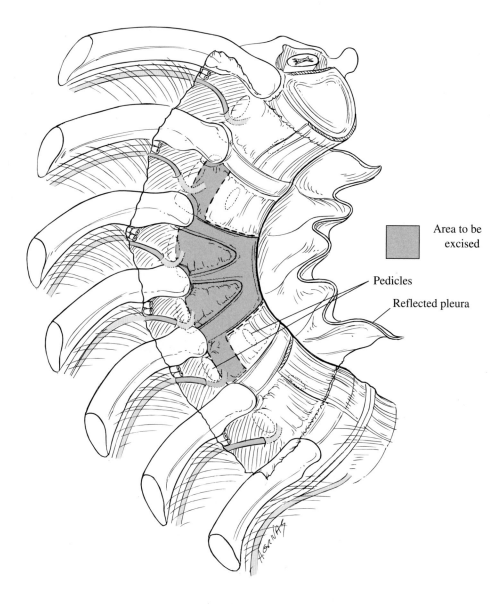

Area to be excised

Pedicles

Reflected pleura

*Figure 6–57*

three or four rib heads at the apex of the kyphus are excised. The disks are removed if present in the deformity. Finally, the bone is removed to give the decompression. Although it is tempting to follow the intercostal nerve roots into the foramen and begin chipping away posteriorly, it has been well demonstrated that this is not an ideal procedure. A large cavity is created in the vertebral bodies (Fig. 6–58). This may necessitate resecting all or most of the apical vertebra. The dissection, not unlike a thoracic disk excision, is carried to the opposite cortex. The resection always involves the vertebrae above and below the apical vertebra leaving finally only the posterior cortex of the three vertebrae. At this point, this bone cavity should be well defined to the opposite cortex and it should be clean and dry, with adequate bone waxing of any exposed surfaces. The spinal canal has not been entered at any point.

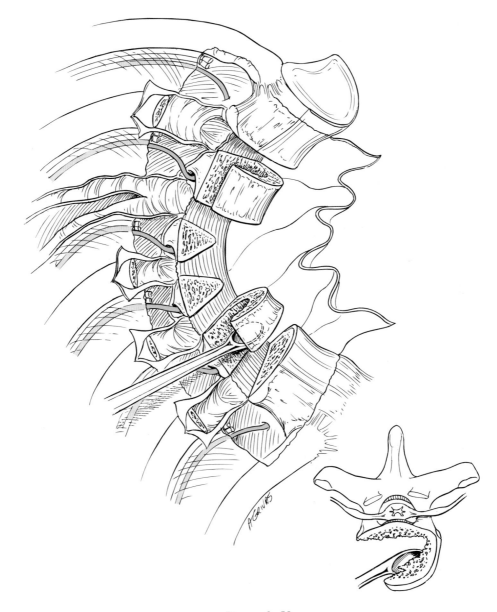

*Figure 6–58*

At this point, the spinal canal is entered and the dura identified. This should *not* be done at the apex of the deformity but either above or below or preferably both. The canal is identified and the opening enlarged so that the dural sac is clearly visible across the vertebral body from one pedicle to the other. The bone is removed toward the apex of the deformity from above and below and from the far side toward the near side. If the near side bone is removed first, the spinal cord will roll toward the surgeon obscuring a ledge of bone behind it. The last bone removed should be the bone at the apex. The bone is removed with burrs, curettes, or fine Kerrison rongeurs. Usually all three are used at one point during the procedure (Fig. 6–59).

At the completion of the procedure, the dura must have visibly sagged forward into the space created. One needs to cut out through the foramina, otherwise the cord becomes suspended under the nerve roots. This is a complex and difficult procedure and blood loss may be significant. Bleeding should be controlled as best as possible with thrombin-soaked Gelfoam, bipolar cautery, and tincture of time. Hypotensive anesthesia is not recommended, since the spinal cord is already at great risk and hypotensive anesthesia intensifies the risk.

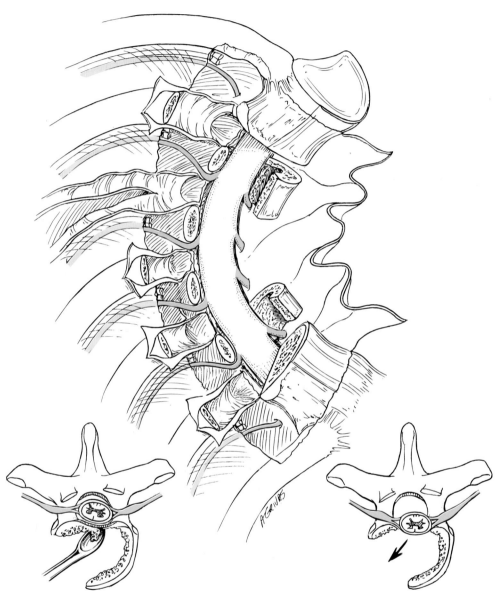

*Figure 6–59*

# Anterior Vertebrectomy and Tricortical Iliac Bone Graft for a Burst Fracture

For a T12 burst fracture, the approach is a thoracolumbotomy through an eleventh rib, which provides an excellent visualization of the burst and the correct approach angle for instruments for decompression (Fig. 6–60). The segmental vessels in front of T11, T12, and L1 are ligated and the posterior part of the burst vertebra approached. At this stage, an x-ray should be taken to ensure that you are at the correct level, unless the anatomy, in particular the presence of the twelfth rib, demonstrates your level.

An excision of the annulus fibrosis between T11–T12 and T12–L1 is made. This is done without damaging the anterior longitudinal ligament. A curette is used to remove the cartilage from the lower end plate of T11 and the superior end plate of L1 (Fig. 6–61). At this stage, it is not possible to reach the posterior point where the retropulsed fragment is pressing on the neuroelements.

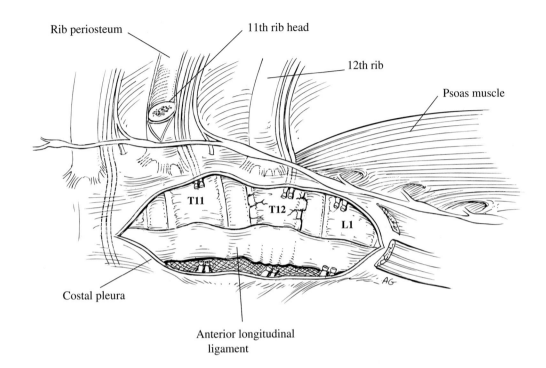

Figure 6–60

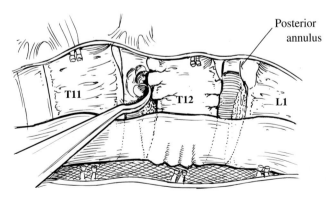

Figure 6–61

Some further fragments may be removed to the contralateral annulus fibrosis with a pituitary or Leksell rongeur (Fig. 6–62).

The most anterior part of the pedicle of the burst vertebra should be exposed, and it may be necessary to excise the head of the twelfth rib, which is overlying the pedicle (Fig. 6–63). Some bone wax may be used to stop the bleeding on the stump of the twelfth rib.

With visualization of the corner between the anterior part of the pedicle and the posterior vertebral body, it is possible to estimate the location of the retropulsed fragment and the direction of the vertebrectomy. In the absence of excellent visualization, the neural elements are at greater risk. For the vertebrectomy, use a Leksell rongeur to remove the posterior aspect of the vertebral body of T12 down to the far cortex (Fig. 6–64).

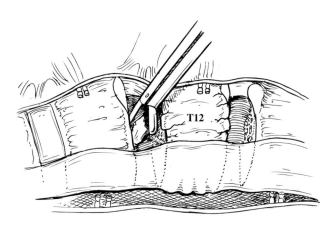

*Figure 6–62*

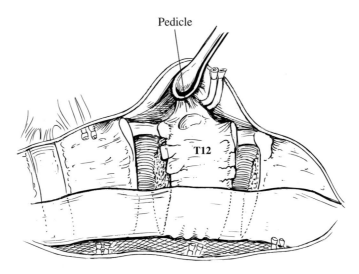

*Figure 6–63*

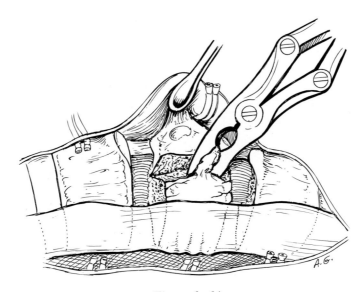

*Figure 6–64*

By using a large laminar elevator between the lower end plate of T11 and the superor end plate of L1, it becomes possible to identify the retropulsed fragment. Distraction applied between the two end plates allows some ligamentotaxis on the posterior longitudinal ligament (PLL), which pushes the retropulsed fragment forward making it more obvious to the surgeon doing the decompression. The use of the large laminar spreader allows the initiation of decompression and protects the neuroelements from the manipulations of that fragment (Fig. 6–65).

The retropulsed fragment has been identified and the decompression proceeds using a Leksell rongeur to remove the posterolateral corner of the vertebral body, directing it toward the junction between the pedicle and the vertebral body itself (Fig. 6–66).

A curette may be used to rotate the fragment further out of the spinal canal (Fig. 6–67).

Figures 6–68 and 6–69 illustrate the effect of ligamentotaxis during anterior decompression. Figure 6–69 demonstrates that it is necessary to remove some of the vertebral body to allow the retropulsed fragment to rotate around its annular hinge and decompress the spinal canal. The ligamentotaxis is best obtained by placing the Inge laminar spreader between the vertebral body of T11 and the vertebral body of L1.

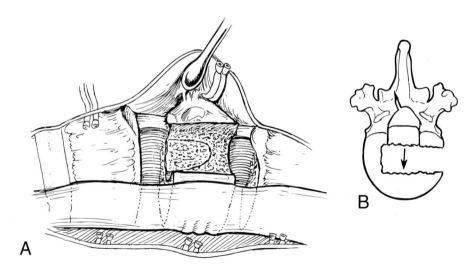

*Figure 6–65*

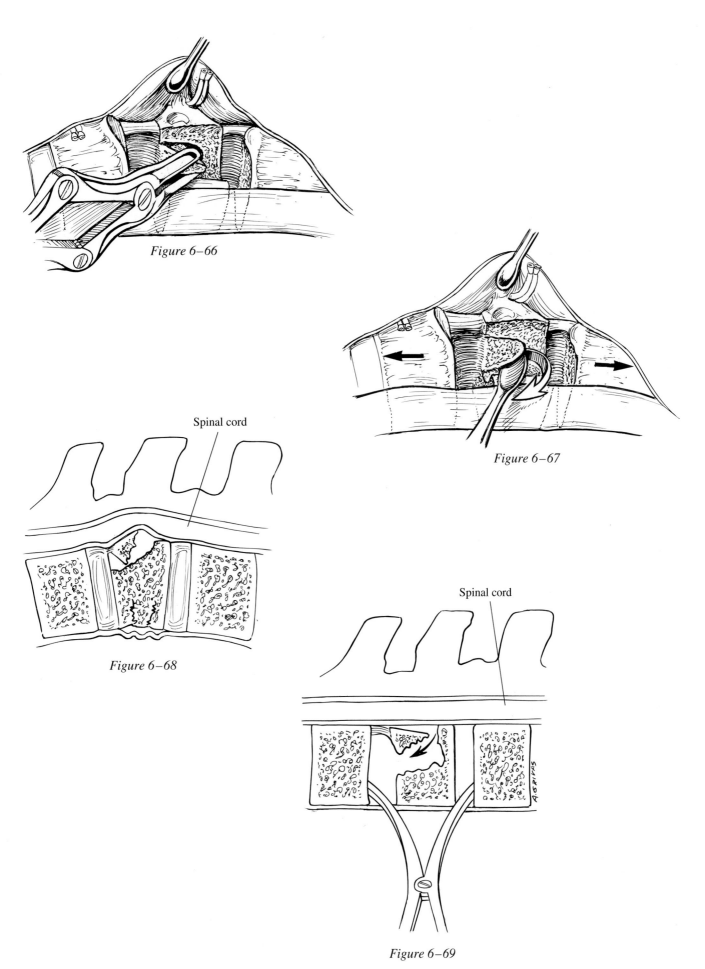

Figure 6–66

Figure 6–67

Spinal cord

Figure 6–68

Spinal cord

Figure 6–69

181

The retropulsed fragment has been removed in parts and the use of a Kerrison rongeur will allow decompression of the ipsilateral recess (Fig. 6–70).

The decompression should extend to the pedicle and actually expose the exiting nerve root at that level. Any significant bleeding in front of the dura may be taken care of with bipolar cautery or with Gelfoam with topical thrombin. The decompression also will extend to the contralateral recess, decompressing the contralateral exiting nerve root. The PLL, generally, is intact and does not have to be removed. It is actually a protective layer to the dura. This is possible only in acute fractures. In chronic fractures, it has to be removed because it does not dissect off of the bone, making it more difficult to estimate the quality of decompression (Fig. 6–71).

After careful exploration of the four corners of the decompression, the end plates are prepared for strut grafting (Fig. 6–72).

Large tricortical grafts, or fibula grafts, will be strutted under maximal distraction between the vertebrae above and below the fracture. The strut grafts have to be anterior to resist actual loading. A posterior graft would have less mechanical strength and be more likely to displace into the spinal canal. It may be necessary to use the large laminar spreader for insertion of the grafts in the maximally distracted position (Fig. 6–73).

After placement of those struts, add some of the cancellous chips that have been removed during the vertebrectomy to provide bone grafts that are more likely to incorporate rapidly when compared to the fibular grafts (Fig. 6–74). The anterior fusion is completed and is covered with Gelfoam for final hemostasis. The thoracolumbotomy is closed in the usual manner.

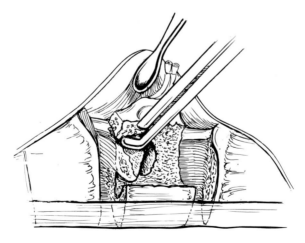

*Figure 6–70*

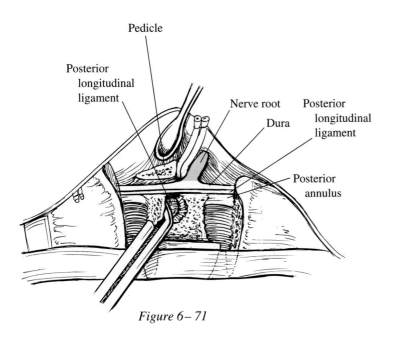

Figure 6–71

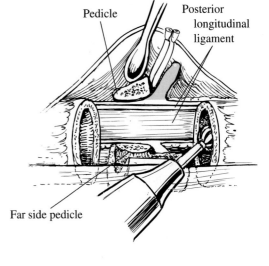

Figure 6–72

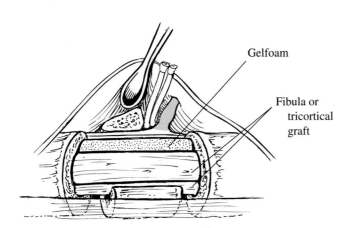

Figure 6–73

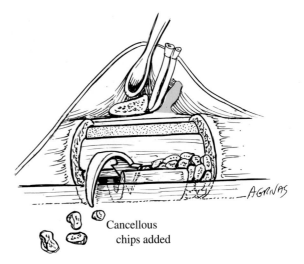

Figure 6–74

183

# Kaneda Instrumentation

Figure 6–75 illustrates a burst fracture type A with intrusion of bone into the spinal canal from the upper and lower end plates. Neurologic deficit at this level justifies proceeding with an anterior decompression and fusion. The Kaneda instrumentation may be helpful in stabilizing the spinal motion segments between the vertebra above and the vertebra below the fracture, which in this case are T12, L1, and L2.

Following anterior decompression, an anterior fusion is carried out with strut grafts placed under maximal distraction of the vertebra above and against the vertebra below. The strut grafts have to be strong in actual loading resistance and will be further stabilized by the Kaneda instrumentation. The spinal plates are positioned on the vertebra above and the vertebra below the fracture. The ideal position is on the lateral to anterolateral corner of the vertebral body. The position of the plates is in the middle of the vertebra, so as to prevent penetration of the screw through the end plates. The posterior rod is short, and the anterior rod is long. The plates have to be positioned with their anterior holes away from the vertebrectomy and posterior holes close to the vertebrectomy. The screws are inserted through the spinal plates to a length calculated from the width of the vertebra in which the screw is inserted. It is appropriate for the screw to penetrate the far cortex. The two screws are typically convergent in the axial view but remain parallel in the coronal plane (Figs. 6–76, 6–77, and 6–78).

The paraspinal rods are inserted and the screws connected. Some compression should be applied against the strut graft to preload the bone and prevent shielding of the bone graft. The basic biomechanical principle of anterior instrumentation is that of a tension band. Providing distraction with the Kaneda system in the hope of obtaining further correction of the local kyphosis would be a poor choice for using the system. It would lead to (1) bending of the screws, (2) likely failure of the metal, and (3) likely pseudoarthrosis, until finally, the metal breakage would allow bone-to-bone opposition, collapse, and healing of the bone graft. The use of two transverse rod couplers also will help further stabilize the Kaneda instrumentation and should be applied away from each other so as to maximize the effect of the couplers. Following insertion of the Kaneda device, it is possible to add some bone chips anteriorly and laterally to the bone struts (Fig. 6–77).

Note in the axial plane the position of the screws and their convergence. Note also the position of the plates in relationship to the vertebral body, avoiding the risk of directing the screws toward the spinal canal (Fig. 6–78).

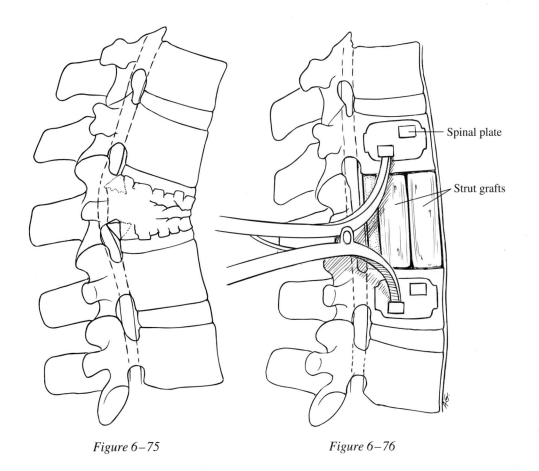

*Figure 6–75*

*Figure 6–76*

Spinal plate

Strut grafts

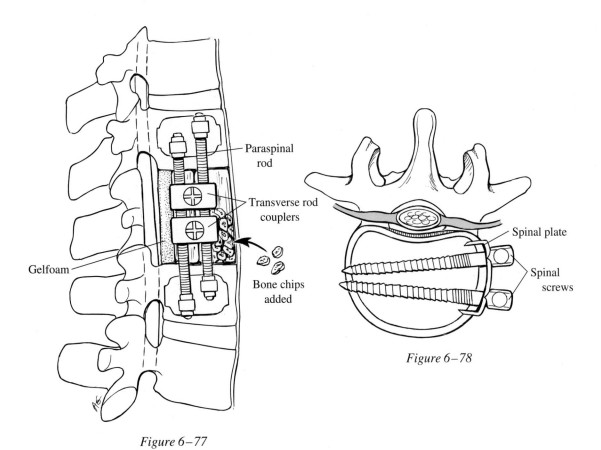

Paraspinal rod

Transverse rod couplers

Gelfoam

Bone chips added

*Figure 6–77*

Spinal plate

Spinal screws

*Figure 6–78*

# Zielke Procedure

For the Zielke procedure, only the disks lying between the vertebral bodies to be included in the fusion area will be removed. Thus, the rib is removed which goes to the most superior vertebra to be included in the fusion area, or one above it. For example, if the upper end of the fusion is to be T11, then the 10th rib is usually removed and a thoracolumbar approach is done. If the lower vertebra to be included in the fusion area is L3, the segmental vessels of the involved vertebra, not going below L3, are ligated. It is important not to violate the disk below the last vertebra in the fusion or above the last superior vertebra in the fusion. Once the segmental vessels have been ligated, the disks are excised. There is no need to remove the anterior longitudinal ligament, but all of the disk material immediately beneath the anterior ligament should be removed to the far side and to the posterior annulus. Failure to remove all of the posterior disk is the most common cause of failure in the Zielke operation. For this reason, it is necessary to reflect the psoas muscle back extremely carefully until the base of the pedicle is palpated with the periosteal elevator and to know precisely where the foramen is but not injure the exiting nerve root in this area. Only a few fibers of the posterior annulus should be left intact. All of the disk must be removed in the posterolateral corner to allow a posterior and lateral closure of the disk space. The anterior disk space should not close completely. Either place a little plug of rib bone just underneath the anterior longitudinal ligament or leave a little extra cartilage in this area to prevent anterior closure. After thorough disk excision, the screws are placed absolutely transversely across the vertebral body from convex to concave side. The surgeon should place his finger on the opposite side of the vertebral body and should definitely feel the tip of the screw coming through the opposite cortex. Failure to penetrate the opposite cortex is one of the major failures of this procedure. All screws must penetrate both cortices (Fig. 6–79). The screws must go absolutely transversely across the vertebral bodies totally parallel to the disk space and must start posteriorly and angulate just slightly forward, particularly at the apex of the curve and a little less so at the ends of the curve. The screws should not be in a straight line but rather in an arcuate manner with the apical screws posteriorly and the end screws more anteriorly (Fig. 6–80).

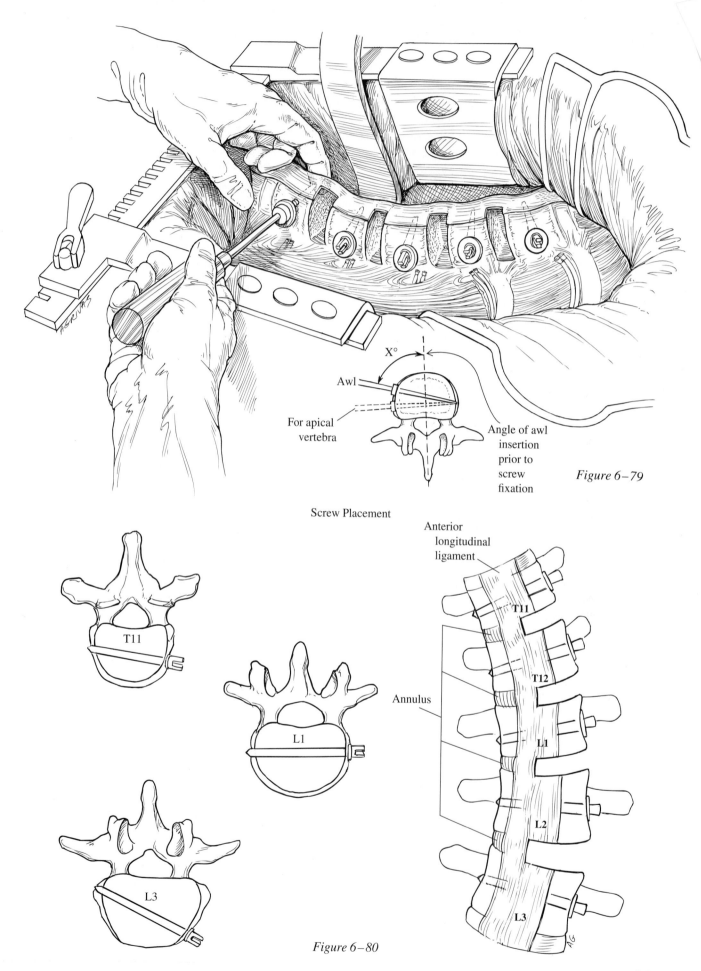

X°

Awl

For apical
vertebra

Angle of awl
insertion
prior to
screw
fixation

Figure 6–79

Screw Placement

Anterior
longitudinal
ligament

Annulus

T11

L1

L3

T11

T12

L1

L2

L3

Figure 6–80

The proper length of Zielke rod is then selected and cut if necessary after the nuts have been added to the rod. Ideally there should be two nuts for each screw head. The rod is slightly crimped at one end and the final nut brought up against this crimping. This end of the rod is placed in the lowermost screw head. It is then placed into the socket of the screw head and the nut above tightened down on it and locked very snugly. This secures the most distal screw; then work proximally one vertebra at a time, placing the rod into the screw head and bringing the nuts against the screw head. The inferior nut remains loose until the disk space is closed, then it is tightened.

As the rod is being placed into the screw heads, the patient is being manually corrected either by the hands of the surgeon on the back of the patient or by blunt screwdriver against the head of the screw so that the arcuate alignment of the screw heads translates into a straight or slightly anterior bowed contour of the rod. Before any disk space is closed, bone chips are packed into the disk space. After the final disk space has been closed, any excess rod is cut off as flush as possible. There is usually very little bleeding from the Zielke procedure, since it is not necessary to strip the vertebral bodies prior to inserting the screws and the decorticated bone ends usually stop bleeding fairly quickly after the disk space has been filled with bone chips and then compressed.

If it is necessary to take an x-ray on the table, the patient should be placed in a purely lateral position and a cross-table x-ray obtained to get a true anteroposterior view. Because the Zielke device is so powerful, overcorrection is possible, which often is not desirable. Occasionally one may wish to overcorrect a small segment of the apex of a curve and the x-ray will determine whether or not the desired goal has been achieved.

At the completion of the procedure, the psoas muscle is then brought forward and often will cover much of the Zielke device except at T12 and higher. The diaphragm is then reapproximated and the chest closed in the standard manner. It has not been necessary to drain the retroperitoneal space. Zielke has designed a derotator device, which this author has not found necessary to use (Fig. 6–81).

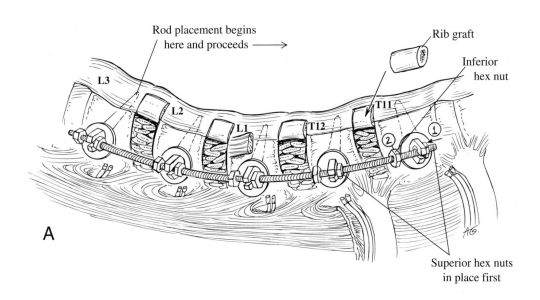

Rod placement begins here and proceeds →

Rib graft

Inferior hex nut

L3

L2

L1

T12

T11

② ①

Superior hex nuts in place first

A

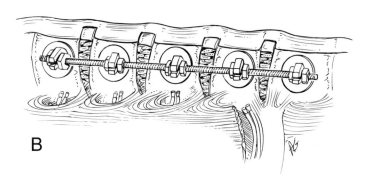

B

*Figure 6–81*

# Vascular Pedicled Rib Grafts

Indications for this procedure are:

1.   Strut grafts in kyphosis
2.   Inlay graft in pseudarthrosis, malunion, resorption, osteoporosis, and infection
3.   Intervertebral graft after vertebrectomy in trauma, tumor, and infection

In preparing a vascular, pedicled rib graft, the initial steps for thoracotomy down to the rib level are the same. The rib chosen for the vascular pedicled rib graft is usually the rib that lies over the apex of gibbosity, leads to the site of the vertebra to be removed, or leads to the pseudarthrosis area to be attacked. If this rib has been removed, the rib above or below can be chosen. If necessary, two adjacent ribs can be prepared as vascular pedicled grafts. Subsequent closure of the chest wall poses no problem. Approximation of the ribs for chest closure can be accomplished using Parham bands pericostally. Even if the intercostal space remains partly separated, chest wall muscles fill in and seal the opening.

The periosteum of the vascular pedicled rib graft is incised with electrocautery longitudinally in the middle from the costochondral junction to the posterior angle of the rib. The periosteum of the rib is then elevated in the upper half and around the upper edge of the rib (Fig. 6–82A) and down to the middle of the rib on the posterior aspect where a longitudinal incision is made in the periosteum and parietal pleura entering the chest. In making this posterior periosteal incision, do not get close to the lower edge and groove of the rib with its vascular bundle (Fig. 6–82B).

The rib is then divided anteriorly at the costochondral junction with electrocautery. This cut is extended halfway into the width of the intercostal muscles, staying 1 to 2 cm beyond the lower edge of the rib. The incision through the intercostal muscles is then carried back to the posterior angle of the rib, where the lower edge of the rib is denuded of its periosteum with a periosteal elevator for about 2 to 3 cm, avoiding injury to the vascular bundle (Fig. 6–82C). The rib is divided. The vascular supply and half of the intercostal muscles remain attached to the lower edge of the rib. The intercostal artery previously ligated at the anterior costochondral junction may be checked for patency by temporarily removing the ligature to allow bleeding, making certain that the vascular supply has not been compromised. It may then be clipped, again. To get more mobility of the rib, it may be necessary to tease the vascular bundle off the groove for additional length before fashioning the rib to fit into the grooves prepared in the vertebrae (Figs. 6–83A and 6–83B).

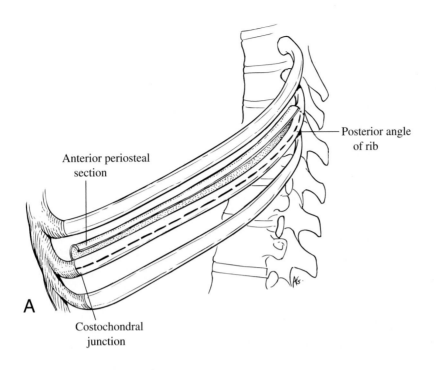

Anterior periosteal section

Posterior angle of rib

Costochondral junction

A

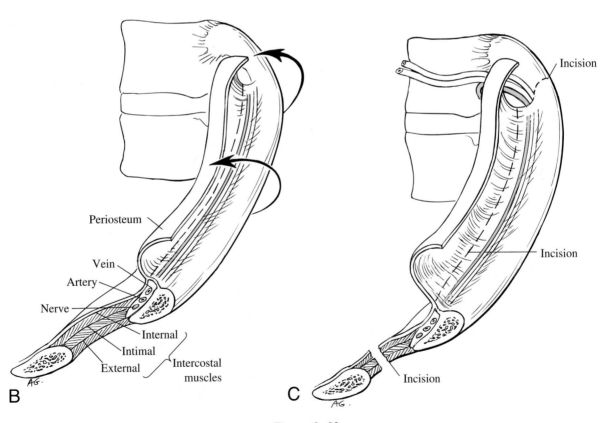

Periosteum

Vein
Artery
Nerve
Internal
Intimal
External
Intercostal muscles

B

Incision

Incision

Incision

C

*Figure 6–82*

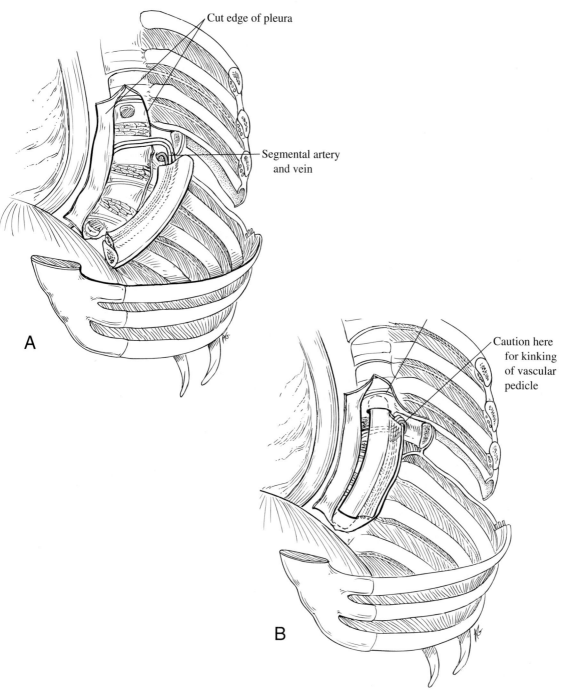

Kyphotic Spine

Cut edge of pleura

Segmental artery
and vein

Caution here
for kinking
of vascular
pedicle

A

B

*Figure 6–83*

192

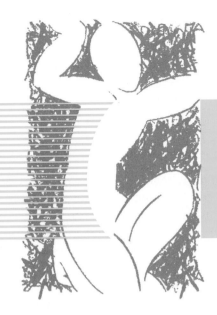

# 7

# POSTERIOR
# THORACIC AND
# THORACOLUMBAR
# PROCEDURES

# *Basic Exposure*

## POSITIONING THE PATIENT

Following induction of anesthesia, intubation, and placement of appropriate monitors and Foley catheter, the patient is turned prone onto a four-poster frame. This frame (Hall-Relton) is designed to allow the abdomen to hang freely and thus not impede the venous return to the heart. With unimpaired venous return, the intra-abdominal pressure is low and thus the pressure in the vertebra and the veins posteriorly also will be low (Fig. 7–1). Support is on the thorax lateral to the breasts and on the anterior iliac spines. Care must be taken in positioning the proximal bolsters to avoid pressure against the brachial plexus. The arms should be appropriately padded and supported.

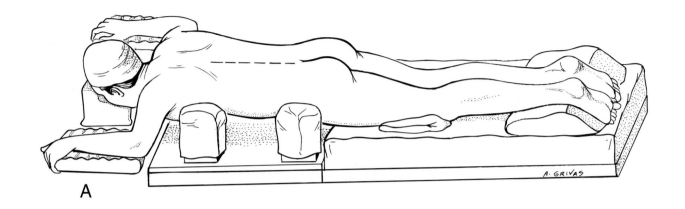

A

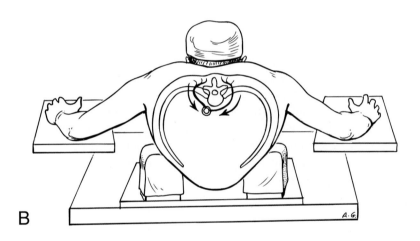

B

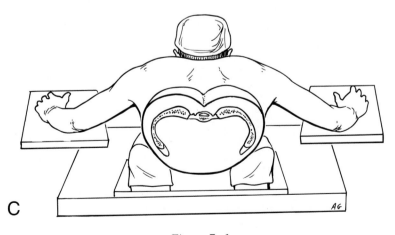

C

Figure 7–1

195

# SURGICAL INCISION

After appropriate skin preparation and draping, a vertical incision is made from one vertebra above the proximal fusion level to one vertebra below the distal fusion level. Except for extremely severe curvatures, a straight incision is used. After bleeding is controlled in the skin and subcutaneous area, the incision is extended to the deep fascia level at the tips of the spinous processes. The cartilage cap on top of the spinous process is sharply divided with the scalpel (Fig. 7–2A). Then with a periosteal elevator, the lateral sides of the spinous processes are dissected subperiosteally (Fig. 7–2B,C).

Once all of the spinous processes and interspinous ligaments have been cleared out, the dissection is carried to the lamina. If the dissection of the tougher fibers from the inferior margin of the spinous processes and the lamina is not done subperiosteally, there will be a large amount of soft tissue remaining attached in these areas. The spinous process and laminae can be stripped rather quickly with an extremely minimal amount of blood loss, as there are no significant bleeders in this area (Fig. 7–2D).

In the thoracic spine the dissection must then be carried out laterally to the tips of the transverse processes. When doing this, the surgeon will encounter a significant small arterial bleeder one millimeter lateral to the capsule of the facet joint. This is a constant finding and should be anticipated and either cauterized before transecting or immediately thereafter. The transverse processes will strip easily with the exception of their cranial surface to which small tendons are attached that must be sharply divided from the bone. We find this can be accomplished easily using electrocautery (Fig. 7–2E).

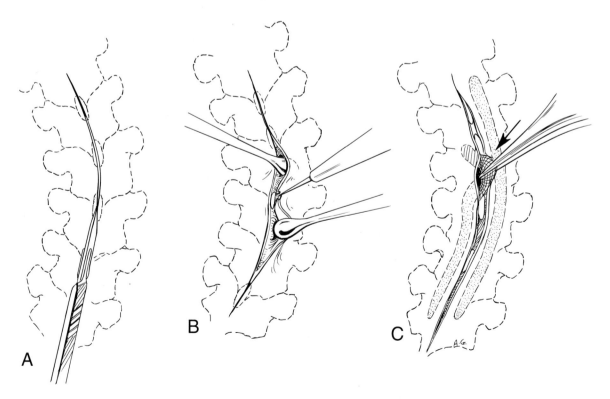

*Figure 7–2*

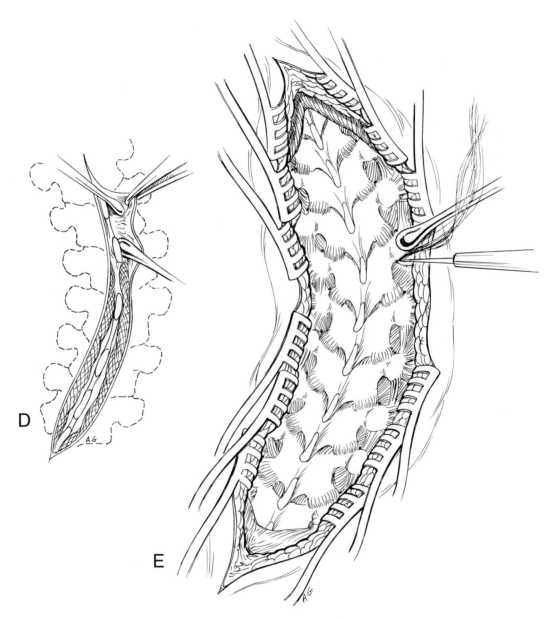

D

E

*Figure 7–2 Continued*

Once the paraspinal muscles have been moved laterally to the tips of the transverse processes of the thoracic spine, the surgeon removes the remaining soft tissue clinging to the bone surfaces (Fig. 7–3). The areas of the capsular tissues in the areas of the facet joint capsules are thoroughly removed down to the bone and joint (Fig. 7–4). This is the most common area to leave some soft tissue even for the experienced surgeon.

In the lumbar spine, the capsules of the facet joints must be resected with a rongeur or reflected with the muscle mass to allow a full view of both the superior and inferior articular processes and pars interarticularis area. There is usually some soft capsular tissue in the tight interval between the inferior articular facet of the vertebra above and the pars articularis of the vertebra below. This should be removed with a sharp curette.

Whether or not the transverse processes are exposed in the lumbar spine is an individual decision depending on the nature of the curvature and the planned surgical procedure. This is usually not necessary for adolescent idiopathic scoliosis.

When the exposure has been completed, the surgeon will be looking at the posterior aspect of the laminae, spinous processes, transverses processes, and facet joints. All capsular tissue and interspinous ligament tissue has been removed, and the bone surfaces will be bare and clean. Any areas bleeding from the bone itself can be controlled with bone wax. All soft tissue bleeders can be electrocoagulated. At this point, there should be no bleeding from the wound. The ligamentum flavum will be visible between each vertebra with no overlying soft tissue.

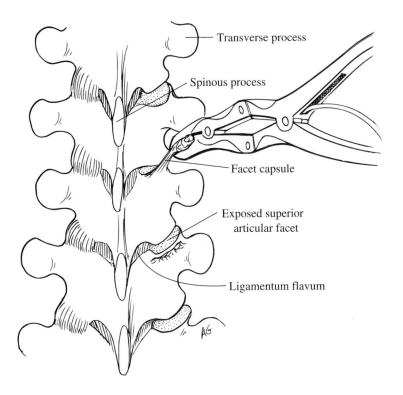

Transverse process

Spinous process

Facet capsule

Exposed superior
articular facet

Ligamentum flavum

Figure 7–3

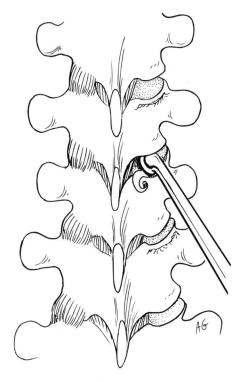

Figure 7–4

199

# *Basic Posterior Arthrodesis*

## FACET JOINT ARTHRODESIS

The facet joint cartilage must be removed at all levels both concave and convex. In the lumbar spine, this is done by two cuts with a thin osteotome just beyond the subchondral bone removing the subchondral bone and cartilage with a rongeur or curette or both or with a small burr. In the thoracic spine the inferior articular facet is excised with a gouge, and the cartilage of the superior articular facet removed with a curette. The subchondral bone of the superior articular facet is very lightly decorticated with a sharp gouge, osteotome, or air-driven burr (Fig. 7–5A–D).

Many techniques have been described for a facet joint fusion. They all, however, have certain factors in common: (1) thorough and complete removal of the joint, (2) removal of the cartilage cutting back to raw bleeding bone, and (3) placement of a bone graft in the area (Fig. 7–5E).

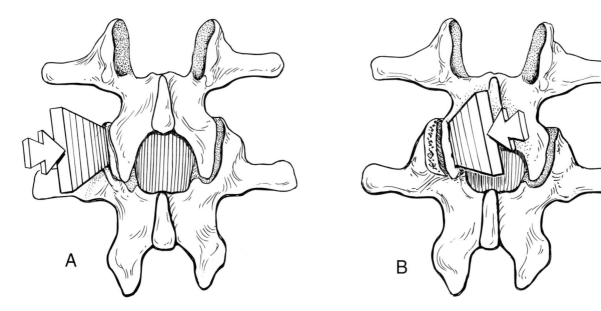

*Figure 7–5*

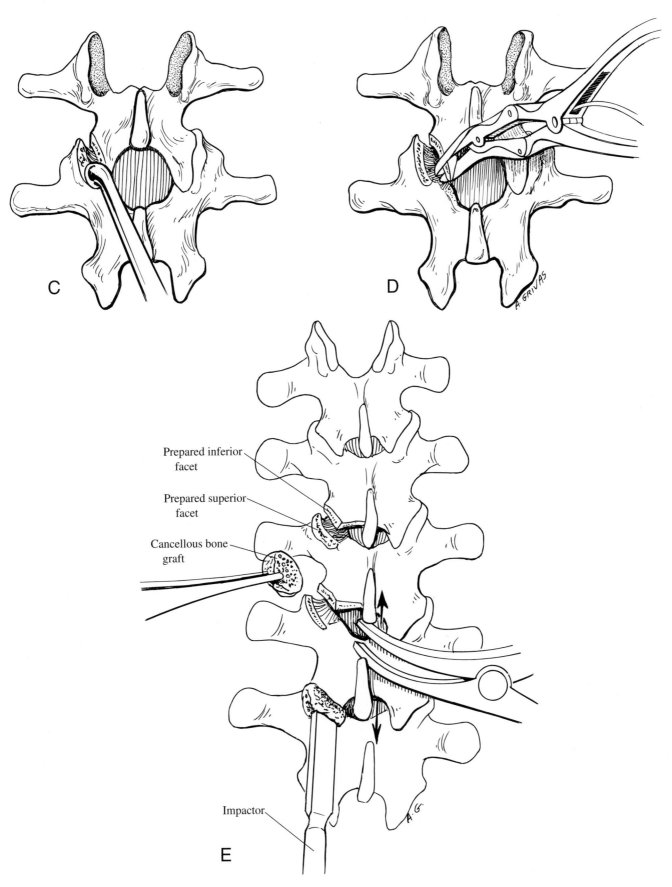

Prepared inferior
facet

Prepared superior
facet

Cancellous bone
graft

Impactor

C

D

A. GRIVAS

E

A. G.

*Figure 7–5 Continued*

201

In Moe's technique for facet fusion in the thoracic spine, a sharp gouge is used to decorticate the lamina. This cut is carried into the base of the transverse process and left attached, and then the bone fragment is levered downward toward the more inferior transverse process (Fig. 7–6A). A second cut is made to remove the deep subchondral bone and inferior facet cartilage, and this piece is removed and discarded (Fig. 7–6B). A third cut is made on the next inferior vertebra starting in the transverse process proceeding medially then superiorly into the facet, leaving the facet attached on the transverse process and levering the bone laterally where it lies in contact with the flap of bone superiorly. The hollow space left in the region of the facet joint is packed with a piece of autogenous cancellous bone from the iliac crest (Fig. 7–6C).

Hall's technique differs slightly in that the entire inferior articular facet is removed with a single cut of a sharp gouge exposing the superior articular facet (Fig. 7–7A). The cartilage is removed with a curette or burr (Fig. 7–7B,F) and the superior articular facet decorticated with a Cobb gouge (Fig. 7–7C). The autogenous iliac bone plug is then inserted (Fig. 7–7D,E).

Harrington and Dickson have described a technique utilizing a dowel cutter that excises the inferior articular facet and cuts into the lamina below in a circular fashion. The bone is removed from the superior articular facet and a matching size dowel graft is obtained with a similar cutter from the iliac crest and placed in the facet area.

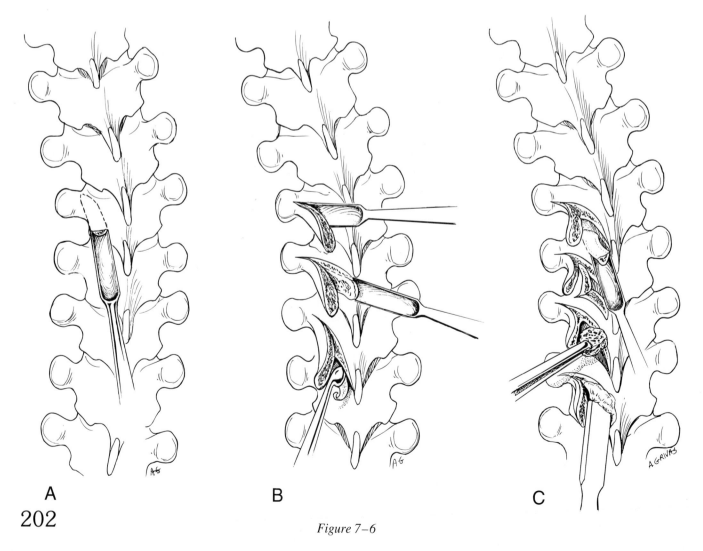

A

B

C

*Figure 7–6*

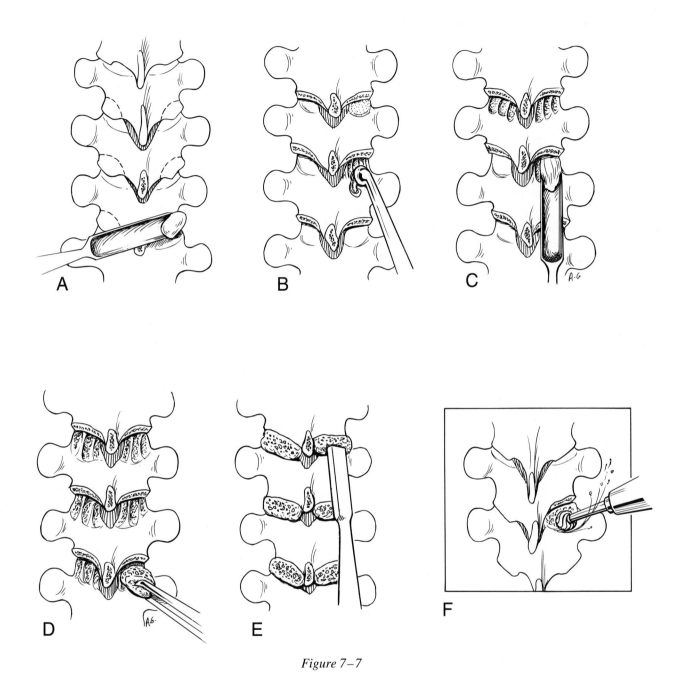

*Figure 7–7*

## Decortication

Once the facet joints have been excised and bone grafted, the remaining bone surfaces of the spinous processes are decorticated with a gouge. The detached bone strips are retained in the wound. An additional bone graft is obtained from the iliac crest and added to the primary fusion area (Fig. 7–8).

## Closure

The wound is closed using a running suture in the fascia just above the paraspinal muscle mass. No attempt should be made to suture the muscle together. A suction drain is placed just above the fascia and brought out through a separate puncture wound. The subcutaneous tissue is closed by a second layer of running suture and the skin with an intracuticular running suture. Adhesive strips are used on the skin. With this technique there are no stitch marks on the skin and no sutures to be removed later. The authors prefer synthetic absorbable sutures at all levels.

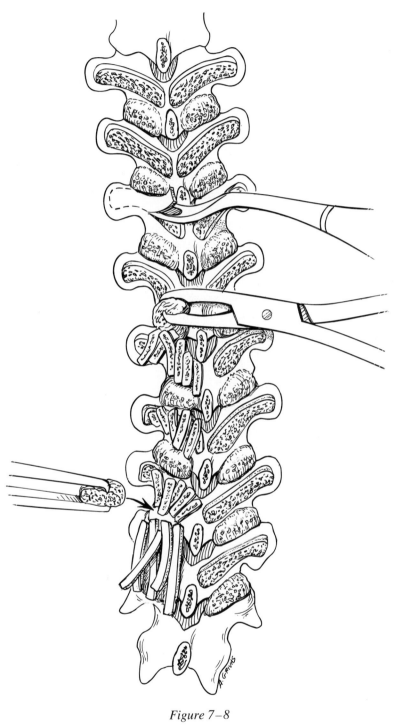

*Figure 7–8*

# Harrington Instrumentation

Harrington instrumentation was developed in the 1950s by Dr. Paul R. Harrington of Houston, Texas. Its worldwide use began in 1960 and rapidly became the treatment of choice for many different scoliosis problems. It must be remembered that the instrumentation used in conjunction with arthrodesis is a supplement to the arthrodesis and never replaces it.

## Placement of the Inferior Hook

A strong bone margin on which the hook can seat firmly is required. In preparing the placement site, the inferior articular facet is removed from the next proximal vertebra to the site (Fig. 7–9A,B). Cartilage should be removed from the superior articular facet of the vertebra on which the hook is placed, and the vertebra very lightly decorticated for the acceptance of a bone graft later. To place the inferior hook, the ligamentum flavum is carefully dissected from the superior laminar margin of the selected vertebra, which exposes the dura and epidural fat (Fig. 7–9C). It may be necessary to use a Kerrison rongeur to prepare the margin of the bone for hook placement (Fig. 7–9D). A #1254 hook, with either a round or square hole depending on the instrumentation system selected, is inserted under the lamina on the superior laminar margin of the most inferior vertebra in the fusion area. Insertion of the hook may be facilitated by using a spreader between the spinous processes (Fig. 7–9E,F).

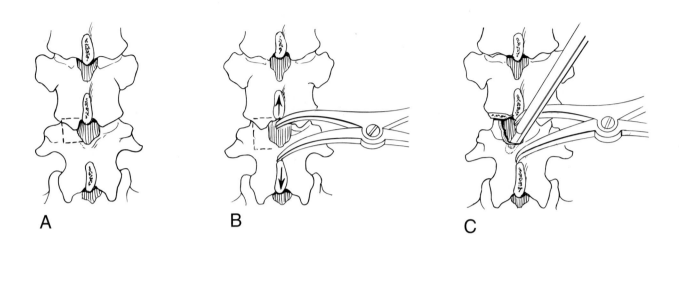

A

B

C

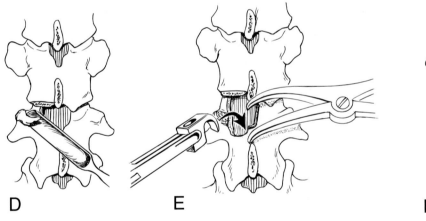

D

E

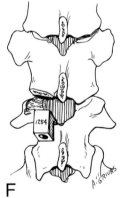

F

*Figure 7–9*

207

## Placement of the Superior Hook

The superior hook is placed in one of two ways. The first is the use of a bifid hook, a hook with a blade designed to engage the pedicle. If this hook is used, it must be placed accurately in the pedicle region. This requires removal of a portion of the inferior articular facet and lower edge of the lamina (Fig. 7–10A–D).

The second technique is to place the hook under the lamina in the facet joint or partially in the facet joint and partially in the spinal canal. In this technique, the medial portion of the box of the hook lies against the base of the spinous process that should be left at least partially intact to help support the hook (Fig. 7–10E).

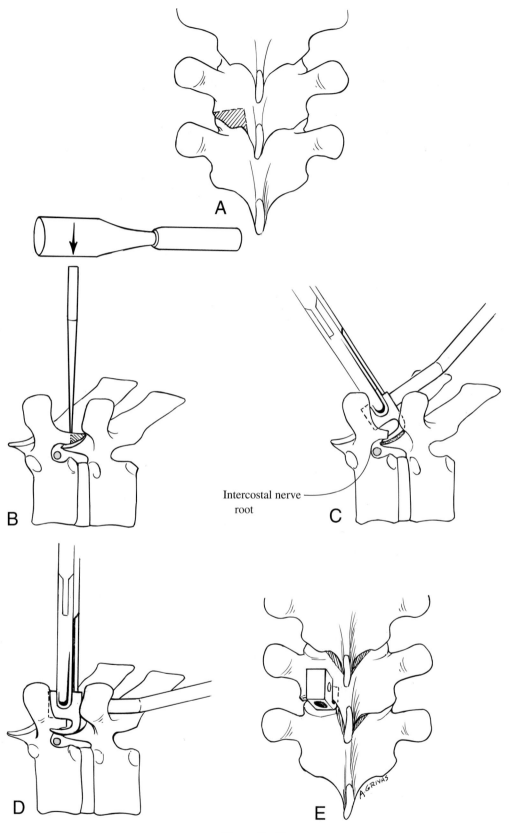

Intercostal nerve
root

*Figure 7–10*

## Harrington Outrigger

After placement of the superior and inferior hooks on the concave side of the curve (Fig. 7–11), the outrigger is inserted. This can be placed directly into the hooks, but by doing so the rods cannot be placed in the hooks in the distracted position. To facilitate this, Zielke clamps are placed on the hooks and the outrigger is placed into the Zielke clamps (Fig. 7–12). The outrigger is gently lengthened taking care to avoid over-distraction of the spine. Usually the facet joints are done after distraction so that the bone grafts are inserted with the spine in the corrected position. Once the outrigger has been tightened and the facet joints done, appropriate decortication of the bone surface is done in the area where the rod will be placed. The rod is inserted, gently tightened, and then the outrigger is removed. This completes the concave side of the surgery. A C ring is inserted just below the upper hook to prevent loosening of the distraction rod (Fig. 7–13). If a C ring is not available, a twist of heavy wire can be utilized to do the same thing.

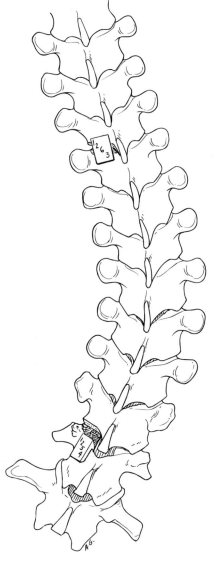

*Figure 7–11*

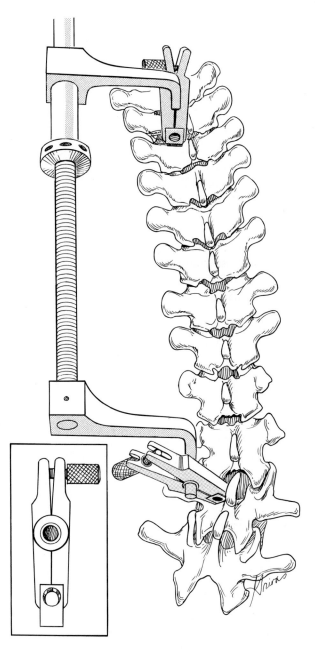

*Figure 7–12*

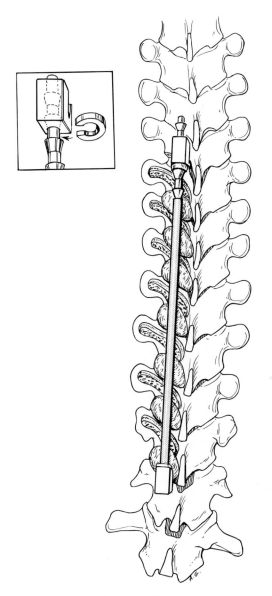

*Figure 7–13*

## Compression Assembly

To insert the compression assembly, the convex transverse processes throughout the length of the fusion area must be fully exposed (Fig. 7–14A). Once exposed, a #1256 hook in a hook holder is inserted around the transverse process of the bone near its base taking care not to dissect into the bone (Fig. 7–14B). The tip of the hook is placed into the costotransverse joint and one can usually feel the ligaments give way as the hook penetrates the joint (Fig. 7–14C). The preliminary use of the #1256 hook greatly facilitates the later insertion of the #1259 hook.

One by one the hooks are inserted around the transverse process, the hooks superior to the apex of the curve are placed over the superior margin of the transverse process, and the hooks distal to the apex of the curve are placed around the inferior margin of the transverse process (Fig. 7–15A–E).

Once all the hook sites have been prepared, which may include the placement of the most distal hook under the lamina of $T_{11}$, $T_{12}$, or $L_1$ rather than on the transverse process, the small (1/8") compression rod is assembled with all of the hooks in place and a nut behind each hook. The number of hooks selected depends on the number of vertebrae to be included in the fusion area.

Prior to placement of the compression assembly, the facet joints should be removed taking care not to penetrate into the transverse process, as it is important not to weaken the base of the transverse process.

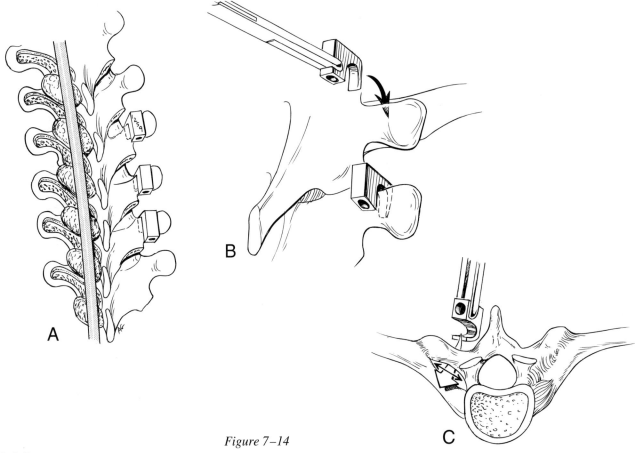

*Figure 7–14*

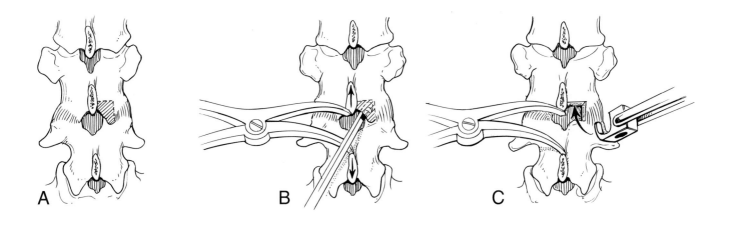

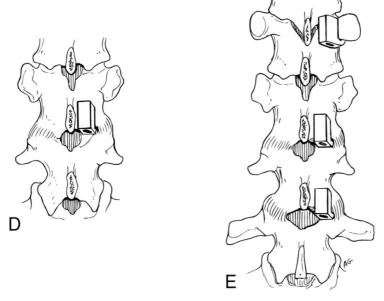

Figure 7–15

If the patient has a kyphoscoliosis, it is often desirable to place the compression rod first to reduce the kyphosis, and then place the distraction rod into the concave hooks after the compression rod has reduced the kyphosis. This lessens the amount of bend needed in the distraction rod.

When placing the compression assembly it is usually easiest to start at the most superior hook and proceed distally, placing one hook at a time (Fig. 7–16). After the compression assembly has been fully inserted (Fig. 7–17), the nuts are tightened carefully to apply compression force to the convexity of the curve providing both a shortening of the convexity and segmental fixation (Fig. 7–18).

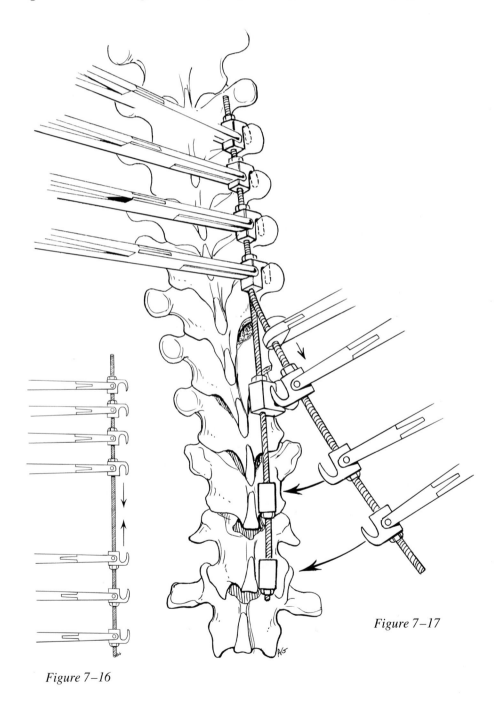

Figure 7–16

Figure 7–17

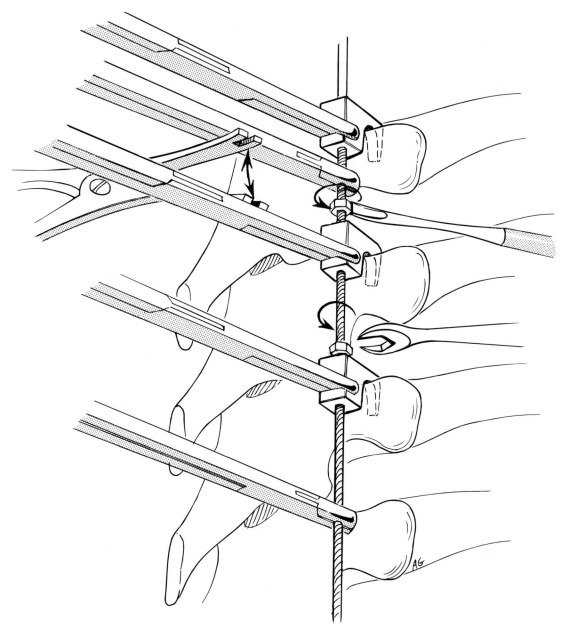

Figure 7–18

After insertion of the compression assembly, the basic instrumentation has been completed but the operation has not been finalized. There are still two steps remaining. First, it is ideal to couple the compression rod to the distraction with a device for transverse traction (DTT). This will pull the compression assembly slightly toward the distraction assembly giving a few degrees more correction, but more importantly adding additional internal stabilization. The DTT should be tightened but not to the point where there is any danger of dislodging the compression assembly (Fig. 7–19A,B).

All exposed cortical surfaces should be decorticated either with a gouge or a rongeur; all the bone chips from this decortication are placed back into the incision; and additional bone graft material, regardless of where it is taken, should be added prior to closure (Fig. 7–19C). The decortication should be done carefully so as not to weaken the bone in an area where a hook purchase is important.

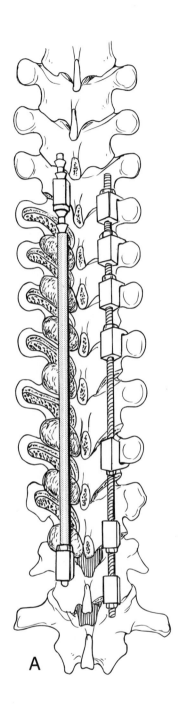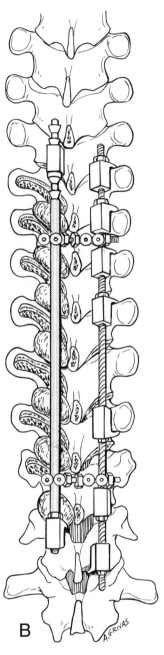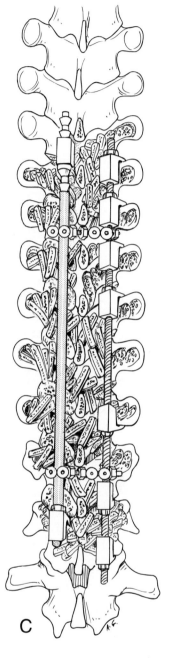

A

B

C

*Figure 7–19*

217

# HARRINGTON RODS TO THE SACRUM

It is the authors' belief that Harrington rods should never be placed to L5 or the sacrum in a distraction mode. The loss of lumbar lordosis by this posterior distraction technique is a significant problem that is best prevented by avoiding posterior distraction.

# HARRINGTON INSTRUMENTATION FOR LARGE CURVES

In dealing with very large curves, particularly 90° or greater, it is often advantageous to place two distraction rods in the concavity of the curve and a compression assembly on the convexity. The extremes of the area of the fusion are determined, hooks are placed in the standard fashion in the vertebrae, and an outrigger applied. Once the outrigger has been lengthened, the shorter rod is inserted. This usually is placed about three vertebrae distal to the proximal hook, three vertebrae proximal to the distal hook, and parallel with the longer rod. The shorter rod is then tightened. The outrigger can be lengthened slightly. At this point, the compression assembly, which should consist of as many hooks as possible with the long system, should be applied. Finally, the longer distraction rod is inserted, and the outrigger removed.

# HARRINGTON INSTRUMENTATION FOR DOUBLE CURVES

There are two double curve patterns—the double thoracic and the double major right thoracic left lumbar. For the double thoracic curve, a single distraction rod should be used with the uppermost hook at T2 on the concave side of the upper curve and the lowermost hook on the concave side of the lower curve. It is usually appropriate to reverse the direction of the rod; that is, the ratchet section is distal and the base of the rod proximal to avoid excessive amount of metal high in the thoracic spine where it can be more bothersome to the patient.

When dealing with the double major right thoracic left lumbar pattern, a single rod should be used. If separate rods are used in the concavity of each curve, there is a greater likelihood of pseudarthrosis and also a significant tendency for kyphosis at the junction of the two rods.

## SPECIAL COMMENTS REGARDING THE LENGTH OF THE RATCHETS

In all situations in which the Harrington distraction rod is used, the fewest number of ratchets as possible should be used between the hook and the shank of the rod (the long smooth part). Each ratchet is a potentially weaker spot in the rod than the strong central part. Thus there is a greater likelihood that the rod will eventually fracture when a greater number of ratchets between the shank and the hook are used. This is one of the reasons the outrigger is advantageous in Harrington instrumentations, since the perfect selection of rod length is possible and any extra portion of rod that may project beyond the upper hook can be cut off. A centimeter of rod projecting above the hook should remain so the hook will not come off of the rod.

# HARRINGTON INSTRUMENTATION WITHOUT FUSION FOR THE TREATMENT OF CURVATURES IN YOUNG CHILDREN

Harrington tried several cases but failed due to a combination of events: (a) the failure to constantly protect the patients with an orthosis, (b) the use of a subperiosteal exposure for placement of the rod, which in young children often led to spontaneous fusion, thus denying the patient the desired longitudinal growth, and (c) lack of a plan for periodic lengthening and/or replacement of the rod.

In the early 1970s, Marchetti once again began to treat children with this technique but added the concept of constant postoperative support in a Milwaukee brace plus periodic lengthening and/or replacement of the rod as necessary. This technique was modified by Moe in 1973 with the placing of the rod in the soft tissues avoiding subperiosteal exposure of the spine except in the areas of hook placement. This technique then became known as the "subcutaneous rod technique."

## TECHNIQUE

The position is the same as for any type of posterior scoliosis surgery. The skin and subcutaneous areas are opened throughout the region of the curve requiring instrumentation (Fig. 7–20A). The use of two small incisions and subcutaneous passing of the rod is not recommended. Metallic markers are placed *both* at the top and the bottom of the planned area and an x-ray is taken to identify the proper levels. It is necessary to mark the top and bottom levels, since it is very difficult to count the unexposed vertebrae.

The vertebrae are exposed only at the levels involved in the hook placement area at each end of the curvature. The periosteum is stripped on the one side, the ligamentum flavum area identified, the flavum removed, and a pediatric-sized hook gently inserted under the lamina into the spinal canal at each end (Fig. 7–20B). The facet joint is fused at this level to aid in the stability of the hook. A rod is inserted and gently distracted, leaving enough rod for lengthening, a C ring or wire is used to prevent incidental shortening of the rod, and the wound is then closed. A ratchet type of rod or Moe rod, which is designed for this purpose and has a 6 mm unthreaded shank with threadings at both ends to allow for distraction, is used (Fig. 7–21A,C). The patient is then placed in a previously made Milwaukee brace. The brace is appropriately adjusted to the new length of the child and pad position tightened. This should be done before ambulating the patient. Underarm braces are not advisable.

When dealing with a double structural curve, the rod is placed in "S" fashion. At the point where the rod crosses over the junction of the two curves, it is necessary to remove one spinous process allowing the rod to lay adequately deep below the skin. It is usually necessary in all cases to divide the deep fascia and some of the muscle just where the rod enters the hook (Fig. 7–21B,D). Subperiosteal exposure will inevitably lead to spontaneous fusion because of the young age and the constant immobilization of these children.

220

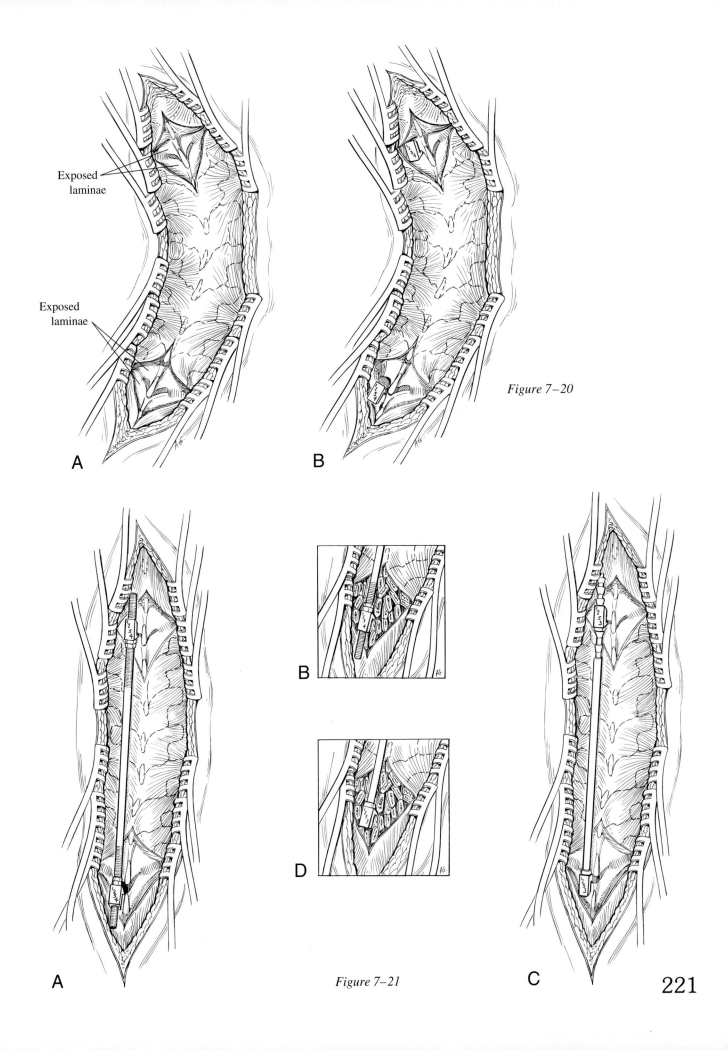

Exposed laminae

Exposed laminae

*Figure 7–20*

A

B

A

B

D

*Figure 7–21*

C

221

### LENGTHENING

The rod is periodically lengthened, usually every six months. At the time of lengthening, only the hook and ratchet or threaded area of the rod are exposed. This is almost always placed so that only one end of the rod needs to be exposed. At time of lengthening, the ratchet or threads are cleared of any soft tissue, a hook holder is placed on the hook, a rod clamp is placed on the rod, and a distractor used between the two clamps to lengthen gently (Figs. 7–22 and 7–23). There is no fixed rule about how much lengthening can be obtained, since each case is totally different. Once the lengthening has been accomplished, a new C ring or wire is used to lock the rod in the lengthened position.

### ROD REPLACEMENT

After one or two lengthenings, it is usually necessary to replace the rod. For replacement, the entire length of the incision is reopened. The hook position should be carefully checked for stability, and the old rod is removed and the new one inserted.

### FINAL FUSION

At some point in time, the arthrodesis will have to be done. If the hooks are totally stable, they can be used at the time of the final fusion, but a new, strong rod should always be used. Rods that have been in place for several months have had stress applied to them and may be close to the breaking point. Selection of the time for fusion is beyond the scope of this atlas, but generally is determined by the progress of the curvature. In a practical sense, the children usually reach a point at which periodic lengthenings no longer are of any benefit and at that point the fusion should be done. This is usually when the adolescent growth spurt begins and growth is more rapid and the curves cannot be controlled by this technique.

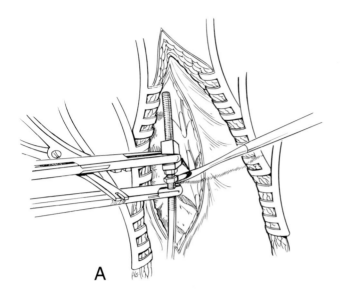

A

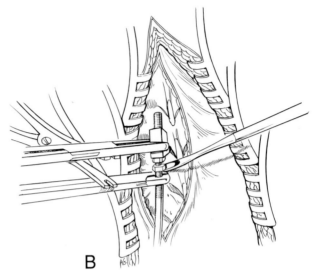

B

*Figure 7–22*

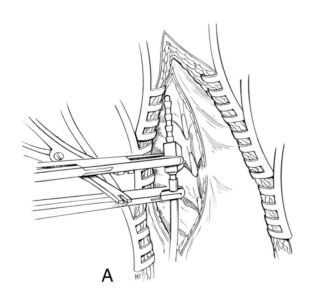

A

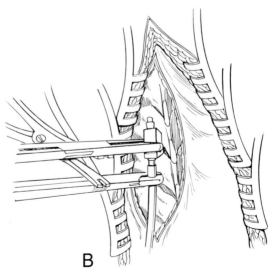

B

*Figure 7–23*

# HARRINGTON INSTRUMENTATION FOR KYPHOSIS

The standard subperiosteal exposure described previously is done, carefully exposing the thoracic spine to the tips of the transverse processes bilaterally and in the lumbar spine just beyond the capsules of the lumbar facet joints if the dissection goes into the lumbar spine. Do not destroy the capsule at the junction distally or proximally, since this is important for the prevention of late deformity at the junctional area. Similarly, the supraspinous and intraspinous ligaments are left intact at the junctional areas.

When the basic exposure has been completed and all soft tissues cleaned from the spine, the facet joints are prepared by the Hall technique, in which the inferior articular facet is cut off, the cartilage of the superior articular facet removed, and the superior articular facet lightly decorticated with a gouge or burr (Fig. 7–24A). Care must be taken not to destroy the strength or integrity of the base of the transverse process when doing the facet joint surgery. Since the transverse processes are not as strong as the lamina, it is important to use as many hooks as possible on each rod to allow force distribution so that no one process is carrying an excessive load (Fig. 7–24B).

Hook placement is usually started superiorly. First place a #1256 hook in a hook holder and dissect around the superior aspect of the transverse process in the upper half of the kyphosis to prepare the area for a #1259 hook insertion. Several passages of the #1256 hook are necessary to properly dissect the costotransverse process ligament, which lies ventral to the transverse process. On the final pass, the hook should be held in such a manner that it is pushed ventrally and then downward around the transverse process rather than simply curving it around the transverse process. When the hooks are on the rod, they are more difficult to insert than if they are free within the hook holder.

The hooks are inserted one at a time starting with the uppermost hook. A rod holder is always placed on the apex of the curve pulling caudally, so that once a hook is in place it will not become dislodged. While longitudinal tension is being held on the first hook, the hook holder is placed on the second hook, which is slid around the top of the transverse process. The nut proximal to the hook is spun down against the top of the hook to prevent displacement (Fig. 7–24C). This procedure is followed for the remaining downgoing hooks in the upper half of the kyphus.

The rod holder is then switched to the lowermost end of the rod to continue to maintain caudal traction. A hook holder is then placed on the first of the upgoing hooks, the one nearest the apex of the curve, and it is placed around the inferior surface of the transverse process, these areas having been previously prepared by the #1256 hook. Once in place, the nut is spun upward securing the hook. When this is done the system will not dislodge, and it is not necessary to have the constant caudal traction on the distal end of the rod.

The next hook is placed below the transverse process. At this point the surgeon will be nearing the lower end of the thoracic spine. In this area the transverse processes become smaller and more obliquely oriented and the hooks become less effective. At T12, there is no longer a transverse process for hook placement, and the hooks are inserted underneath the lower edge of the lamina. When the final most distal hook is reached, it is important that the facet joint capsule at this junctional area or the interspinous ligament is not destroyed. Once all the hooks have been placed, all the nuts are tightened with a wrench, working always to correct the kyphosis. The authors usually set all the upper nuts and then tighten from bottom up.

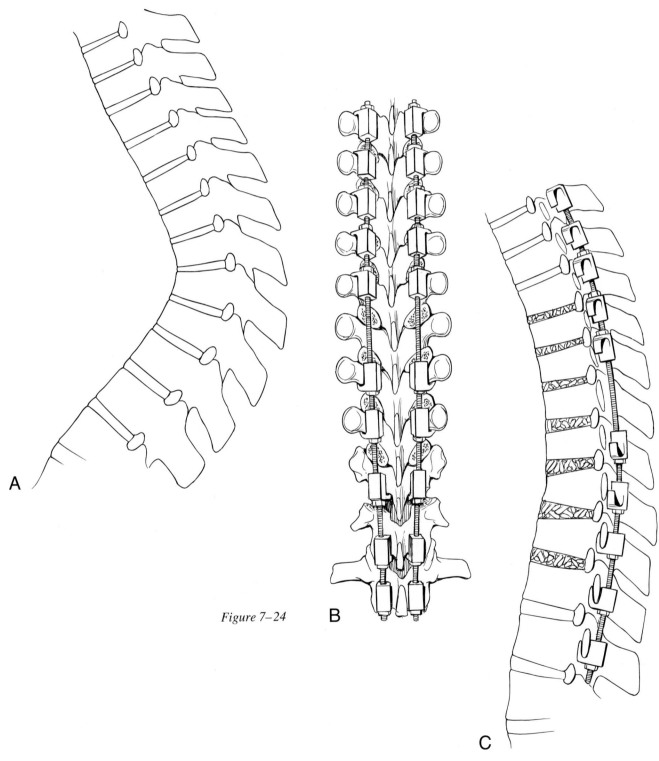

A

*Figure 7–24*    B

C

After the first rod is inserted, the second rod on the opposite side is inserted in a similar fashion. Tightening is done going back and forth from right to left so as not to produce a scoliosis by over-tightening one rod compared to the other rod. When full tightening and the desired correction is obtained, score or mark the threads just above or below each nut to damage the threads in such a way that the nut cannot loosen. An ordinary screwdriver and mallet can be used. If necessary, particularly at the ends of the system, a small piece of #18-gauge wire can be wound around the rods burying it into the threads and twisting it firmly to prevent the nut from becoming loose.

Once all of the instrumentation is completed, the midline spinous processes and available laminae are very lightly decorticated and an abundant autogenous iliac bone graft applied. The spinous processes should not be cut off, but rather decorticate their sides lightly. Because this is a kyphosis problem, it is important that the bone graft be as thick from front to back as possible, which is why the height of the spinous processes is not cut down. Similarly, it is not vital to have a wide fusion. The authors do not wish to weaken the transverse processes so it is not decorticated nor is a wide bone graft placed.

# Harri–Luque Procedure (Harrington Instrumentation with Luque Wiring)

## TECHNIQUE

After exposure of the spine as described above, the ligamentum flavum is removed at all levels between the upper and lower Harrington hook placement sites (Fig. 7–25A,B). The technique of ligamentum flavum removal is described in the section on Luque instrumentation on page 240. Next a doubled loop of stainless steel wire is passed under each lamina and is bent to conform to the lamina to avoid penetration into the spinal canal (Fig. 7–25C). The wire loop is not cut. After all of the wires are inserted, the Harrington rod is placed in the usual manner and moderately tightened (Fig. 7–25D). Beginning at the distal end of the system (the end away from the ratchets), the Luque wires are brought around the Harrington rod and twisted down (Fig. 7–25E). After one half of the wires are twisted down, the Harrington rod usually can be lengthened another ratchet proximally. The remaining wires are then tightened. When all of the wires are tightened, check if any further distraction is possible. Avoid excessive force in the distraction component because some of the correction comes from the lateral translation force of the wires. Each wire is then retested for appropriate tightness of the twist and, if satisfactory, is then bent down along the Harrington rod.

The facet joints must be excised and bone grafted before the rod is inserted, but the laminae should be decorticated extremely lightly or not at all, so the laminae on which the wires are placed are not weaken. Once the rod and wires are placed in the concavity of the curve, the facets in the convexity of the curve should be removed, the facet joints packed with bone, and the convexity fully decorticated (Figs. 7–25F and 7–26A–F).

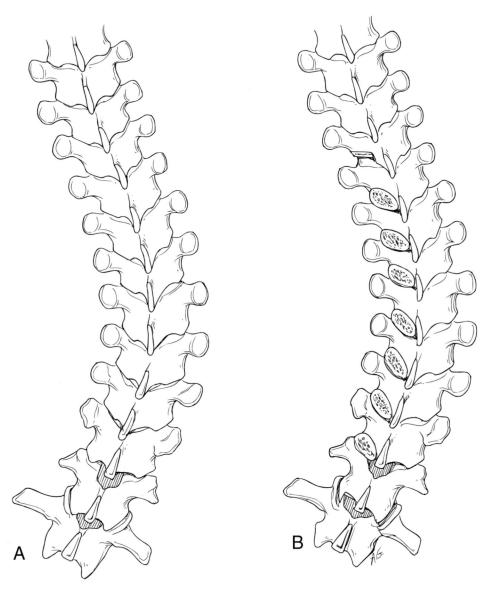

Figure 7–25

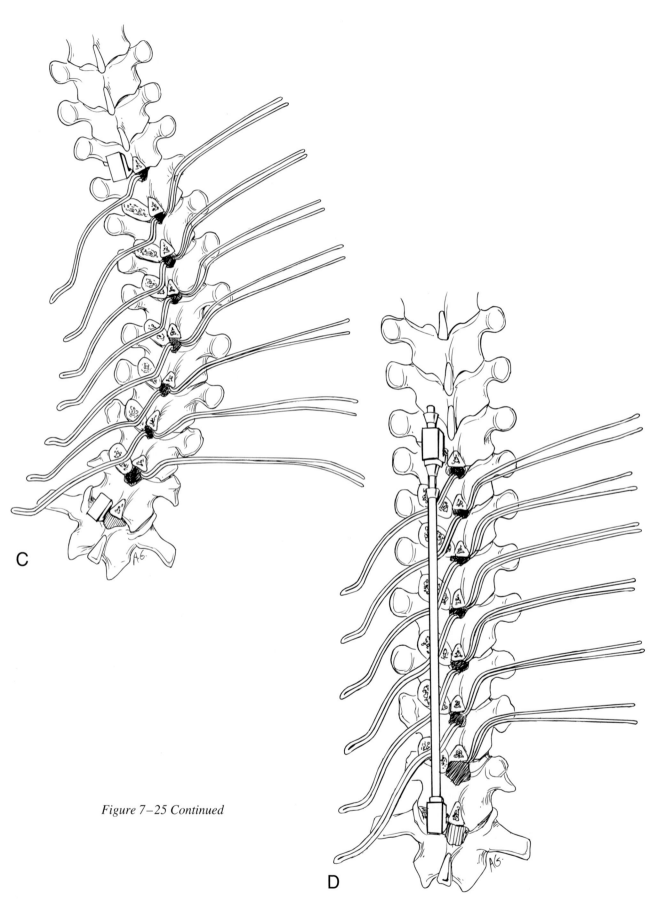

C

*Figure 7–25 Continued*

D

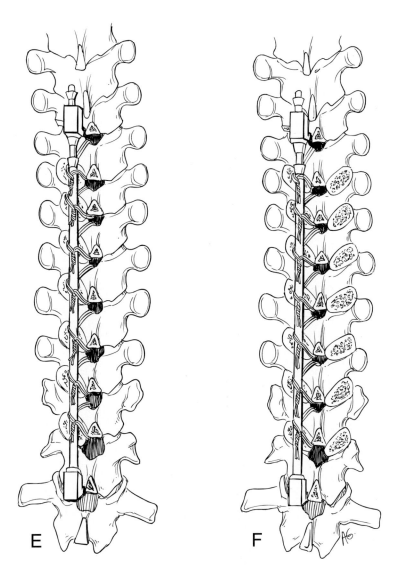

E

F

*Figure 7–25 Continued*

# POSTERIOR THORACIC AND THORACOLUMBAR PROCEDURES

### PLACEMENT OF THE HARRINGTON DISTRACTION ROD IN THE LUMBAR SPINE

When a Harrington rod is placed in the lumbar spine, it must be contoured to fit the normal sagittal contours, that is, the normal lumbar lordosis must be preserved. The use of a square-holed Harrington hook and a square-ended rod greatly facilitates the performance of this maneuver since rotation of the rod is prevented.

Harri-Luque for Double Thoracic Curve Pattern

Harri-Luque for Double Major Curve Pattern
Preoperative

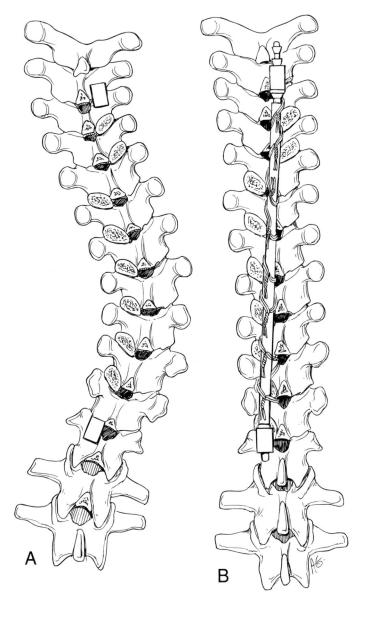

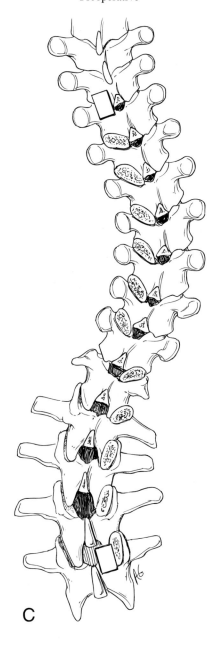

*Figure 7–26*

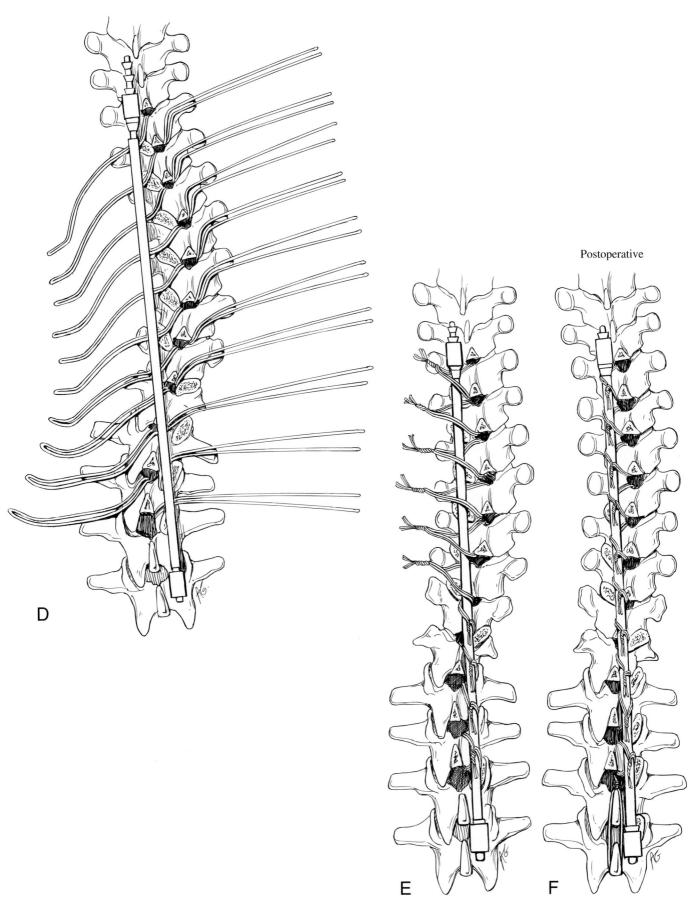

Postoperative

D

E          F

*Figure 7–26 Continued*

The authors have found it extremely helpful to utilize a special technique when inserting the distal hook into the lumbar spine in order to totally preserve lumbar lordosis. The hook, always square holed, is first placed on the lamina according to the technique described above and the wires passed. The spinous process of the most distal vertebra to be included in the fusion (the vertebra onto which the hook is inserted) has its spinous process wired to the spinous process of the next proximal vertebra. For example, if the most distal hook is on L4, then the spinous process of L3 and L4 are wired together. The purpose of this technique is to prevent distraction of these two vertebrae as tension is placed on the rod. Using a square-ended, lordotically contoured rod in the lumbar spine, not only can distraction to correct the scordliosis be provided, but lumbar lordosis also can be simultaneously maintained because the convexity of the lordotic curve of the rod lies against the laminae in the concavity of the curve (Fig. 7–27).

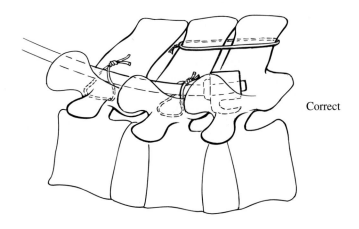

Correct

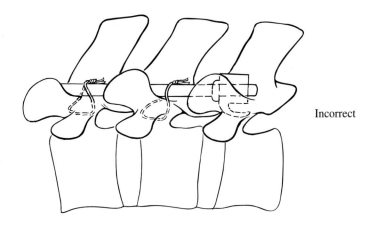

Incorrect

*Figure 7–27*

## THORACIC LORDOSCOLIOSIS

The Harri–Luque procedure is particularly effective for the treatment of thoracic lordoscoliosis where the desire on the part of the surgeon is to create kyphosis in the thoracic spine. In performing this procedure a square-ended rod and a square-holed distal hook are used.

A kyphosis is placed in the rod corresponding to a normal 20 to 25° of thoracic kyphosis. The most distal 2 to 3 cm and the upper end of the rod should not have this kyphosis. Minimal distraction should be used at first and then the wires sequentially tightened making two or three passes up and down the spine to slowly correct the lordosis. A space between the laminae and the rod of up to 3 cm can be readily corrected in the typical flexible, adolescent idiopathic scoliosis patient. If one elongates the rod maximally the ligaments are placed in such a degree of tension that it is difficult to correct the lordosis, which is the reason for the minimal lengthening of the rod at first. For more rigid deformities, preliminary anterior discectomy will allow better and easier correction (Fig. 7–28).

Harri-Luque Procedure (Lateral View)

Preoperative                                    Postoperative

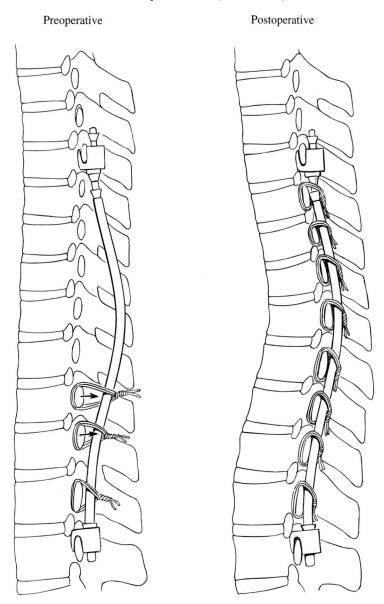

*Figure 7–28*

# Wisconsin Procedure (Drummond Operation)

This procedure combines a Harrington distraction rod in the concavity of the curve with a Luque rod on the convexity (Fig. 7–29). A wire is passed through the base of the spinous process connecting the two rods with each other and segmentally fixating the spine.

With a curved awl, a hole is made through the base of the spinous process taking care to not penetrate the spinal canal but simultaneously to be very deep in the base of the spinous process to be just above the internal cortex of the spinal canal (Fig. 7–30A). Special wires are passed through this hole, which have small stainless steel buttons that abut the base of the spinous process to prevent cutting through by the wires (Fig. 7–30B). After removing the facet joints in the concavity and decorticating the concavity, the deep parts of the wires are laid out from the midline toward the side of the patient (Fig. 7–31).

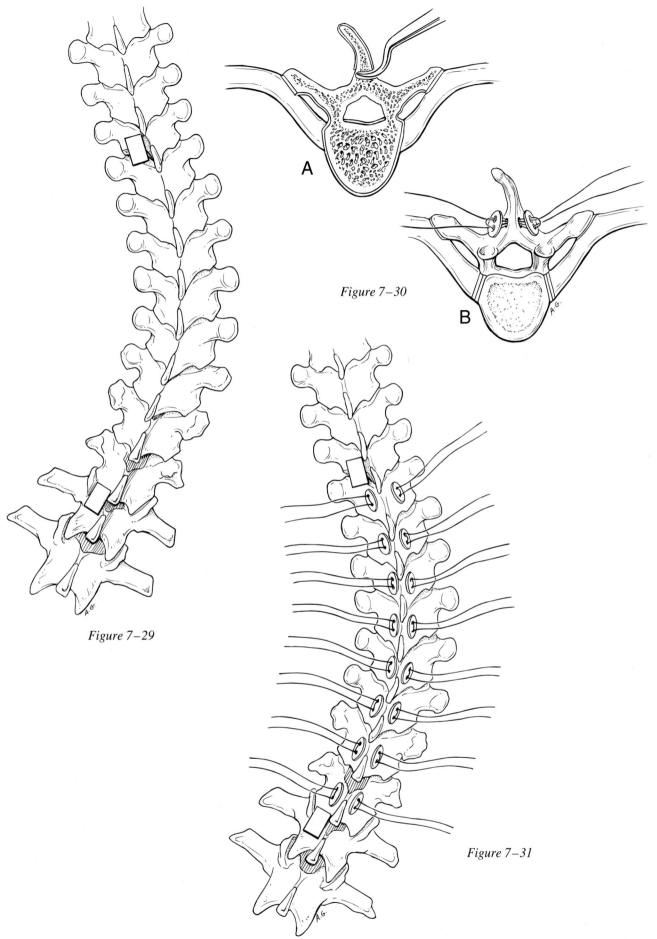

*Figure 7–30*

*Figure 7–29*

*Figure 7–31*

237

The distraction rod is inserted and lengthened, the superficial portions of the wires are brought over the rod, and the two parts of the wire are twisted down against the rod (Fig. 7–32). The Luque rod is then appropriately shaped so that there is an "L" at *both* ends of the rod at the ends of the fusion (Fig. 7–33). This rod is contoured to slightly less curvature than the scoliosis. The convex facet joints are excised and bone grafted, the convex laminae decorticated, and the deep parts of the wires are laid out. The Luque rod is inserted, the superficial portion of the wires is placed over the rod, and the two halves of the wire are brought together and twisted.

Starting in the center and working distally, the wires are tightened going back and forth between the concave and convex side, and, if necessary, gently distracting the rod further.

This procedure provides the benefit of both Harrington distraction and segmental stabilization with a rod on each side and avoiding the necessity of passing wires into the spinal canal. It has excellent lateral correction and fixation powers, but because the forces are purely translational, does not address well the correction of either kyphosis or lordosis. When dealing with a double major curve, a long, central single distraction rod and two separate Luque rods are used, one for the convexity of each curve.

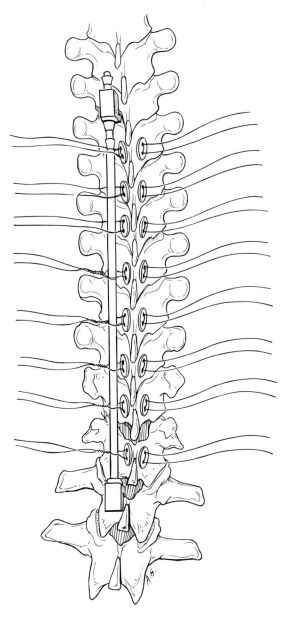

Figure 7–32

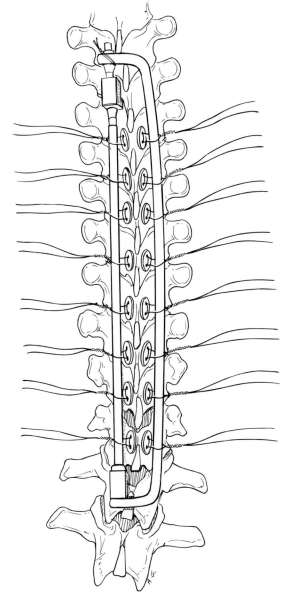

Figure 7–33

239

# Luque System

The spine is exposed from one vertebra proximal to the proximal fusion level to one vertebra caudal to the caudal fusion level preserving the facet joints proximal and distal to the proposed fusion limits. Exposure is to the tips of transverse processes in the thoracic and lumbar spine with removal of all the facet capsules with a curette.

To minimize blood loss, the best sequence of the procedure is excision of the facets, laminotomy, passage of wires, rod bending, rod insertion, and wire tightening.

### EXCISION OF FACETS

The facets are excised at each level and a curette is used to remove the cartilage of the superior articular process. Facet excision is necessary at this stage, since once the laminotomy has been performed facet excisions are difficult and dangerous. At this stage, the facets are best fused with insertion of bone plugs. If the plugs are inserted after the laminotomies have been performed, care must be taken to direct the bone impactor or drift laterally away from the open interlaminar space and spinal canal.

### LAMINOTOMY

Laminotomies are performed throughout the extent of the fusion area from cranial to the upper extent of the fusion to the interspace caudal to the lower extent of the fusion. The procedure is usually performed starting caudally and working cranially. A wide, double-action rongeur is used to remove the spinous process at its base with bone wax applied to the cut bony edge to minimize blood loss (Fig. 7–34). The double-action rongeur is next used to carefully remove the superficial portions of the ligamentum flavum until the midline portion of the spinal canal with a small amount of epidural fat is visualized. The remaining portion of the ligamentum flavum is removed using a Kerrison rongeur or narrow, double-action rongeur working away from the midline on both sides (Fig. 7–35). The majority of the ligamentum flavum has to be removed so that sufficient space is available for the insertion of wires at each interlaminar space. In the thoracic area there is normally an overlapping of laminae, similar to shingles on a roof. Because of this, additional bone is removed at the base of the spinous process and inferior edge of the lamina of the cranial vertebra to adequately visualize the interlaminar space and ligamentum flavum. In addition, the medial edge of the superior articular process may need to be removed with the Kerrison rongeur to give sufficient space for wire passage. Laminotomies are performed throughout the length of the fusion area and any bleeding encountered from the epidural space at the corners of the interlaminar space is controlled with a Gelfoam pledget soaked in thrombin.

240

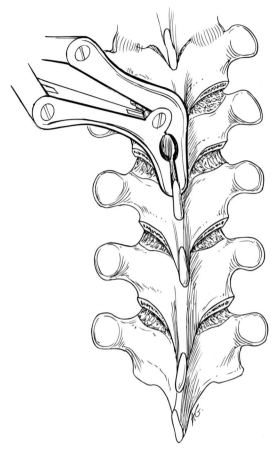

Figure 7–34

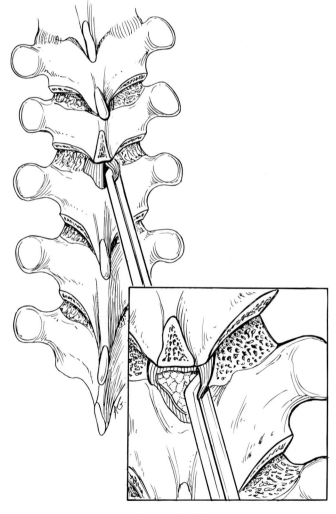

Figure 7–35

241

WIRE PASSAGE

Depending on the laminar contour and length of the lamina, the wire loop is bent into an appropriately shaped "L" so that the wire can be easily passed under the lamina (Fig. 7–36A). In shorter laminae or in the lower lumbar area, the wire is more efficiently bent into a "C" shape to pass under the lamina. The wire is passed under the lamina in the midline where there is more anteroposterior canal space. The wire is slowly passed and controlled so that the tip of the wire is held against the undersurface of the lamina so that when it reaches the cranial end of the lamina it pops into the interlaminar space (Fig. 7–36B,C). A #16-gauge (1.2 mm) wire is used in most cases even with soft osteopenic bone. The thicker wire is less likely to cut the softer bone.

The end of the wire in the interlaminar space is grasped with a wire holder and gradually advanced, pulling up away from the spine while maintaining tension on both ends of the wire to avoid penetrating the spinal canal (Fig. 7–36D). The wire loops are pinched over the lamina, the cranial wire is bent caudally and the caudal wire is bent cranially (Fig. 7–36E). In cases where a single wire is used at each side, the double-wire loop is split and one wire is moved to each side of the lamina and pinched over the edges of the lamina (Fig. 7–37A). In cases where a double loop is used at each side at each level, the double loop of wire is pinched over the lamina and is moved to the side being instrumented first (usually the concave curve) (Fig. 7–37B).

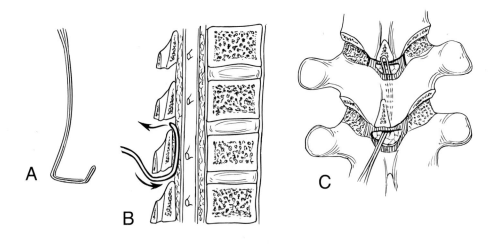

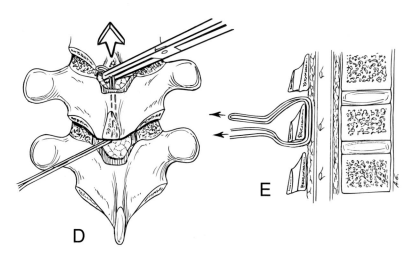

Figure 7–36

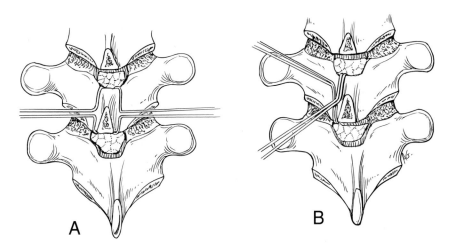

Figure 7–37

243

### Determination of Rod Bend

Determination of the rod bend is made in a number of ways. The upright radiograph shows the amount of curvature present and the end vertebrae to be fused (Fig. 7–38). The correctability of the spine can be shown in a number of ways. In patients able to actively side bend, the supine side-bending view will demonstrate the correctability of the curve and the rod contour can be taken from this (Fig. 7–39). In patients unable to actively side bend, a preoperative distraction view taken on the Risser table with a lateral localizer strap will show the curve's correctability and can be used for rod contouring (Fig. 7–40). Gen-

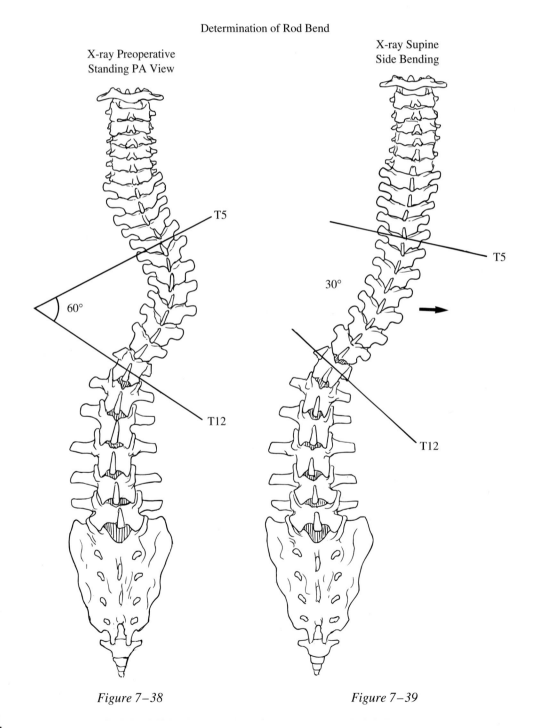

Determination of Rod Bend

X-ray Preoperative
Standing PA View

X-ray Supine
Side Bending

*Figure 7–38*

*Figure 7–39*

erally, a better estimation is obtained at the time of surgery where, with the patient in the prone position under anesthesia, curve correction is already partially present. The curve correctability is seen with the addition of a manual lateral force over the apex of the scoliosis, thus showing the maximum correctability of the spine (Fig. 7–41). The rod is contoured a little straighter than the spine with correction.

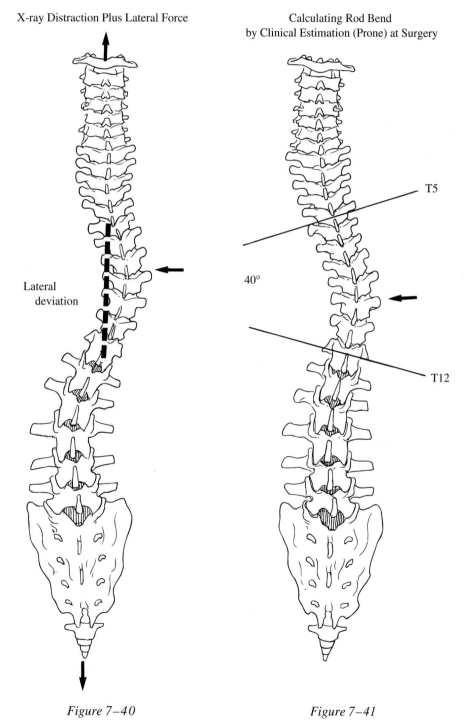

Determination of Rod Bend

X-ray Distraction Plus Lateral Force

Calculating Rod Bend
by Clinical Estimation (Prone) at Surgery

T5

Lateral
deviation

40°

T12

*Figure 7–40*

*Figure 7–41*

### INSTRUMENTATION (ROD INSERTION AND WIRE TIGHTENING)

The wires are passed at each level to be instrumented. Both the concave and convex wires can be passed at this stage (Fig. 7–42). If this is done, cover one set of wires with a towel to prevent the wires from being mixed up, while the second set is being used in the instrumentation (Fig. 7–43). The authors' preferred method is to pass one set of wires and use these to secure the first rod, with a second set of wires being passed after that.

Instrumentation commences at one end of the fusion using the "L" portion of the Luque rod, which is contoured to the corrected spinal shape while also maintaining the appropriate kyphosis and lordosis. A notch is made in the upper end of the upper vertebra to be fused (or below the spinous process of the lower vertebra to be fused) for placement of the L portion of the rod. With fusion to the lumbar spine with a large spinous process it is sometimes possible to make a hole in the spinous process to accept the L portion of the rod. The wires are sequentially tightened from the L portion of the rod toward the apex of the curve at the first stage of the instrumentation so that the wire is tightened opposing the rod to the lamina (Fig. 7–44). During handling of the wire and the wire tightening process it is essential to maintain traction on the wire at all times so that inadvertent anterior motions of the hands and wire are prevented from impinging on the contents of the spinal canal.

The exact sequence of wire tightening depends on the instrumentation technique being used. The first rod is inserted either on the concavity (concave technique) or convexity (convex technique) of the curve. For scoliosis the concave technique is more commonly used.

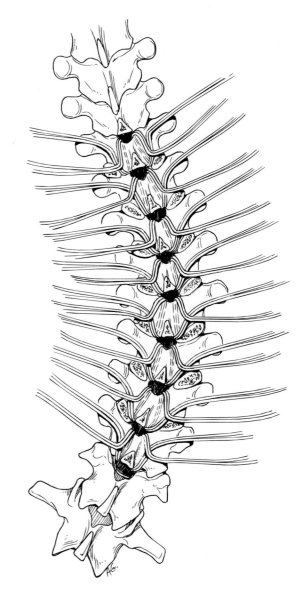

Figure 7–42

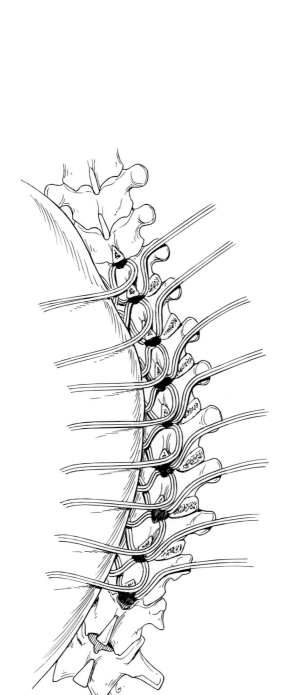

Figure 7–43

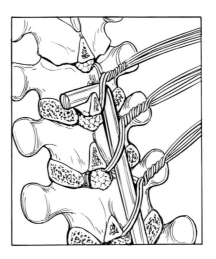

Figure 7–44

247

In the *concave technique,* the concave rod is inserted first. The L end of the rod is secured to the spine with two or three loops of wire followed by securing the other end of the rod to the spine with two or three loops of wire. The wire tightening then proceeds toward the center portion of the curve by tightening one wire from each end sequentially (Fig. 7–45A). At the same time as the central wires are tightened, pressure is applied over the convexity of the curve to approximate the curve to the rod during the tightening process (Fig. 7–45B). Care should be taken not to overtighten the wires and cut into the bone. Tightening ceases at a specific level when each wire is tight on the rod. Initially there will be a gap between the rod and the bone and as the tightening moves toward the apex of the curve the previously tightened wires will become loose. Once the central wires are tightened the wires are again tightened moving from the ends of the curve toward the apex. At this stage it will be seen that the bone is approximated to the rod, and at the end of the tightening procedure, the rod and bone are in contact. The convex rod is now inserted after checking the rod contour so that the rod lies exactly on the spine. The convex wires are now passed (if they have not been passed initially). The convex rod is inserted and wired to the spine at each level; the L portion of the convex rod is at the opposite end of the fusion area to the L portion of the concave rod.

In the *convex technique* the rod on the convexity of the curve is inserted first. The L end is secured to the spine with two or three loops and then sequentially the wire loops are tightened away from the L end of the rod to the apex of the curve and beyond it (Fig. 7–45C). Once the tightening occurs past the apex of the curve, the wire loops are not completely tight with approximation of the spine to the rod. A second sequence of tightening is again necessary to approximate the spine to the bone (Fig. 7–45D). Once all the convex wires have been tightened, the concave rod is checked so that it is contoured exactly to the spine. The concave wires are now passed (if they have not been passed initially) and the concave rod inserted and wired in place.

In the case of kyphosis all the wires on the right and left of the spine are passed at the initial stage. Two rods are contoured, one with the L portion cranially and the other with the L portion caudally. A "double" convex technique is used. The rods are undercontoured so that correction of the kyphosis can occur with rod insertion. Each rod is fixed to the spine with 3 to 4 loops of wire, the L portion of one being fixed to the cranial end of the curve and the L portion of the other rod fixed to the opposite side of the spine at the caudal end. Once the rods have been secured to the spine, sequential tightening of each set of wires away from the L portion occurs with the rods being forced toward the spine, correcting the kyphosis (Fig. 7–45E).

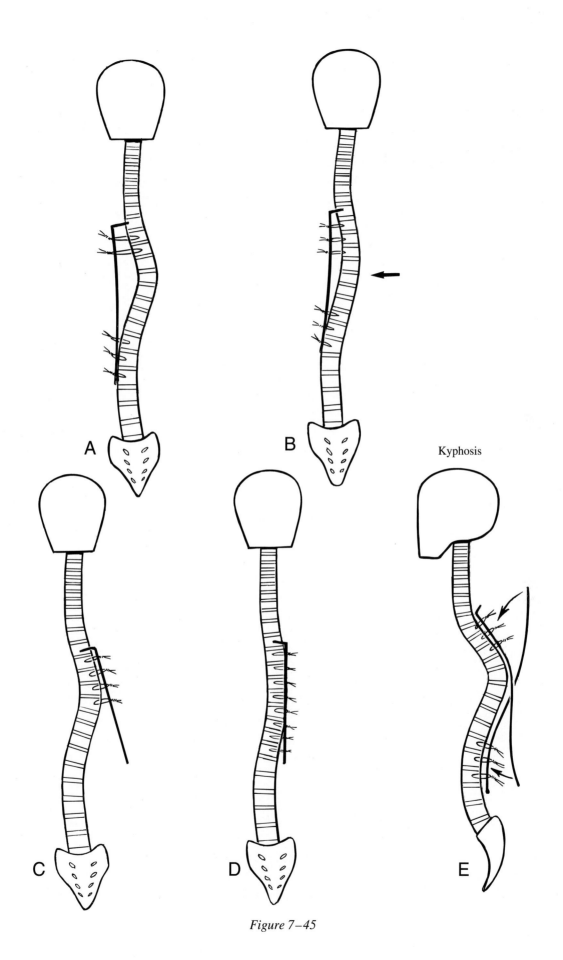

A

B

Kyphosis

C

D

E

*Figure 7–45*

249

Where possible, at the ends of the rods, the L portion of one rod is fixed deep to the straight portion of the opposite rod with a single wire securing both rods. All the twisted wires are bent toward the rod and spine, the bend and direction being set with a drift. Whenever possible, cross-linking devices are added cranially and caudally to stabilize the rods and form a strong, closed loop. The cross-linking device is being added at the end of instrumentation or during instrumentation, depending on the type of device being used (Fig. 7–46). Decortication is performed over each transverse process and in the midline over each lamina with the addition of autologous or bank bone for the fusion.

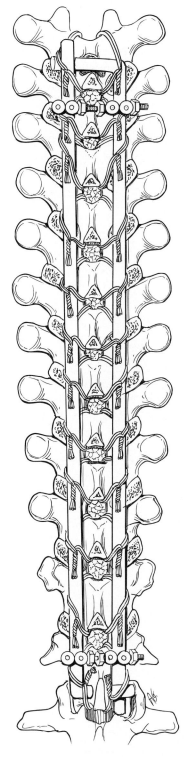

*Figure 7–46*

## LORDOSIS

In cases of lordoscoliosis, the double concave rod technique is best. DD had a 48 degree right thoracic idiopathic scoliosis (Fig. 7–47A) accompanied by severe lordosis (Fig. 7–47B) that was flexible as shown with forward flexion. Exposure and laminotomies were performed as described above, and both wire loops inserted at each level throughout the area to be instrumented. The rods were contoured to restore the thoracic kyphosis and inserted fixing the ends of the rods to the spine, firmly applied to the laminae by three wire loops.

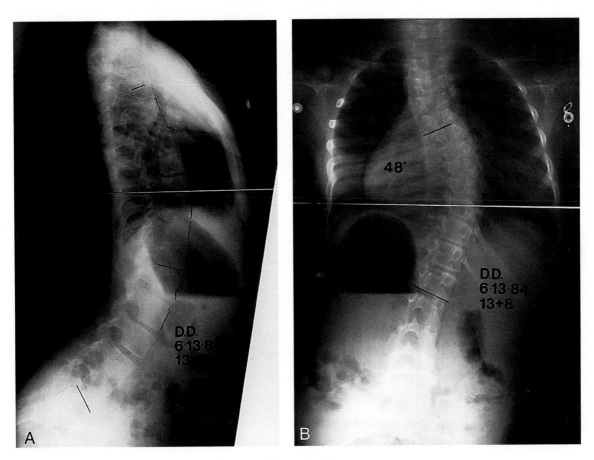

*Figure 7–47*

The loops were then tightened working toward the apex of the deformities (scoliosis and lordosis), the wires on the concave (left) rod being tightened first followed by the convex wires at the same level and then repeating the sequence (Fig. 7–48A,B). During the first wire tightening sequence the rod and laminae are not in contact. The wire is tensioned (with pressure over the apex of the scoliosis in lordoscoliosis) until it is tight. Once all the wires are tightened, it is

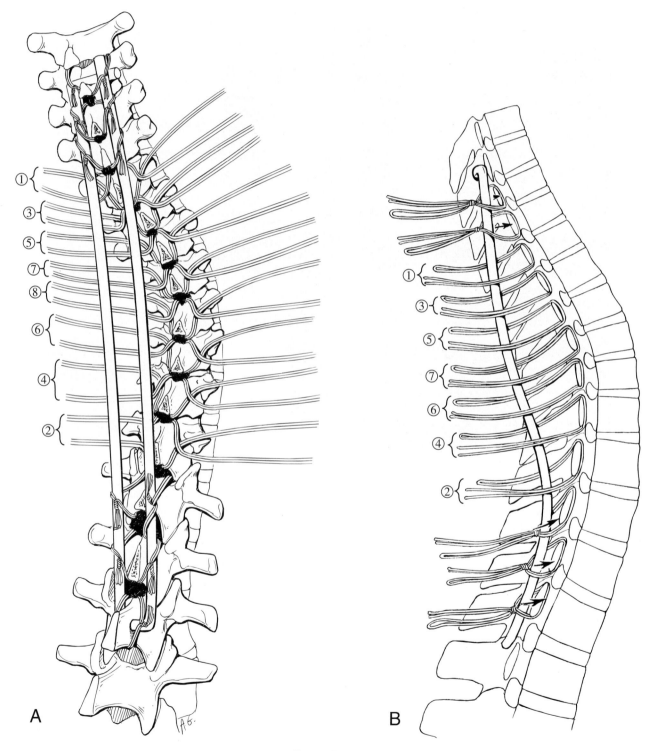

A

B

*Figure 7–48*

seen that the wires away from the apex are loose. The tightening is repeated a number of times until the laminae are in contact with the rod throughout its length, with each sequence. The distance between bone and rod decreases. This double concave technique corrects the scoliosis and kyphosis (Fig. 7–49A,B).

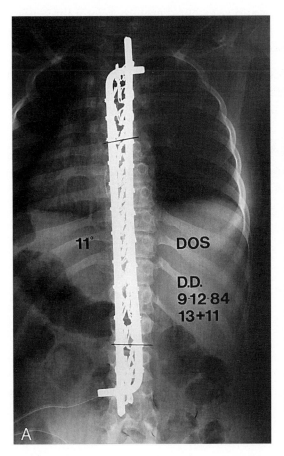
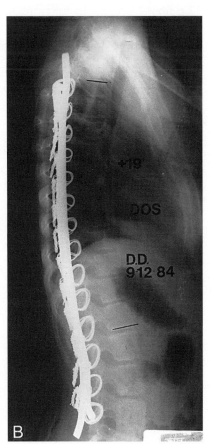

*Figure 7–49*

255

# Cotrel–Dubousset Instrumentation

The conception of Cotrel–Dubousset instrumentation (C–D) took place between 1978 and 1983. This system has increased the number of purchase points on the spine as compared to the Harrington system in that it provides a reliable enough fixation allowing most patients to go braceless postoperatively without significant loss of correction.

The rod is a knurled rod with toric notches (Fig. 7–50). It comes in two versions: (1) the standard rod with a greater ductility than the Harrington rod allowing complex bending in severe deformities and (2) a cold rolled rod with increased stiffness allowing it to resist bending forces.

The hooks present in different shapes and sizes but there are mainly three types of hooks—the pedicle hook, the thoracic laminar hook, and the lumbar laminar hook. All three hooks come in closed and open varieties (Fig. 7–50).

The pedicle hook gains its purchase on the spine against the strongest part of the posterior arch, that is, the posterior base of the pedicle. The bifid configuration of the pedicle hook increases the rotational strength of the hook by catching the cortex of the pedicle.

The thoracic and lumbar laminar hooks allow safe purchase on thoracic and lumbar laminae, respectively. Hook penetration into the spinal canal is minimized by the use of the appropriate hook.

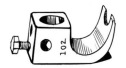

Closed
Pedicular (CP)

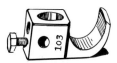

Closed
Laminar
(Lumbar) (CLL)

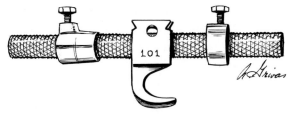

Open Laminar (OL)

Open
Laminar
(Thoracic) (OL)

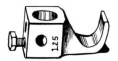

Closed
Laminar
(Thoracic) (CL)

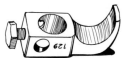

Narrow Box
(4 mm)

Open
Pedicular (OP)

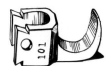

Open
Laminar
(Lumbar) (OLL)

*Figure 7–50*

257

# SINGLE RIGHT THORACIC CURVE

### INSERTION OF THE PEDICLE HOOK

The pedicle hook is applied primarily to the thoracic spine from T1 to T9 or all the way to T11 depending on the anatomy of the patient. A portion of the inferior facet must be removed in order to place the hook directly in front of the pedicle and to have the bifid part of the hook's blade against the base of the pedicle while keeping good contact of the hook against the inferior facet itself (Fig. 7–51). The vertical cut is made at the junction between the convexity of the superior facet and the concavity of its junction with the spinous process. The horizontal cut is made 4 to 5 mm below the inferior transverse process line. A curette is then used to clean up the cartilage of the superior facet of the vertebra below and ascertain that the plane of the facet joint is visualized (Fig. 7–52). A pedicle finder may be used to identify the pedicle, but this should be done very carefully, since cases of paraplegia have been reported in association with "plunging" into the spinal canal with this instrument. The horizontal cut on the inferior facet should be perpendicular to the line of instrumentation or to the anticipated path of the rod. This will provide optimal purchase of the pedicle hook onto the vertebra.

The pedicle hook, held by a hook holder and directed by a hook inserter, is pushed manually into the small joint space (Fig. 7–53). The hook must be directed at an angle cephalad and anteriorly in order to ascertain that both horns of its bifid blade are penetrating in the appropriate plane. The most frequent problem is that the angle of approach to the facet plane is too low and thereby makes the horns of the hook penetrate the inferior facet posterior to the plane of the joint. Do not try to force it in, as this may result in fracture of the inferior facet and, therefore, the purchase point. Particular attention must be directed to the lateral horn of the pedicle hook, which presents the greater difficulties in penetrating the appropriate plane. The Leksell rongeur may be used to remove a portion of the posterior transverse process of the vertebra below in order to facilitate easier insertion.

It is important to realize that the pedicle hook sits on the superior facet from below. This is what provides the safety of that hook. Two situations may arise where the pedicle hook may become a liability to the spinal cord. First, there are situations where due to anatomic variations, the superior facet may be relatively short in comparison to the inferior facet from above. The usual excision of the inferior part of the inferior facet may result in placement of the pedicle hook at the very tip of the superior facet from below. As the hook reaches the pedicle, it may move anteriorly against the neural structures. Second, the superior facet may be fractured during the insertion of the hook or during insertion of the pedicle finder (Fig. 7–54). This is usually accompanied by a pathognomonic cracking sound. The hook should be removed immediately and the superior facet fracture identified. If the fracture line is not displaced, the fragment of superior facet may be left in place. If there is a significant amount of displacement of the fragment of the superior facet toward the spinal cord, a small laminotomy should be done at that level to remove the floating fragment. In no

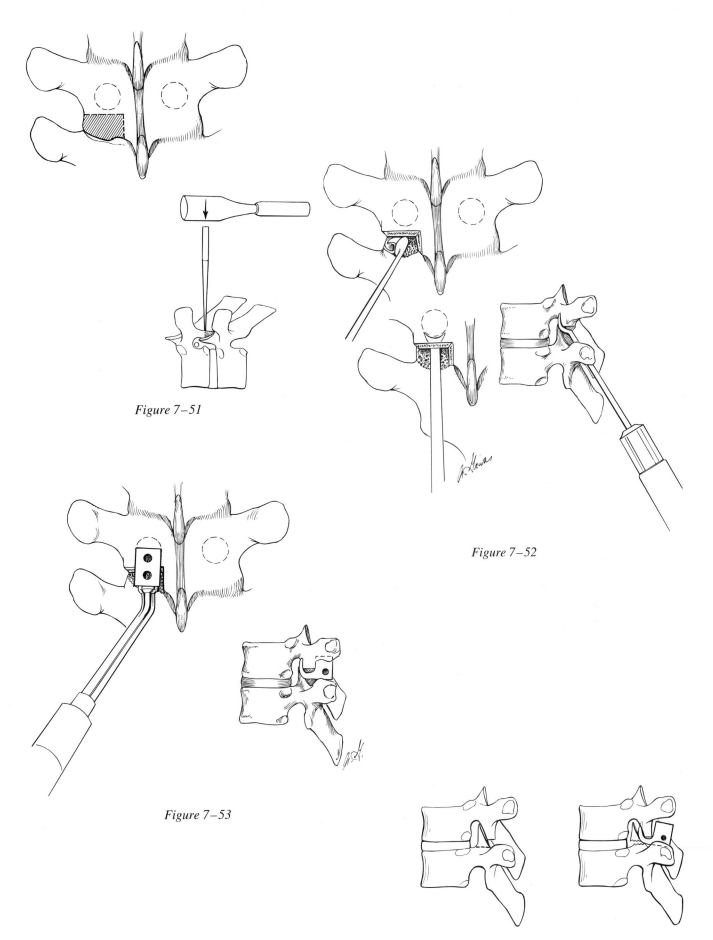

*Figure 7–51*

*Figure 7–52*

*Figure 7–53*

*Figure 7–54*

case should a hook be reinserted at that level. It would not only result in displacement of the hook anteriorly into the canal, but also displacement of the superior facet fragment in front of it.

There are typically four pedicle hooks inserted for a right thoracic curve, two closed pedicle hooks on the upper end vertebra, one open pedicle hook at the apex of the convexity of the curve, and one open pedicle hook one or two levels above on the concavity side. This last hook is called the "upper intermediate concave hook."

### INSERTION OF A LAMINAR HOOK IN THE SUPRALAMINAR POSITION

This mode of insertion applies to the two lower concave hooks in the simple right thoracic curve. It is crucial to keep the laminotomy for hook insertion as small as possible to decrease the risk of an inadvertent "plunging" into the canal during rod insertion. When the upper end of the lamina is perpendicular to the anticipated axis of the rod and when its bone is of good quality, it is left as is. In the event of the superior edge of the lamina being at an angle or the bone being too soft, bone is removed with the use of a Kerrison rongeur until the purchase point on the superior end of the lamina becomes both perpendicular to the rod axis and thick enough to provide good purchase (Fig. 7–55A). The amount of removal of superior lamina also may vary depending on the size of the hook to be used. For instance, if the thoracic hook appears to be too small and the lumbar hook too large, additional bone will have to be removed from the superior end of the lamina until the lumbar laminar hook fits snugly without any anterior or posterior motion when seated. Insertion of the hook in the supralaminar position will be facilitated by removal of the spinous process down to its base. A small laminar spreader may have to be used to enlarge the laminotomy during hook insertion. The hook is usually inserted using a hook holder (Fig. 7–55B). Occasionally the hook holder may come into contact with the lower part of the wound or the self-retaining retractors holding the wound when trying to gain the correct approach angle for insertion. In such instances, switch from a hook holder to a hook inserter and then gain the correct approach angle for safe insertion.

Whenever the laminotomy is too large or when the hook seems to have a tendency to plunge into the canal, extreme care must be taken during manipulation of hooks and rods (Fig. 7–55C,D). The simplest way to stabilize the hook is to have it held in the fully seated position pulled slightly in the caudad direction. This is particularly important during insertion of the rod on the concave side.

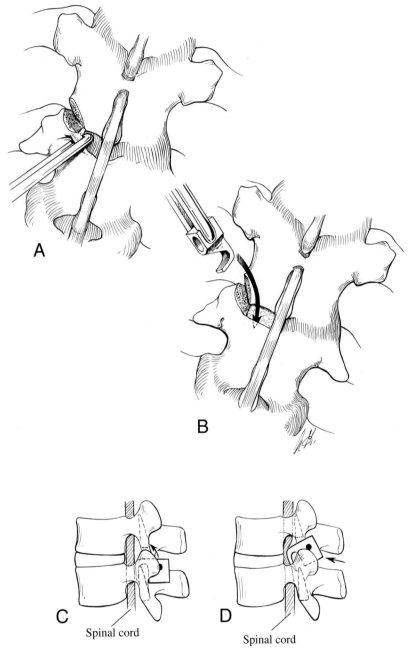

C Spinal cord

D Spinal cord

*Figure 7–55*

# POSTERIOR THORACIC AND THORACOLUMBAR PROCEDURES

### INSERTION OF THE TRANSVERSE PROCESS HOOK

This is carried out primarily on the convex transverse process of the upper end vertebra. The space for the hook is started with a transverse process elevator which hugs the superior aspect of the transverse process and is then rotated around the transverse process cutting some of the ligaments between the rib and the transverse process (Fig. 7–56A). If it is done at the base of the transverse process it does not significantly damage the joint between the rib and the tip of the transverse process. The hook most frequently used in that location is a closed lumbar laminar hook. It is held by a hook holder and follows a circular path similar to the path necessary for the transverse process elevator (Fig. 7–56B).

### INFRALAMINAR HOOK INSERTION

The lower end vertebra receives a hook on the inferior aspect of its convex lamina. This hook is usually a closed lumbar laminar hook. A small inferior laminotomy is carried out providing horizontal purchase for that hook. An effort is made to preserve the adjacent capsule and the stronger bone of the medial aspect of that inferior lamina. Some of the thickness of the lamina may have to be reduced with the help of a rongeur (Fig. 7–57A). The infralaminar hook is inserted with a hook holder and is pushed with a hook inserter into the plane between the anterior aspect of the lamina and ligamentum flavum originating from it (Fig. 7–57B).

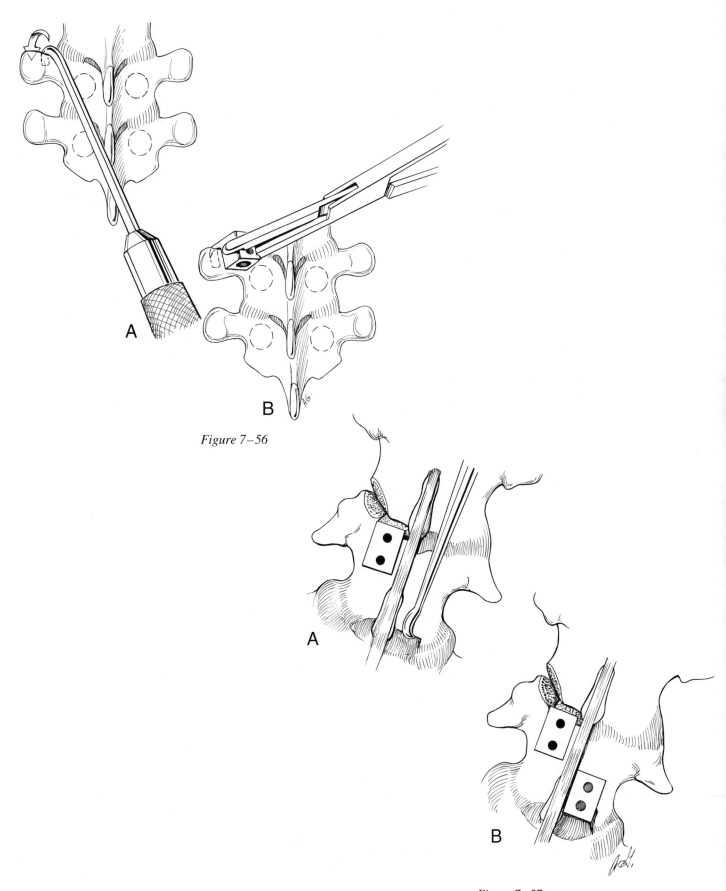

*Figure 7–56*

*Figure 7–57*

### HOOK CHECKOUT

It is important during and just after the insertion of a hook to check other inserted hooks. In particular, pounding on a convex pedicle hook while the lower intermediate hook is in the spinal canal could lead to dangerous motions of that hook against the spinal cord. This is particularly true if the facet fusions are started after all hooks are placed. It may be safer to temporarily remove the hooks in the spinal canal during the pounding required for facet fusions. Fusions are done in a standard fashion with placement of a cancellous bone plug harvested from the patient's iliac crest. Hook placement still allows a facet fusion on at least one side of every motion segment (Fig. 7–58). This is not true, however, at the uppermost segment where two pedicle hooks obliterate both joints. A meticulous decortication of transverse processes, spinous process, and medial lamina will have to be done at that level after instrumentation.

### FACET FUSION

Concave facet fusions are performed just prior to concave rod insertion. Convex facet fusions are done after concave rod insertion and just before the convex rod is set into position. The main rationale for this sequence is blood loss. Facet fusions are done wherever accessible, provided they do not compromise hook purchase.

### CONCAVE ROD CONTOURING, INSERTION, AND ROTATION

The effects of the concave rod are as follows:

1. *Distraction.* Some distraction of the concavity of the scoliotic curve, primarily within the short structural apical segment is effective. There is no question that the C–D rod in the concavity does not apply the same kind of distraction as a Harrington distraction rod. This will reduce the risk of spinal cord stretch.
2. *Sagittal recontouring.* The concave rod does pull the apex of the thoracic lordosis or the thoracic hypokyphosis posteriorly, thereby creating or increasing kyphosis.
3. *Derotation.* By definition, the combination of pulling of the concavity backward and pushing the convexity forward does allow derotation.

Consequently, contouring of the rod will be a happy medium between contouring into scoliosis to allow easy rod insertion (initial rod shape) and contouring into the expected final kyphosis after the rod is rotated 90 degrees (final rod shape).

It is hoped that the initial rod shape and the final rod shape are similar. Otherwise, the discrepancy indicates unbending during the rotation of the rod. The amount of force necessary to unbend the rod is similar to that necessary to bend it. It is, therefore, easy to imagine the forces applied on the hooks and to understand the fracture of the lamina during rod rotation.

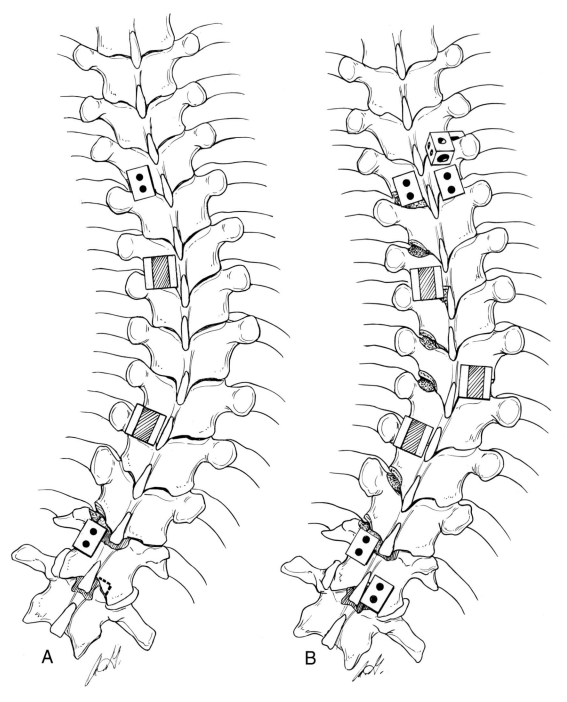

Figure 7–58

4. *After the rod has been contoured to the shape of the scoliosis and to the anticipated sagittal contour, including lordosis in the lumbar spine, it is inserted into the upper pedicle hook first* (Fig. 7–59). Two blockers are inserted on the lower end of the rod; they are back-to-back. Gentle tightening of the hex bolts locks the blockers in the midpart of the rods to prevent their movement up and down during rod insertion, and they are away from the open hooks.

The rod then is inserted into the lower closed hook, and if contouring has been done correctly, the rod will slip into the open box of the open hooks. Again, as the rod is pushed into the upper intermediate hook, check the lower intermediate hook, which may be pushed into the spinal canal. Usually the rod is easily placed into the upper intermediate hook, but occasionally requires the use of the rod introducer for the lower intermediate hook.

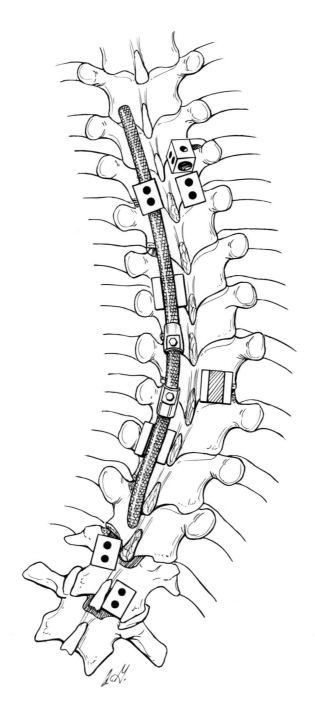

Figure 7–59

When the rod is in the opening of the open hook, the blocker may be unlocked and pushed into the hook box. This should be done with a hook holder aiming the hook down to the blocker. If done with the hook "looking up" to the blocker, the blocker will not penetrate easily and actually will spread the open box making it a weaker purchase point (Fig. 7–60).

The completed rod insertion is shown in Figure 7–61.

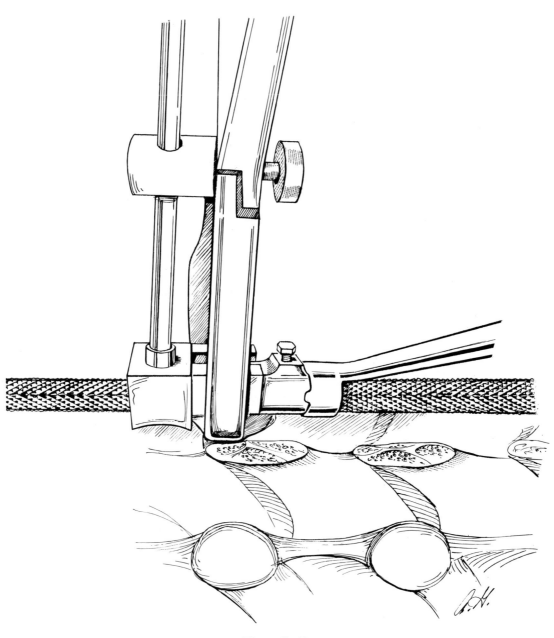

*Figure 7–60*

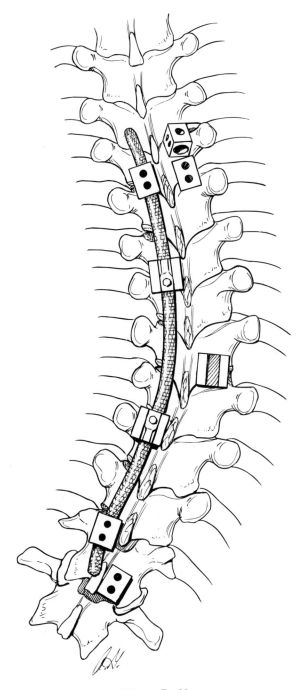

Figure 7–61

There are two tools for blocker manipulation that are used both for hooks and blockers. The *hook driver* has rotational control on both hook and blocker owing to its lateral flanges. The *hook and blocker pusher* is flat and, therefore, without rotational control.

The C rings then are placed over the rod between the intermediate hooks. They allow some distraction of the apical vertebrae without blocking rotation. When appropriate distraction has been applied between a rod holder and the C rings on either side, the intermediate hooks are well seated and under minimal to moderate distraction. The upper and lower hooks should be checked for position (Fig. 7–62).

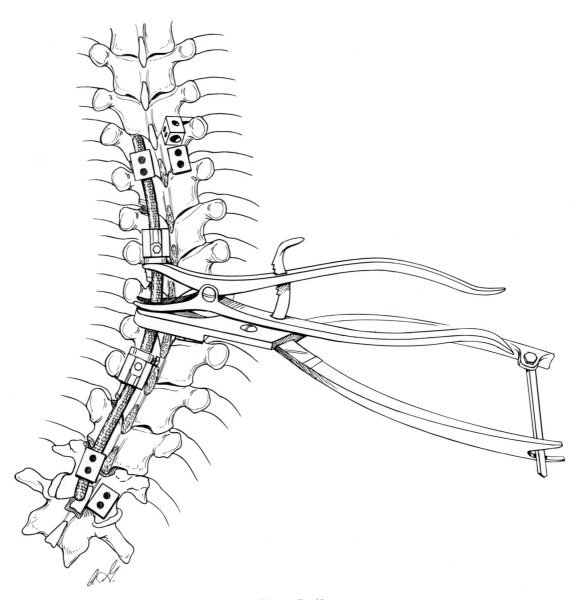

*Figure 7–62*

271

Two large rod holders then are used to rotate the rod 90 degrees from its scoliotic configuration to a kyphotic configuration (Fig. 7–63). This maneuver may be easy in supple curves when rod contouring is adequate, but it may be difficult when the curvature is more severe and when rod contouring is too kyphotic. In this situation, "forcing the rotation" unbends the rod with the unexpected result, when reaching 90 degrees of rotation, that the rod is not providing the expected kyphosis (Figs. 7–64 and 7–65).

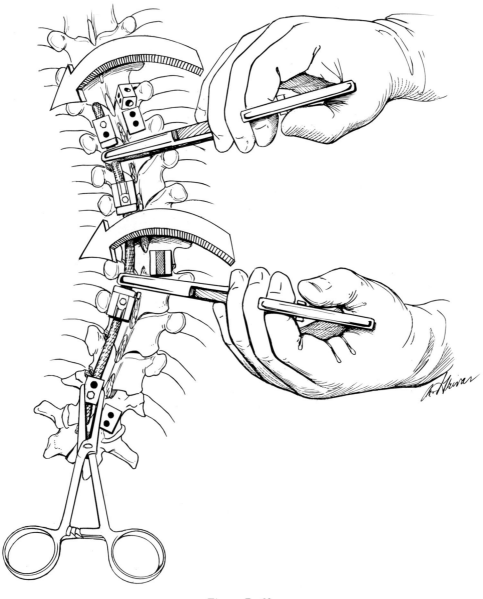

*Figure 7–63*

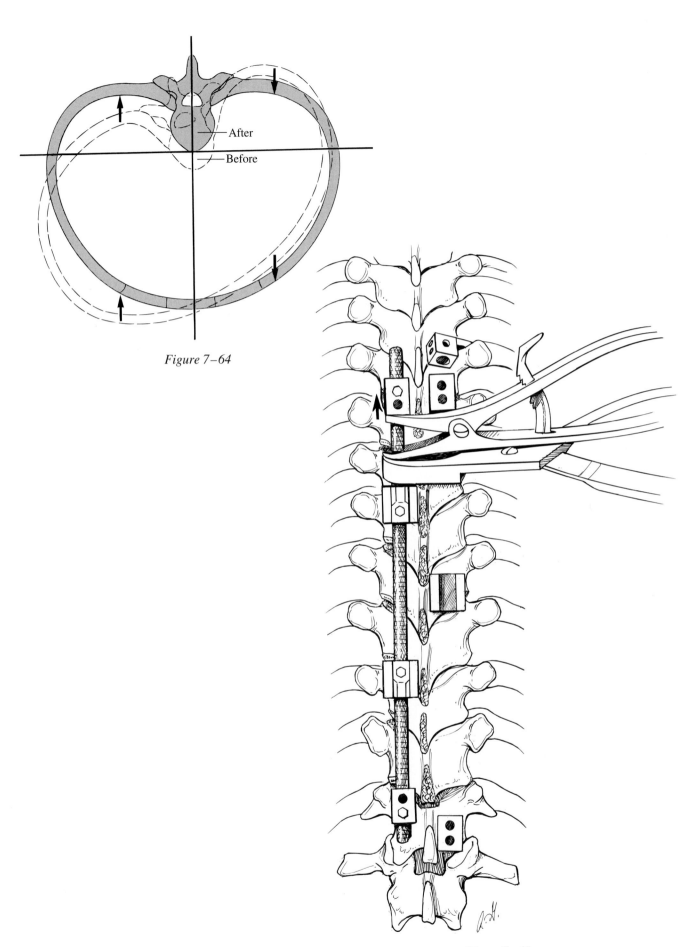

Figure 7–64

Figure 7–65

273

After derotation the upper intermediate hook may displace laterally. It should be immediately repositioned by pushing the apex of the curve back toward the rod and resecuring the upper intermediate pedicle hook against the pedicle (Figs. 7–66 to 7–69).

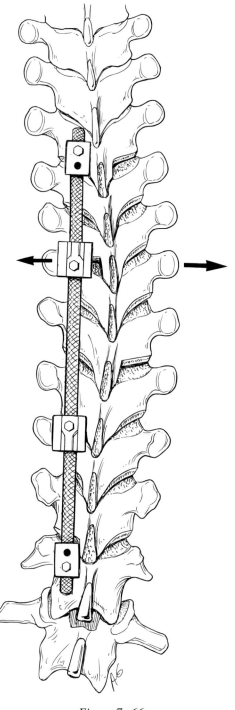

*Figure 7–66*

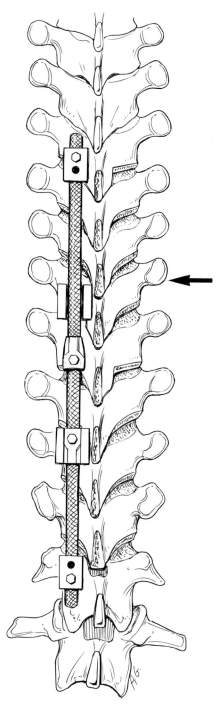

*Figure 7–67*

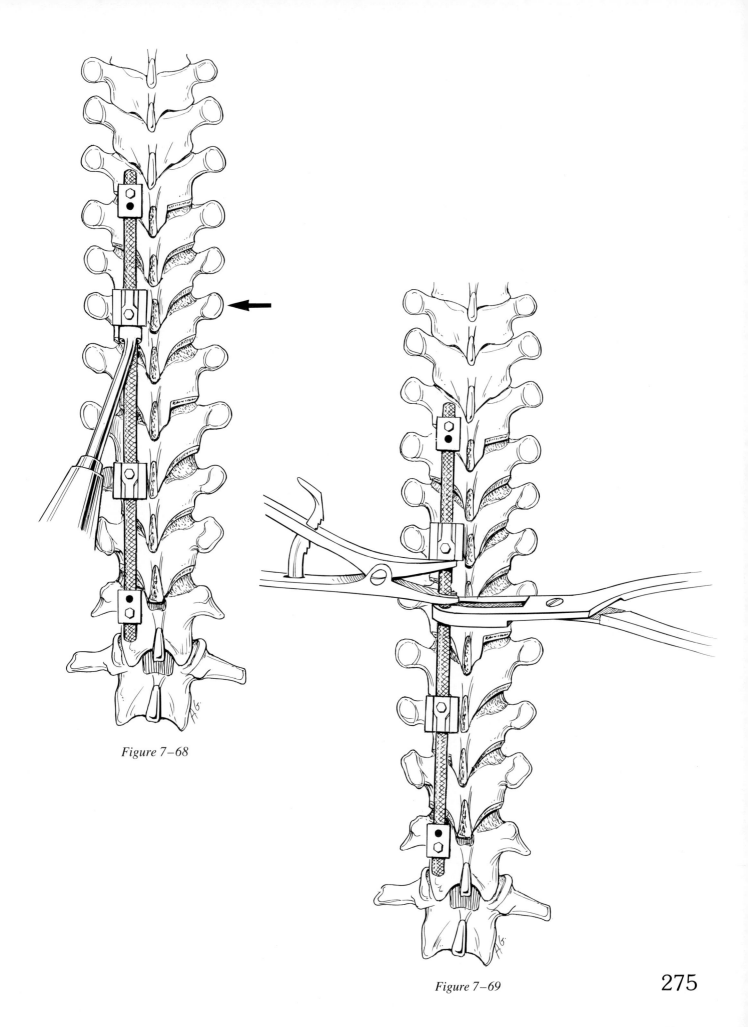

Figure 7–68

Figure 7–69

### CONVEX ROD CONTOURING

The convex rod is undercontoured in less kyphosis than the patient's so as to push the convexity forward during instrumentation. The bottom of the rod (the last 4 or 5 cm) accounts for some lordosis, as seen physiologically at the thoracolumbar junction.

The convex rod is inserted in its upper claw first and pushed down into the apical open hook. The blocker then is moved cephalad into the apical hook. The rod holder is placed approximately 3 to 5 cm from the lower end, allowing the rod to slip into the lower hook. The lower hook may have to be repositioned; its purchase on the lower lamina must be seated properly, otherwise the hook will pull out posteriorly (Fig. 7–70).

The upper claw is tightened against itself (Fig. 7–71), the convex apical hook is compressed against the upper claw (Fig. 7–72), and the lower hook then is compressed against a rod gripper with a hook compressor (Fig. 7–73).

Some further compression loading takes place on the convex rod when additional distraction is produced on the concave rod. At this point, ascertain that all hex bolts have been tightened onto the rod and the rod is stable within all eight hooks.

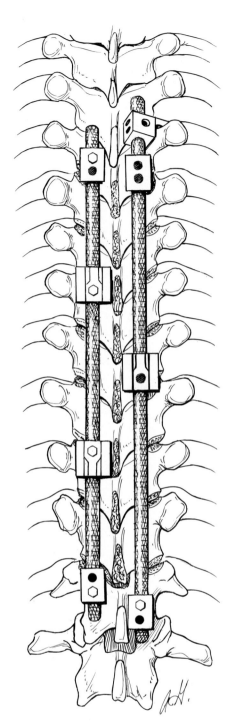

Figure 7–70

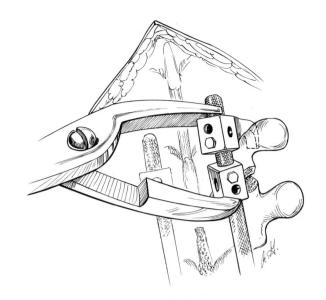

Figure 7–71

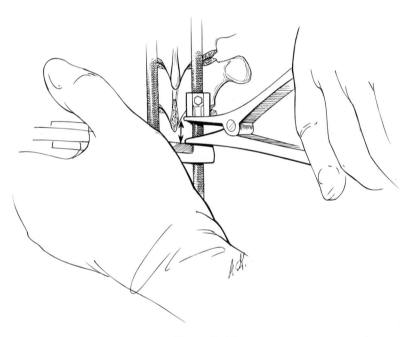

Figure 7–72

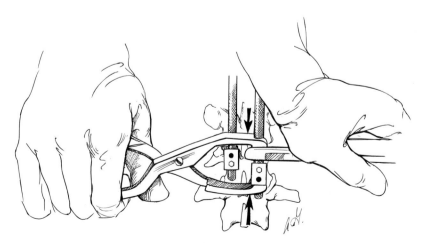

Figure 7–73

277

### DECORTICATION

At this point, the decortication of the available parts of posterior arches throughout the entire length of instrumentation should be started. Decortication should not jeopardize the stability of the hooks.

### DEVICE FOR TRANSVERSE TRACTION INSERTION (DTT)

In the case of a right thoracic curve, two DTTs are inserted at each end of the rods just below the upper hooks and just above the lower hooks (Fig. 7–74). This provides a rectangular configuration to the spinal montage, enhancing its overall strength.

### WAKE-UP TEST

Spinal cord monitoring is checked after full instrumentation. Because of some reported false-negatives, we still ask the anesthesiologist to do a formal wake-up test. If the wake-up test is negative (patient moves his lower extremities and toes), then proceed with adding the remaining autogenous iliac bone grafts. All hex screws are tightened to shearing. Second hex screws are inserted and sheared on all closed hooks.

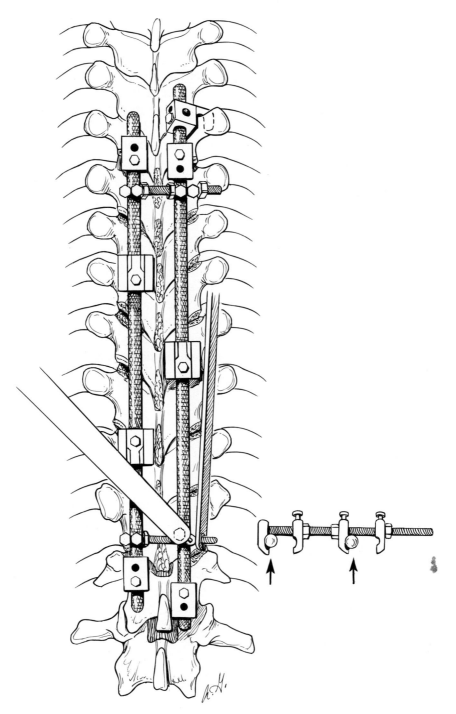

*Figure 7–74*

# RIGHT THORACIC SCOLIOSIS WITH MILD THORACIC LORDOSIS

There are no significant changes in the case of thoracic lordosis. The concave rod is contoured and inserted in scoliotic and lordotic curvature and is rotated more than in standard scoliosis. For example, instead of 90 degrees, it may be rotated 120 degrees before the bend in the rod reaches its kyphotic configuration. The convex rod is not significantly underbent and little pressure, if any, is applied over the apex because of the risk of increasing thoracic lordosis.

# RIGHT THORACIC SCOLIOSIS WITH SEVERE LORDOSIS

Thoracic lordosis itself may be an indication for surgery owing to the incidence of respiratory dysfunction. The purpose of surgery is to try to reduce the lordosis and, if possible, create some kyphosis to increase the chest volume for lung expansion. The problem initially encountered when attempting to create a kyphosis in the thoracic spine was the ductility of the rod, which did not provide enough force to pull the apex of the lordosis posteriorly. There is no question that posterior distraction in itself tends to reduce the lordosis and starts to create some kyphosis. The extent of instrumentation in thoracic lordosis usually will be longer than for a typical right thoracic curve.

### CORRECTION OF THE LORDOSIS

The fusion is from T2 to L1. The T2 vertebra is equipped bilaterally with a pediculotransverse claw. The inferior anchor of the instrumentation is a two-level claw with a supralaminar hook on T12 and a closed lumbar laminar (CLL) hook in the intralaminar position under L1. Open pedicle (OP) hooks will be placed on T4 and T6 and an open lumbar laminar (OLL) hook on T10. If the blade of the OLL hook is penetrating too deeply into the spinal canal, additional bone is removed to allow a greater level of safety for the hook. The advantage of the OLL hook over the open thoracic laminar is that it has a wider blade, which provides less risk of breaking the lamina when pulled posteriorly. A cold rolled rod must be used to prevent the likelihood of unbending as the reduction forces are applied (Fig. 7–75). In order to facilitate creation of kyphosis, two Luque wires are passed under the laminae of T7 and T8 bilaterally (Fig. 7–76). This will allow pulling the apex of the lordosis back to the cold rolled rod and facilitate the insertion of the blockers into the open hooks.

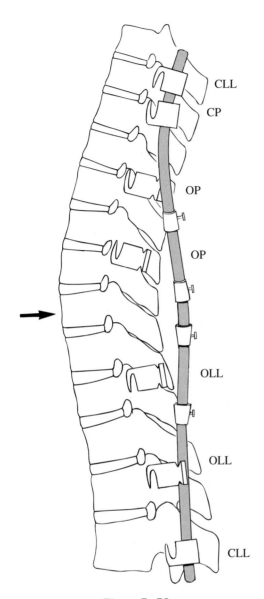

Figure 7–75

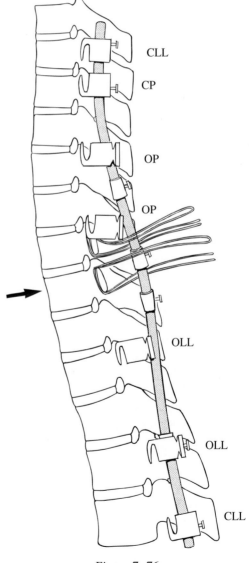

Figure 7–76

281

A moderate amount of distraction is applied between T2 and T12. The contour of the rod places its midportion at about 4 to 5 cm posteriorly to the posterior arches of the apex of the lordosis. The Luque wires are tightened onto the rod (Fig. 7–77). As the apex of the lordosis starts to get reapproximated to the rod, the T4 and T6 blockers are pushed into the hooks (Fig. 7–78). The pedicle hooks are reseated to make sure that they are not pulling posteriorly. After full tightening of the Luque wires, the final blocker on T10 is inserted. When all of the open hooks are loaded with their blockers, additional distraction between T2 and T12 may be applied. The claw at T2 is then secured and finally the intralaminar hook at L1 is reapproximated toward the T12 supralaminar hook. These two last maneuvers secure the ends of the rod.

# Right Thoracic Scoliosis with Thoracic Kyphosis

The convex rod is inserted first. It is significantly underbent and is fastened at the upper claw before it is pushed down into the para-apical open hooks and then against the lower-end vertebra lamina.

The lower hook should be a closed hook. If the upper claw is tight, it is not possible to slip the rod into a closed lower hook that is positioned on its lamina. Therefore, the surgeon must slip the hook up onto the rod and under the lamina at the same time. This is difficult, particularly if the bottom part of the rod is straight. However, if the last 4 cm of the rod are contoured in a 10 to 15 degree lordosis, it will redirect the closed hook right under the lamina as it glides up the rod.

When the kyphotic component is severe, a preliminary anterior release and anterior interbody fusion may be required. Posterior osteotomies may be necessary if optimal correction is sought. In this situation, the convex apical hook may become a tremendous liability to the system. The convex apical hook is really the fulcrum on which you push to reduce the kyphosis. If the kyphosis is supple enough or has been made more supple by multiple osteotomies and if the bone stock of the patient allows, the fulcrum will hold and the convex apical hook will stay where it should.

Conversely, if the kyphosis is severe and rigid and/or the surgeon tries too hard and/or the bone stock is porotic, a catastrophe may be pending with the sudden fracture of the superior facet of the underlying vertebra, fracture of the inferior facet of the instrumented vertebra, and major penetration of the hook into the thoracic spinal canal with the expected neurologic results.

In short, do not try too hard. If you want to push hard against the kyphus, do it with the rod, not with the convex apical hook. If you have to push hard on the kyphus, then place two intermediate hooks as on the convexity: one above the kyphus (on a transverse process) and one, the pedicular type, facing cephalad below the apex. This will allow better distribution of the fulcrum and less risk of "plunging" of the apical hook into the spinal canal and avoids hook prominence at the kyphosis apex.

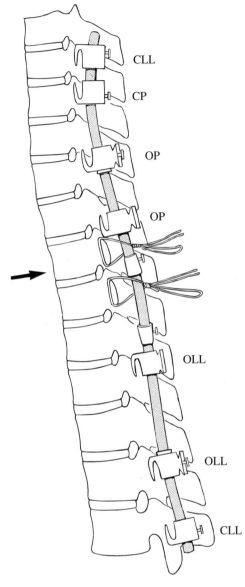

CLL

CP

OP

OP

OLL

OLL

CLL

Figure 7-77

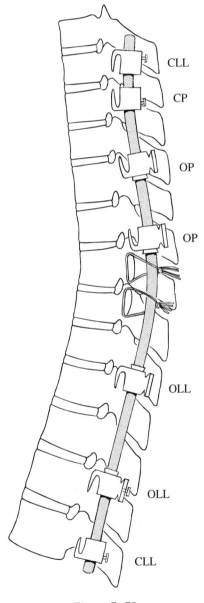

CLL

CP

OP

OP

OLL

OLL

CLL

Figure 7-78

283

## SEVERE CURVES

A short, apical rod is inserted in the concavity of the most structural portion of the curvature. A long rod bridges from the upper-end vertebra to the lower-end vertebra (Fig. 7–79). It should be a cold rolled rod.

Two apical DTTs approximate the two concave rods to maximize transverse correction (Fig. 7–80). The convex rod is applied after maximal correction on the concave side. Two additional DTTs then are applied at the end vertebrae and improve the correction further (Figs. 7–81 and 7–82).

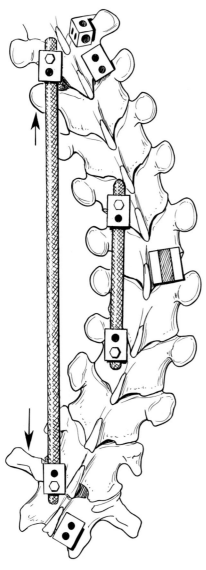

*Figure 7–79*

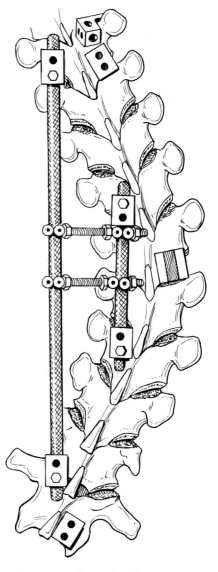

*Figure 7–80*

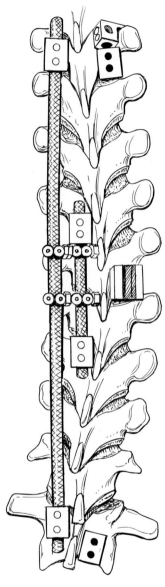

*Figure 7–81*

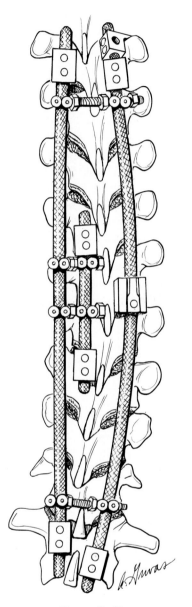

*Figure 7–82*

# DOUBLE THORACIC SCOLIOSIS

## HOOK PLACEMENT (Fig. 7–83)

The upper-end vertebra, usually T2, is instrumented with two closed pedicle hooks and a supratransverse hook on the side of the convexity, usually on the left. The lower-end vertebra, often but not always T12, is instrumented with a closed thoracic or closed lumbar laminar hook in the supralaminar position on the concave side and a closed lumbar laminar hook in the intralaminar position on the convex side of the lower curve. The junctional vertebra, usually T5, is equipped with two open hooks, a pedicle hook on the convexity of the upper curve, and a supratransverse hook on the opposite side. The apical vertebra of the lower curve, usually T9, receives an open pedicle hook on the right. T10 is chosen for the sole intermediate hook on the concavity of the right thoracic curve because it is next to the apical vertebra and the right thoracic component of the double thoracic idiopathic scoliosis is usually shorter than the simple right thoracic idiopathic curve, thereby requiring fewer hooks in its concavity (3 instead of 4). Facet fusions are carried out in the usual manner.

A short temporary rod is inserted in the concavity of the upper thoracic curve allowing some precorrection of the curve (Fig. 7–84). This will permit insertion of the left rod in its optimal shape.

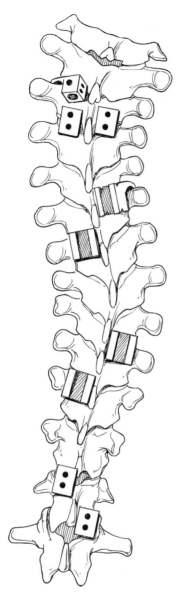

Figure 7–83

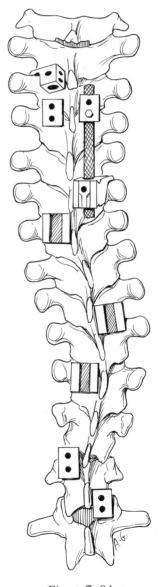

Figure 7–84

The left rod is precontoured in some kyphosis as required for the specific patient (Fig. 7–85). Some lordosis is added at the bottom of the rod whenever instrumentation goes into the lumbar spine. The rod is inserted into the upper claw first. It is then pushed into the open T5 hook and its blocker is inserted into the hook. While an assistant holds the blocker in T5, the surgeon pulls the rod into the T12 supralaminar hook. The rod usually misses the T10 open hook. Avoid pushing the T10 hook into the spinal canal with the rod. The rod is not inserted in a fully scoliotic position as it is in the classic right thoracic instrumentation. The reason is that the required kyphosis in both the upper and lower thoracic curves prevents the double scoliosis contouring. Consequently, the rod is inserted in a plane intermediate between sagittal and coronal. The T10 hook has to be taken to the rod by applying a force on the convexity of the curve. For instance, an assistant may apply pressure on the lateral aspect of the chest to permit the insertion. The blocker is then pushed into the T10 hook. Another method is to use the rod introducer.

The short rod is now removed; the right rod will be contoured into a kyphotic curve just short of the kyphosis noted in the patient (Fig. 7–86). It is inserted into the T2 pedicle hook first, then pushed down into the T5 and T9 open hooks, and pulled down into the T12 closed laminar hook held firmly with a hook holder. The T5 and T9 blockers are pushed into place. Distraction is applied in the concavity of the upper thoracic curve and compression on the lower thoracic curve.

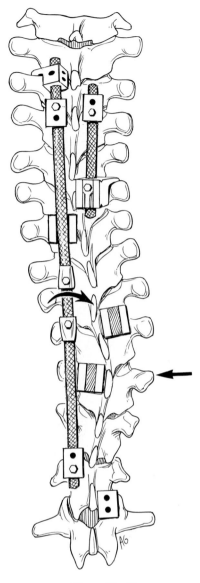

*Figure 7–85*

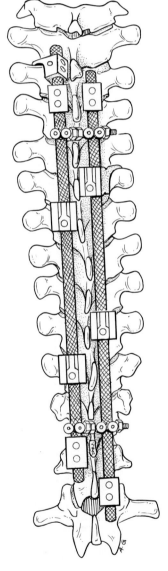

*Figure 7–86*

289

# DOUBLE MAJOR RIGHT THORACIC AND LEFT LUMBAR CURVES

The right thoracic curve is instrumented in a standard fashion, although both of its lower hooks are open. The left lumbar curve will be equipped with a supralaminar closed lumbar hook on the concavity of its lower-end vertebra (Fig. 7–87).

The infralaminar hook on the opposite side will be a closed lumbar laminar hook. The convex apical hook has to be an open lumbar hook placed in a supralaminar or infralaminar position. The left rod contouring will be S-shaped, as the scoliosis (Fig. 7–88). On rotation, it will provide kyphosis in the thoracic curve and lordosis in the lumbar curve. It will have a derotating effect on both curves at the same time (Fig. 7–89).

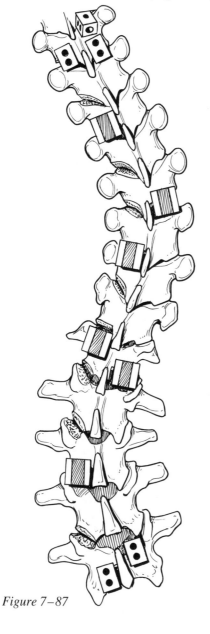

*Figure 7–87*

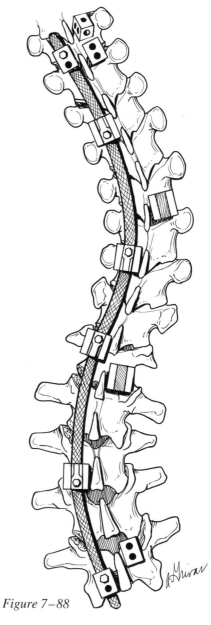

*Figure 7–88*

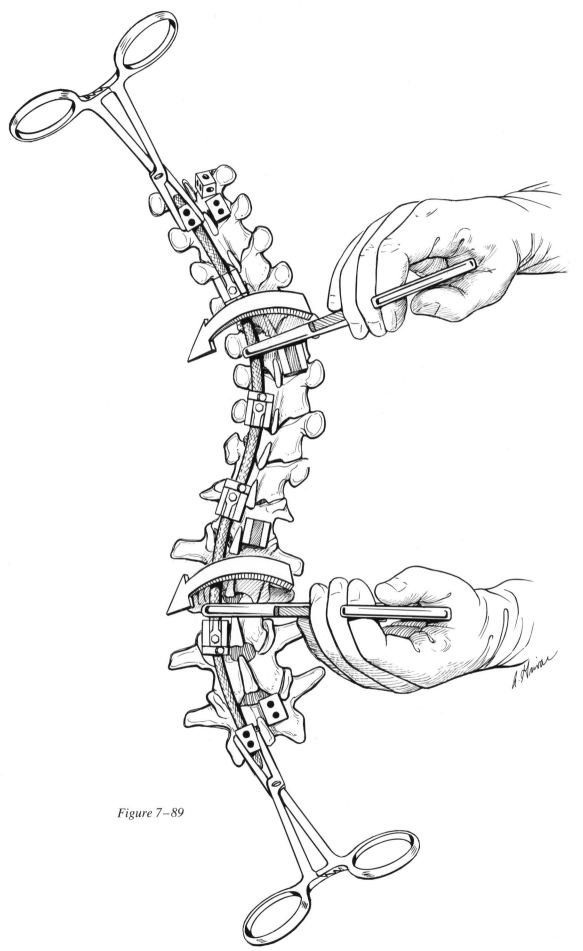

*Figure 7–89*

291

A frequent problem encountered during derotation is the dislodging of the inferior hook. This is due to the shortening of the convexity of the lumbar curve as it is corrected and derotated and to the increased lordosis which results from derotation. A possible solution to this problem is the use of a pedicular screw replacing the infralaminar hook, which allows rotation of the rod without the risks of hook dislodgement. The correction of the two curves should not be maximal at both levels. It should be thought out so as to preserve the balance of the spine both in the coronal and sagittal planes.

If necessary, a posteroanterior roentgenogram should be obtained on the operative table to verify the proper alignment of the spine.

The right rod will be straighter, with hypokyphotic contouring in the thoracic region. The lumbar contouring is in mild lordosis so rotation in that region is not accentuated. Three DTTs usually are necessary to provide maximum rigidity. Excellent correction can be obtained and maintained with this instrumentation (Figs. 7–90 and 7–91).

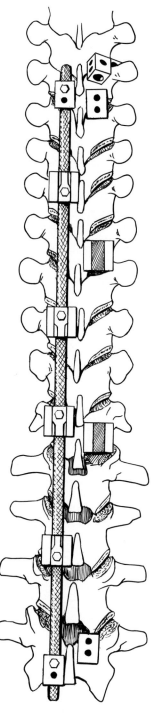

Figure 7–90

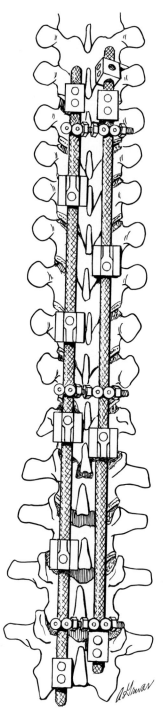

Figure 7–91

## THORACOLUMBAR CURVE

### HOOK PLACEMENT (Fig. 7–92)

The apex is typically at T12 or L1 and the thoracolumbar curve frequently has a component of rotational kyphosis. Therefore, the hook placement will address the need to gain lumbar lordosis in the lumbar vertebrae and to correct some of the apparent kyphosis that is present at the apex of the curve. A typical instrumentation for a left thoracolumbar curve will go from T9 to L3 using a claw between the transverse process and the pedicle on the upper left and a closed pedicle hook on the upper right. On the right side of the L3 vertebra a closed lumbar laminar hook is inserted in the supralaminar position and on the left, a closed lumbar laminar hook in intralaminar position. The convexity is equipped with a supralaminar hook on T12 and an infralaminar hook under L1. Those two hooks are typically open lumbar laminars. An open laminar hook also may be placed on the superior aspect of the lamina of L1 on the right to provide some additional fixation in the concavity.

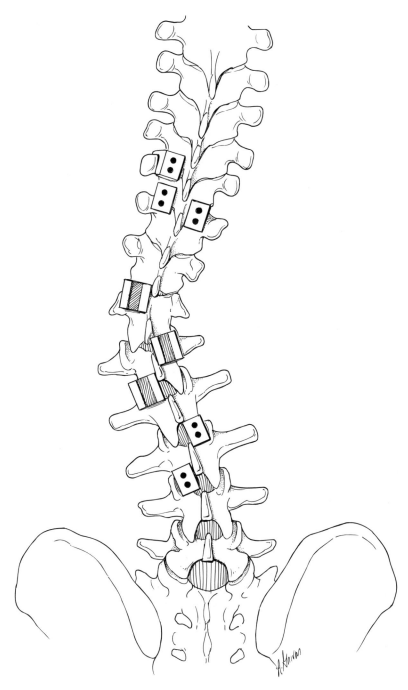

*Figure 7–92*

## ROD INSERTION

Typically the left rod (convexity) will be inserted first. It has to be contoured with some moderate kyphosis for the T9 to T12 segment and some lordosis for the T12 to L3 segment. The rod is inserted starting with the claw on T9 and then pushing the rod into the T12 hook and, if possible, into the L1 prior to inserting the lower portion of the rod into the infralaminar hook on L3 (Fig. 7–93). Some rotation may be exerted, obtaining both lordosis and derotation of the curve. The derotation maneuver may dislodge the lower hook on the infralaminar aspect of L3 as the convexity of the curve is shortened by the correction of the curve, the derotation, and the creation of lordosis. For this reason it is useful in certain cases to replace the infralaminar hook on L3 with a closed sacral screw inserted into the left pedicle of L3, which allows some derotation without the risk of dislodgement of the lower hook. After the rod has reached its derotated position, compression is applied between T12 and L3 and between T9 and L1. The right rod is then inserted between the closed pedicle hook on T9 and the closed lumbar laminar hook on L3. The open lumbar laminar hooks of L1 should be pulled up to the rod after some distraction. This allows further derotation of the thoracolumbar curve (Fig. 7–94).

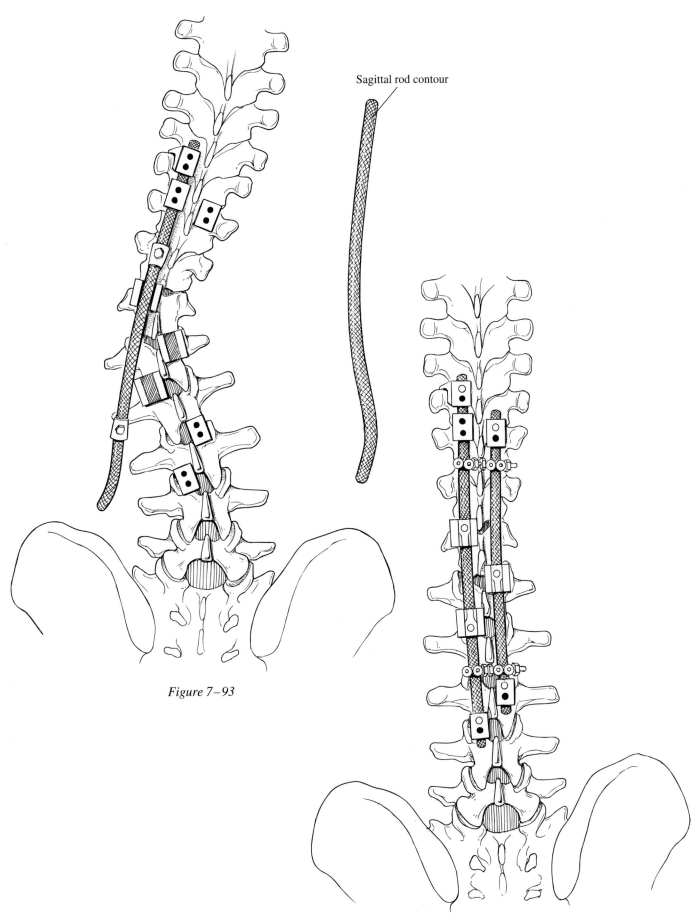

Sagittal rod contour

*Figure 7–93*

*Figure 7–94*

# LUMBAR CURVE

The typical idiopathic lumbar curve has an apex which is below the level of L1, typically L2 or L3.

### HOOK PLACEMENT (Fig. 7–95A,B)

Typically instrumentation in the upper vertebra is T11 and the lower vertebra is L4. T11 cannot receive a claw and is typically instrumented with a closed thoracic laminar hook in the supralaminar position on the left and a closed infralaminar hook on the right. L4 is instrumented with closed lumbar laminar hooks in the supralaminar position on the right and in the infralaminar position on the left. The apical vertebra L2 is instrumented with an open lumbar laminar hook in the supralaminar position, and L3 receives an open lumbar supralaminar hook on the right.

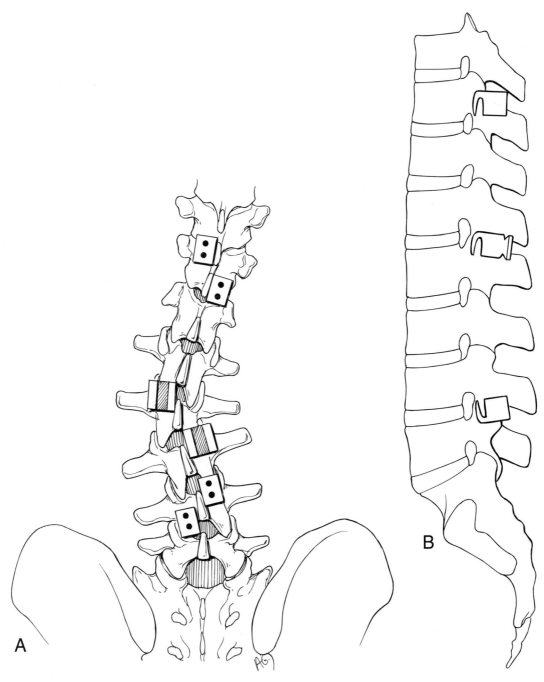

*Figure 7–95*

### ROD INSERTION

Again the contouring of the rod is carried out primarily with lordosis with a slight amount of straightening or kyphosis at the top (Fig. 7–96A,B). The derotation maneuver is carried out on the left rod, which is applied against the convexity. The rod is inserted first in the T11 hook, then pushed into the open hook at L2, and finally pulled into the L4 hook. An assistant should hold the L4 intralaminar hook with a hook holder to prevent its dislodgement. A firm pressure should be applied on the lower aspect of the lamina of L4 to prevent pullout. The rod is rotated 90 degrees, providing both lordosis and correction of the deformity (Fig. 7–97A,B). The concave rod is then applied with a minimal amount of distraction between T12 and L4 (Fig. 7–98A,B). This is carried out after full compression on the convexity to prevent loss of lumbar lordosis.

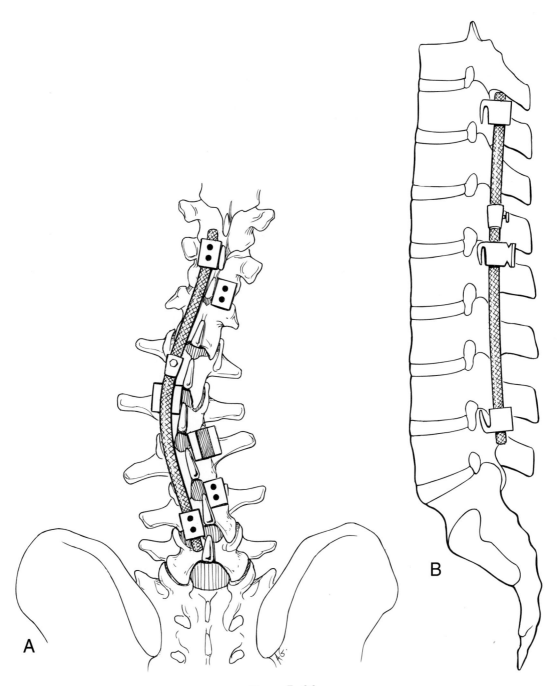

*Figure 7–96*

A

B

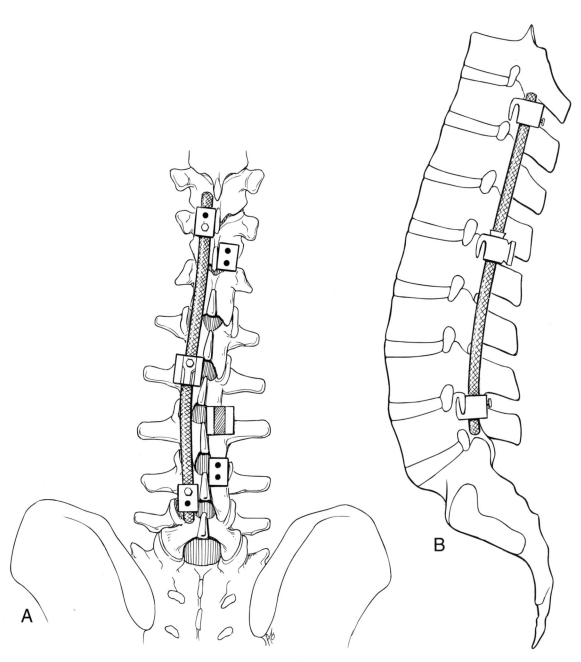

*Figure 7–97*

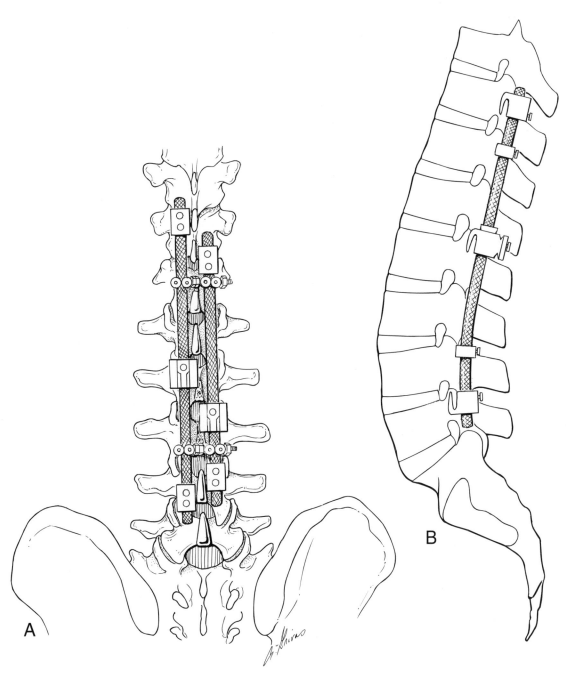

*Figure 7–98*

# FRACTURES

## Compression Fractures

The typical compression fracture without bone retropulsion (burst) in the canal and without evidence of any subluxation presents primarily a problem of kyphosis. Typically for a midthoracic compression fracture, two closed hook claws are placed above the fracture (T4 and T6) and one or two claws below the level of injury (T8 and T10) (Fig. 7–99A). On the two lower claws all hooks are open but for the lowest infralaminar hook, which is a closed hook to be inserted "onto the rod onto the lamina" in the event of the T10 lamina being too thin for proper purchase (Fig. 7–99B). The fusion should extend caudad to a solid lamina. The surgeon may be tempted to use a pedicle hook at the most distal point of purchase; this, however, would be improper as it would violate the integrity of the T10–T11 joint which was not planned to be fused (Fig. 7–100).

If significant persisting kyphosis is present, it should be included in its entirety in the area of fusion, as junctional kyphosis would be the result of short fusion.

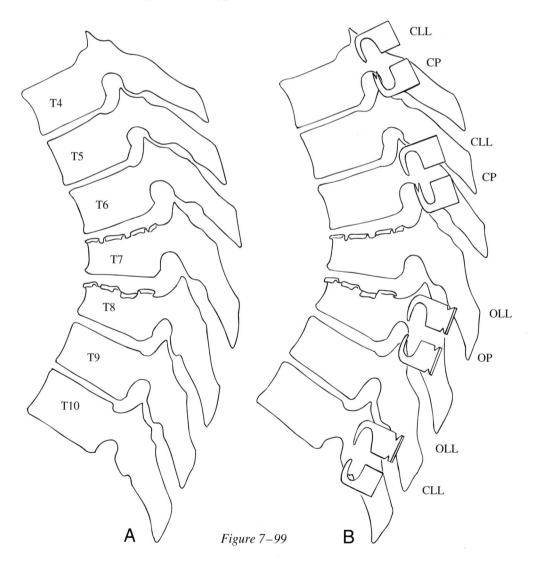

*Figure 7–99*

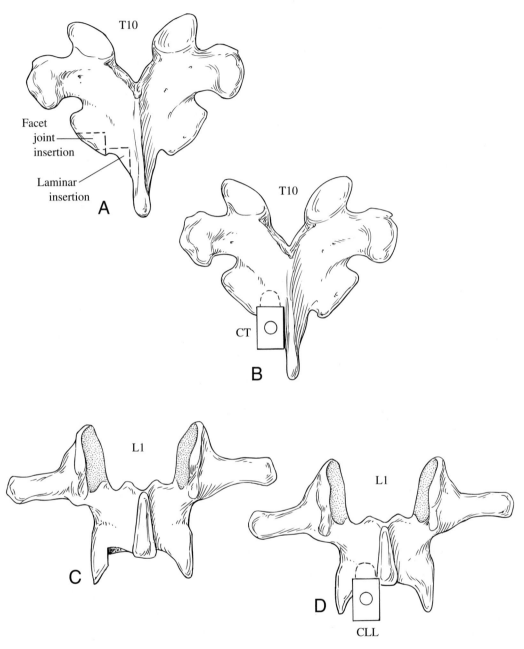

Figure 7–100

### HOOK INSERTION

Closed lumbar laminar hooks are placed on the transverse process of T4 and T6 bilaterally and closed pedicle hooks are placed under the pedicle of T4 and T6 bilaterally taking care not to notch the cortex of the pedicle because of the risk of stress riser leading ultimately to fracture of the posterior arch.

The claw on T8 is an open claw and will be utilized only when the transverse process is intact. If the transverse process is fractured, there would be a risk of penetration of the T8 pedicle hook in the spinal canal when it is used as a fulcrum in the correction process. An open lumbar laminar hook is then placed on the transverse process of T10 if it is large enough. If the T10 transverse process is small, the open thoracic laminar hook is placed in a supralaminar posterior position and the opposite hook is an infralaminar hook on T11. If the T10 transverse process is large and the lamina solid, the entire lower claw is placed on T10 by adding an infralaminar hook to the supratransverse hook. The most caudad hook is closed for a better lock against the shear forces at that level.

### ROD INSERTION

The rod insertion is somewhat similar to that for kyphosis in general (see page 322 for a more thorough discussion). Nevertheless there are some specific details that should be mentioned here.

The rod is inserted into the two cephalad claws. Contouring of the rod is checked at this point and it should be significantly less than the deformity. The rod is then backed into the two upper claws, some compression applied between T4 and T6, and then the rod is pushed down into the T8 claw (Fig. 7–101A). A rod holder is placed below the T8 pedicle hook and distraction between that hook and the rod holder provides some correction. The T8 claw should be tightened before T8 is used as a fulcrum. As the rod is pushed anteriorly it is directed into the open supratransverse hook on T10. The T10 blocker is positioned in the hook without significant force. The infralaminar T10 or T11 hook is then placed "onto the rod onto the lamina" (Fig. 7–101B). It should not be pounded into place but rather should slide into place. The problem with pounding is that the blade of the hook may catch the lamina, split it in the coronal plane, and then push the fragment anteriorly into the canal against the spinal cord, while the surgeon may have the erroneous feeling that it is now in good position.

The contralateral rod is placed in a similar fashion. An intraoperative crosstable lateral x-ray is obtained to assess the realignment and reduction of the compression fracture. Decortication is done with minimal mallet pounding. Two DTTs will be used, one at either end of the rods.

An L1 vertebra is, of course, much easier to instrument as a caudal end vertebra because of its broad lamina medial to the posterior joint.

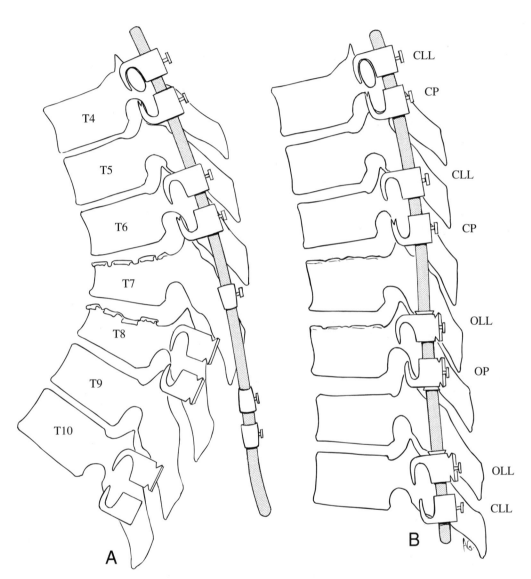

*Figure 7–101*

## Burst Fracture

In the most typical Type B burst fracture of L1, posterior instrumentation with C–D extends from T10 to L3 (Fig. 7–102A).

### HOOK POSITIONING

T10 receives a closed claw with closed lumbar laminar hook on the transverse process and closed pedicle hook under the pedicle. T11 will receive an open pedicle hook or an open thoracic laminar hook depending on the anatomic structure (Fig. 7–102B).

No hooks are placed on T12, particularly an infralaminar hook, because it would be placed right over the retropulsed bone fragment, presenting a risk of iatrogenic paraplegia. A supralaminar hook is placed on L2 when the retropulsed bone comes only from the superior end plate (Type B burst). If retropulsed bone comes from both end plates (Type A burst), the supralaminar L2 hook should be replaced by an open sacral screw (provided the pedicle is large enough). L3 receives a closed lumbar laminar hook in the infralaminar position or an offset hook if a screw has been placed in L2 (Fig. 7–102B).

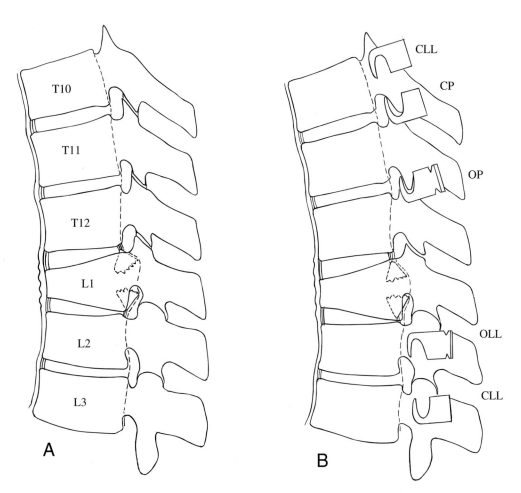

*Figure 7–102*

### ROD PLACEMENT

The cold rolled rod is used because in addition to the distraction force aimed at ligamentotaxis, a three point fixation principle is crucial to the correction. Use of the standard 7 mm C–D rod has led to unbending of the rod and "weakness of the third point" with consequent recurrence of the traumatic kyphosis. The cold rolled rod is inserted into the cephalad claw at T10 and then slipped into the T11 open hook. The blocker is inserted into the hook. Set screws are tightened on the upper claw. Some compression is applied between T10 and T11 (Fig. 7–103A). The lordotic contoured rod is then pushed into and against the open L2 hook. The blocker is pushed into the hook. Distraction is then applied between the upper claw and L2.

The lower end of the rod is still in lordosis and should be about 1.5 cm from the lamina of L3. A rod holder will be used to push the rod against the L3 lamina and the infralaminar hook will then be slipped into position (Fig. 7–103B). Some compression will be applied between L2 and L3. The same process is followed for the contralateral rod. An intraoperative cross-table lateral x-ray is obtained to assess the reduction of retropulsed fragments and the general correction of the traumatic deformity.

The T12–L1 hemilaminectomy is explored to verify and enhance the decompression as necessary. This procedure is done primarily for L1 burst fractures without neurologic deficit, but the spinal canal should still be checked as it tends to be further narrowed by the ligamentotaxis, which is often unable to provide adequate reduction.

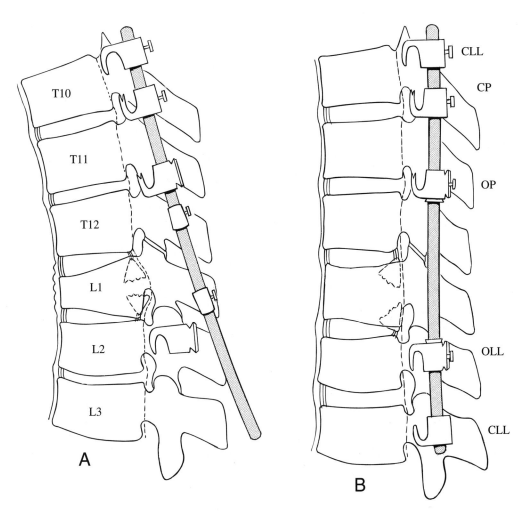

Figure 7–103

## L3 Burst Fracture

An L3 burst fracture with some neurologic deficit is a typical indication for an anterior decompression, anterior fusion at L2–L4, and a posterior stabilization with C–D instrumentation using an L2–L4 intrapedicular fixation (Fig. 7–104) or anterior fixation with a Kaneda device.

### TECHNIQUE

When there is no evidence of entrapment of the cauda equina in the vertical laminar fracture, it is appropriate to do the anterior decompression first and then proceed with the posterior stabilization (Fig. 7–104A).

If there is any significant evidence either clinically or radiologically of entrapment, the posterior approach is done first to free the cauda equina through a wide laminectomy and proceed with the anterior decompression. During the subperiosteal exposure, care must be taken not to push downward over the fragile L3 lamina, which is often fractured vertically and already may be pressing against the cauda equina.

Sacral screws are inserted into the pedicles of L2 and L4 whenever the pedicles are judged to be large enough to receive a 7 mm screw. When the pedicles are smaller, either use smaller diameter vertebral screws or hooks depending on availability. Cross-table lateral and posteroanterior x-rays are obtained for checking screw position (Fig. 7–104C).

The screws may displace an anterior strut graft; it is therefore advisable to direct the screws somewhat away from the strut. Whenever there is a doubt as to its position, the screw should be inserted only halfway, just short of the area of the strut. If the x-ray confirms good positioning of the screw it can then be advanced to its ultimate position.

### ROD INSERTION TECHNIQUE

It is not unusual for the screws to be placed in a kyphotic position (screws are convergent anteriorly). Rod insertion will decrease that kyphotic deformity and produce quite often a lordotic position (screws are convergent posteriorly). Lordosis is obtained primarily by compressing posteriorly (Fig. 7–104D). Actually it is crucial to preload the anterior strut if one desires to avoid postoperative loss of correction. Distraction would be followed almost in every case by loss of correction and delayed bone union. Two set screws should be utilized whenever possible so as to decrease the risk of loosening. A DTT or two will be placed between the rods in a slight amount of compression. Posterolateral fusion and facet fusions are done at L2–L4.

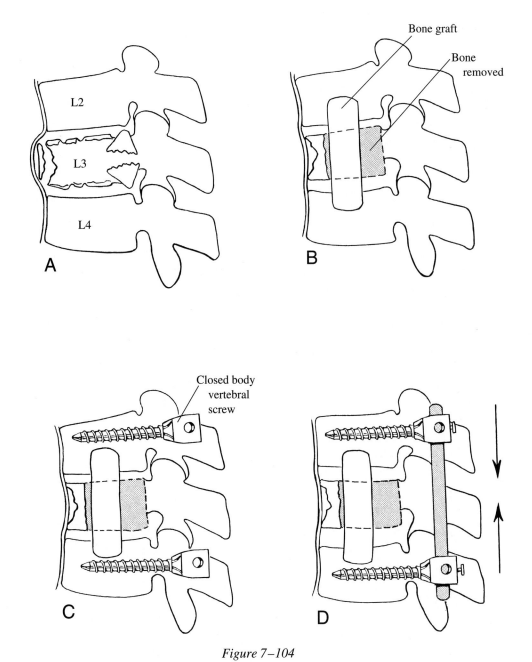

*Figure 7–104*

## Seat Belt Type Injuries (One Level)

The biomechanical principles of reduction and fixation of this injury are very simple and best summarized by the term "posterior tension band" (Fig. 7–105A). The facet joints are cleaned of their capsules and cartilage and screws are inserted in the usual fashion (Fig. 7–105B). The nerves and dural sac are exposed. The interlaminar space is grossly enlarged by the deformity. However, as reduction of the displacement takes place the interlaminar space closes. Several cases of compression of the lateral nerve root or the central dura have been reported to be due to displacement of cartilage and torn annulus fibrosis into the canal. For this specific reason a moderate laminotomy is performed to allow control of the spinal canal and adequate exploration during correction of the deformity, particularly after full reduction when the interlaminar space is closed.

### ROD INSERTION

The appropriate length rod is inserted into the upper screw and then pulled down into the lower screw (Fig. 7–105C). Some compression is applied with moderate force, the canal explored, and an intraoperative crosstable lateral x-ray is obtained to verify the quality of correction (Fig. 7–105D). A simple way of assessing correction is to check the position of opposition of the facets. The ideal position is about 2 to 5 mm beyond full opposition. Jamming the facets and posterior arches is unnecessary for correction of this injury and tends only to promote retropulsion of chondroannular fragments into the spinal canal.

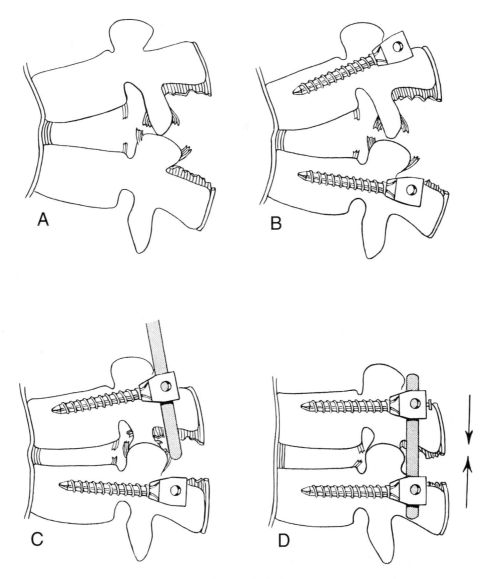

*Figure 7–105*

## Seat Belt Type Injuries (Two Levels)

In this case, screws will be inserted into the upper and lower vertebrae. The middle vertebra frequently presents a failure around the pedicle, which contraindicates screw placement at this level (Fig. 7–106A–D).

The principles of correction are similar to those described in the one level seat belt type injury.

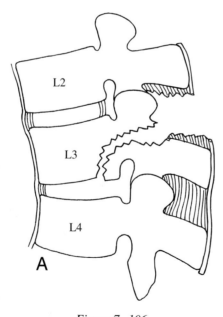

*Figure 7–106*

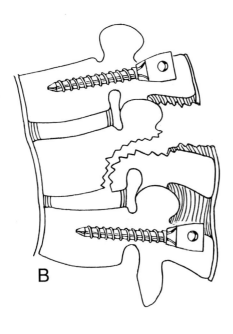

B

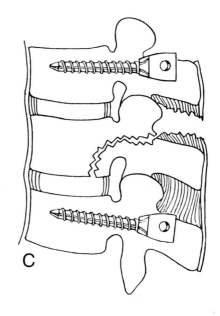

C

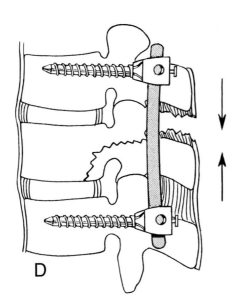

D

*Figure 7–106 Continued*

## Fracture Dislocations

C–D instrumentation in fracture dislocations of the spine provides an excellent device for the purpose of stabilization. However, at times the reduction of the fracture dislocation itself remains difficult and not without risks to the neural elements. This is not a problem for the patient with complete paraplegia where the potential recovery of neurologic function is absent, but it is for the patient with mild paraparesis where the manipulation of the spine may lead to worsening of the neurologic function.

### TECHNIQUE

It is important in fracture dislocations to provide good fixation of both the upper and lower segments of the spine around the level of instability and the use of at least two hooks for each segment is mandatory. Figure 7–107A illustrates a fracture dislocation at T10–T11. The instrumentation is placed three levels above the level of dislocation and three levels below the level of dislocation (Fig. 7–107B). The T8 vertebra will be equipped with a typical claw with a closed lumbar laminar hook installed on the super aspect of the transverse process of T8 and a closed pedicle hook opposing it on the pedicle. An additional hook is placed on the superior aspect of the transverse process of T10 to provide extra control of the superior segment as well as some potential compression at the level of disruption between the hook and the lower claw. The lower claw will consist of a superlaminar hook inserted on T12. This must be an open thoracic or lumbar laminar hook. A great amount of caution is exercised in the choice of this hook because protrusion of the blade of the hook into the spinal canal may have negative effects on the already contused spinal cord just under it. The infralaminar hook on L1 is typically a closed lumbar laminar hook.

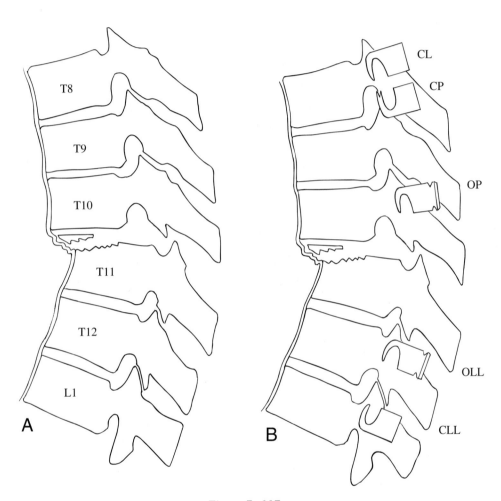

*Figure 7–107*

REDUCTION OF THE DISLOCATION

A reduction of the translational component of the injury is sometimes difficult and it would be hazardous to do it forcefully without a very careful assessment of the potential damage to neurological injuries during broad insertion as well as during the leverage of the segments that is applied by the rod. In a first round, it is important to enlarge slightly the "traumatic laminectomy" so as to free completely the dural sac, both posteriorly and laterally along the exiting nerve roots. One should be certain that there is not a fragment of bone anterior to the dural sac which might displace further as you reduce the fracture. This is particularly risky when applying compression, as that fragment of bone may be popped back into the canal by the compressive force. The reduction will therefore take place with a very meticulous sequence of events.

Some slight distraction of the level of dislocation may be obtained by using a temporary rod between the upper claw on T8 and the T12 open hook. The distraction should be minimal and aimed at unlocking facets. A large amount of distraction would produce the risk of overdistracting the spinal cord. During the distraction phase of the operation it is a good idea to have the anesthesiologist extend the patient's neck to relax the spinal cord. The reduction maneuver is carried out by levering the inferior facets of T10 onto the superior facets of T11. When the opposition of the facets of T10 on the facets of T11 is regained, a small compressive force may be applied with a short rod between T10 and T11 on one side allowing locking the reduction into its anatomic position (Fig. 7–108A). The risk of compression, however, is that it may displace a fragment of posterior wall back into the spinal canal. At maximal reduction, the spinal canal should be explored posteriorly, laterally, and anteriorly around the spinal cord to determine that there is no such fragment in the reduced position. The temporary rod is then removed and replaced with a slightly undercontoured rod, which is placed first into the upper claw at T8, then down into T10, T12, and finally slipped into the closed hook at L1 (Fig. 7–108B). The upper claw at T8 is tightened first. A slight amount of compression is then applied between the infralaminar hook on L1 directed toward the upper claw. The lower claw is tightened by placing a rod holder just above the open T12 hook and applying slight distraction between the rod holder and the T12 hook. The set screw on T12 is then tightened.

Finally, the T10 hook is pushed onto the transverse process with moderate force. The small compression system is removed from the opposite side and a second rod is inserted in a similar sequence as the first.

After completion of instrumentation, the spinal canal is again explored to ensure that there is no compression of the neural elements. The decortication is then carried out while avoiding pounding too hard on the spine, as there may be some potential risks on the spinal cord from the shock wave of the pounding. It is, therefore, preferable to use a Leksell rongeur for decortication or a burr, depending on the preference of the surgeon.

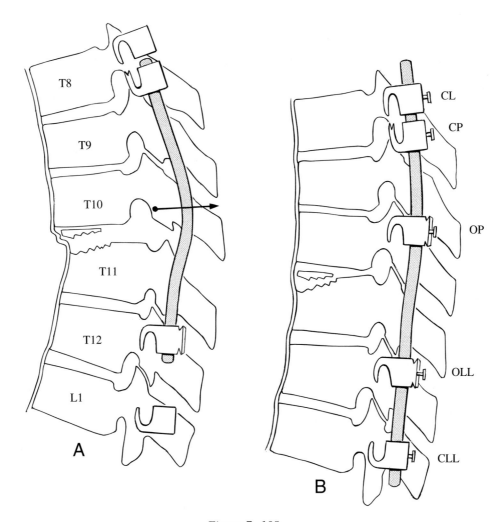

*Figure 7–108*

# Scheuermann's Kyphosis

### Fusion Levels

The basic rule is to include all levels involved in the deformity.

The problem with the basic rule is that it has been shown not to be enough following Harrington and Luque instrumentations. Kyphosis tends to recur just above and below instrumentation in the form of a junctional kyphosis. Cotrel–Dubousset instrumentation is more powerful than the two other instrumentations and tends to maximize junctional kyphoses.

In order to prevent this, the surgeon should not hesitate to extend the fusion one to two levels above and below the upper- and lower-end vertebrae of the deformity. This means including at least the neutral disk on standing lateral and sometimes the first lordotic disk. It is particularly important to do so in the more supple curves where a great amount of correction is expected. Flexion and hyperextension x-rays along with the standing lateral x-ray assist in determining the neutral disk.

Another important point in the prevention of junctional kyphosis is not to damage the motion segments immediately above or below the fusion area. Therefore, the upper and lower spinous process of the fusion area, the supraspinous and interspinous ligaments, the ligamentum flavum, and the capsule will be preserved.

### Hook Insertion

The typical instrumentation for kyphosis will be symmetrical. Its primary biomechanical principle is that of a tension band. The bending strength of the rod is, therefore, not an issue, that is, the use of the cold rolled rod over the regular rod presents a strong disadvantage, because there is a significant increase in difficulty of insertion and rate of postoperative failure of fixation.

The upper-end vertebra is equipped with a closed lumbar laminar hook over the superior aspect of the transverse process and a closed pedicle hook under the pedicle bilaterally. Two additional claws will be placed two and four vertebrae below the upper end vertebra, respectively. These usually consist of closed hooks. The bilateral three-claw configuration gets an excellent hold on the upper segment of the kyphus during intraoperative correction (Fig. 7–109).

The apex of the kyphus should not be instrumented because any hooks at this level will be very likely to slip into the spinal canal compressing the spinal cord as the rod is levered against the spine during correction. Also, they do not provide any useful corrective force or any fixation point of value.

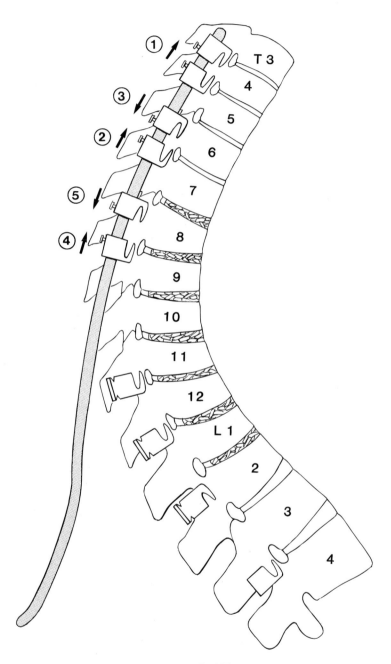

*Figure 7–109*

The lower segment of the kyphus is instrumented with three or four open hooks and a closed hook. The closed hook is an infralaminar hook at the lower end of the fusion. Among the three or four open hooks, two or three will be pedicle hooks and the lower open hook will be a laminar hook placed in a supralaminar position on the vertebra just above the lower vertebra of the fusion (Fig. 7–110). The lower end vertebra receives a closed laminar hook in the infralaminar position.

## TECHNIQUE

Three closed claws are inserted in the standard manner on T4, T6, and T8. There may be an advantage to use a lower profile pedicle hook at each level because it will increase the coaxial fit of the six hooks. Two open pedicle hooks are inserted on T11 and T12. An open lumbar laminar hook is inserted on L2 in the supralaminar position. The lower closed hook on L3 is placed with minimal damage to the ligamentum flavum (without a laminectomy) and with absolute preservation of the supraspinous and interspinous ligaments and the capsule of the posterior joints.

## FACET FUSIONS

The facets are decorticated and plugged with cancellous bone at all levels possible.

## ROD CONTOURING

The rod is contoured into what is felt to be the postcorrection contour of the spine with minimal to moderate kyphosis and lumbar lordosis.

In addition, "rod top kyphus" and "rod bottom lordosis" are added to the primary contouring to facilitate insertion of the rod into the upper claws at the top and the insertion of the closed hook and lower lamina hook onto the rod at the bottom.

## ROD INSERTION

The rod is inserted into the six closed hooks without major difficulty as long as the upper tip is bent into some kyphosis allowing easier passage from one hook to the next (Fig. 7–109). After insertion, a Cobb elevator is placed above the tip to hold the rod at about 5 mm beyond the upper hook.

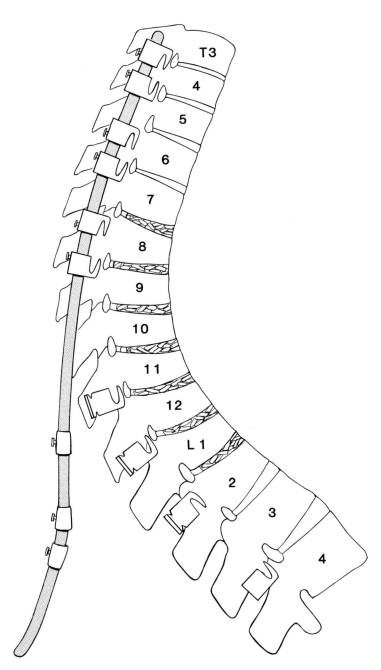

*Figure 7–110*

The sequence of tightening illustrated in Figure 7–109 is typical of that used in a healthy young adult with good bone stock.

1. The upper claw is tightened with moderate force.
2. A rod holder is placed just below the second pedicle hook. Distraction between the rod holder and the T6 pedicle hook provides some compression on the T4–T6 segment.
3. The T6 claw is tightened.
4. A similar compression is applied between T8 and T4.
5. The T8 claw is tightened.

The tightening sequence should be changed if the bone stock is weaker. In the presence of osteoporosis, the T4 transverse process would be likely to break owing to the load concentration. Therefore, the tightening sequence will be aimed at distributing the tension-band load over the T4, T6, and T8 transverse processes but also at minimizing the tightening of the claws. The pedicle hook that is powerfully pounded against or simply compressed too energetically against the pedicle does break its cortex, thereby creating a stress riser likely to facilitate fracture of the posterior arch during correction (Fig. 7–110).

CORRECTION PHASE

The rod is grasped with a rod holder in its lower segment. It is then pushed against the apex, providing a strong lever arm that corrects the deformity. At this point, the surgeon should be keenly observant of:

1. The T4, T6 transverse process integrity.
2. What is the rod doing at the apex (risk of fracture of posterior arches if the force is too concentrated).
3. Appropriateness of contouring and possible need to increase the kyphosis or the lordosis with the in situ benders.
4. The rod has to be directed toward the opening of the T11 pedicle hook.
5. The rod should not be pushing the T12 and L2 hooks into the spinal canal.

The next move consists of pushing the upper blocker into T11 and then placing a rod holder just below it. Distraction between T11 and the rod holder seats the T11 hook better and also participates in the correction by tensioning of the tension band. Similar process is applied to T12 (Fig. 7–111).

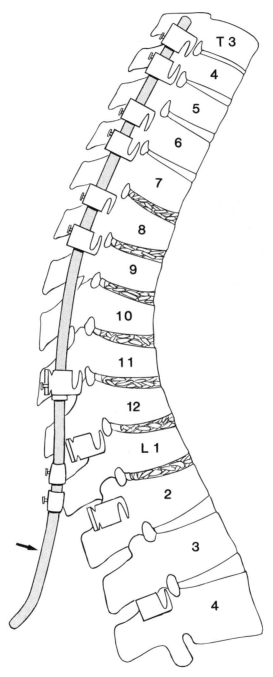

*Figure 7–111*

The rod is then placed on L2, the blocker pushed into the hook but not loaded (Fig. 7–112). The rod length, at this point, should be about 1 cm below the lower edge of the L3 lamina. The in situ bender will optimize the "rod bottom lordosis" allowing relatively easy passage of the closed lumbar laminar hook onto the rod and onto the lamina (Fig. 7–113).

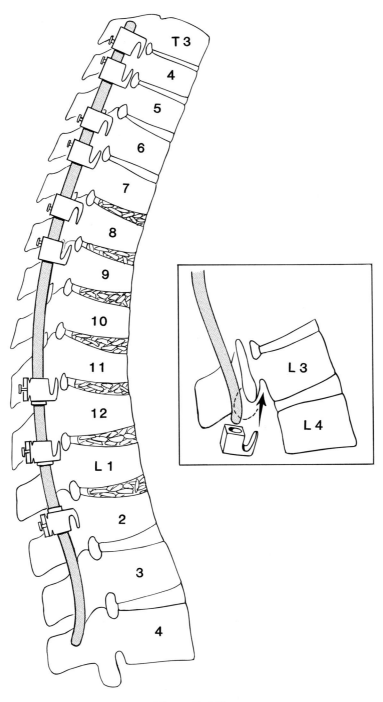

*Figure 7–112*

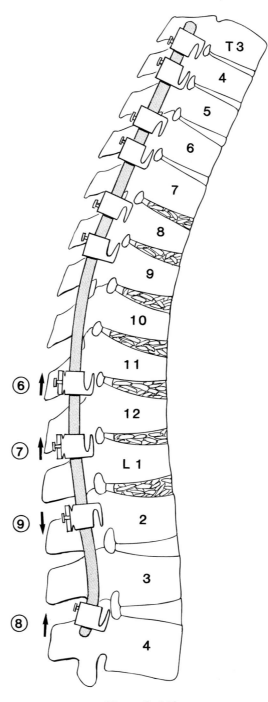

*Figure 7–113*

The rod holder is then placed cephalad to the L3 hook and compression between both will obtain good seating of that crucial hook and further correction. The L2 hook then may be gently compressed toward the L3 hook in order to obtain the lower claw effect. (Fig. 7–114).

A similar procedure is performed on the opposite side. Final tuning of the different hook sites and balancing of the rods is performed. Whenever there is some scoliosis in addition to the kyphus, the convexity of the scoliosis should be instrumented first.

Wake-up test is performed while a gentle decortication is done.

Two DTTs are placed close to the top and bottom of the rods. Bone grafts are added prior to shearing off the set screws.

An alternative to the hook claws at the lower end of the instrumentation has been the use of open sacral screws, which facilitate pushing the rod into the lower instrumentation and prevents overextension of the last segment (Fig. 7–115).

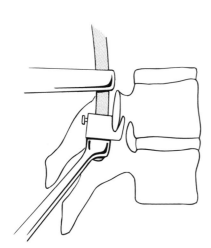
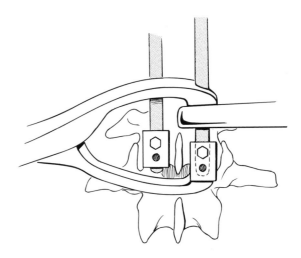

*Figure 7–114*

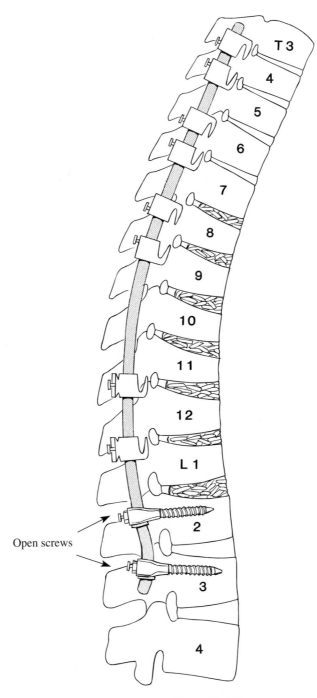

Open screws

*Figure 7–115*

# Pseudarthrosis Repair

## HARRINGTON COMPRESSION INSTRUMENTATION

The Harrington compression system is useful in fixation of pseudarthrosis repairs. The principle is to obtain compression at the level of the pseudarthrosis to enhance the chances of obtaining fusion. Hooks are placed in the fusion mass through holes that are drilled with a burr or made with a small osteotome. The small Harrington compression system utilizes the #1259 hook; the heavy compression system will be carried out with #1256 hooks. Ideally, three hooks are placed on either side of the pseudarthrosis to obtain a significant amount of compression and to maintain axial alignment of the pseudarthrosis. After inserting the rod into the six hooks, the nuts are tightened with an open wrench balancing the amount of force between all the hooks (Fig. 7–116). After compression has been completed, the rod is gently crimped behind the nut to prevent its loosening.

## C–D RODS

The old Harrington concept of applying purely compression on either side of the osteotomy or the pseudarthrosis does not apply. There is an effort to gain mechanical control of the two segments on either side of the defect as securely as possible. The use of claws on longer segments, sometimes both in distraction and compression, may allow excellent control of those long levers of the previous fusion.

### HOOK PLACEMENT

Hooks are placed directly into the fusion mass. Whenever the fusion is too thin, the hook is placed into the spinal canal with particular care not to damage the underlying neural elements. A typical montage would consist of placing three hooks on either side of the defect (pseudarthrosis) (Fig. 7–117). The two extreme hooks are closed lumbar laminar hooks facing toward the defect. The two intermediate hooks will be facing the previous hook and could be an open lumbar laminar hook. The two hooks closest to the defect will be placed in compression to increase resistance of the instrumentation against the tension forces. Rod insertion is performed with moderate bending of the rod.

In cases of multiple pseudarthroses, the principles remain. An attempt is made to place multiple claws on either side of the pseudarthroses. The instrumentation covers the entire length of the previous fusion. This provides better fixation of the pseudarthrosis.

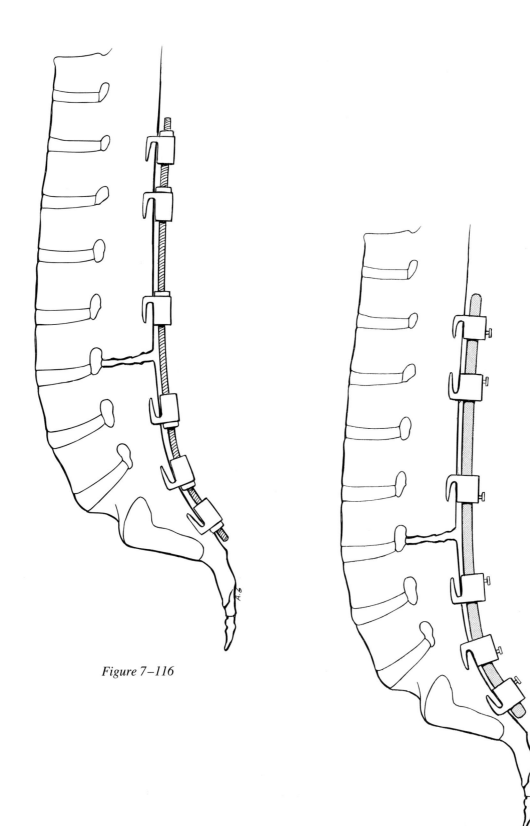

*Figure 7–116*

*Figure 7–117*

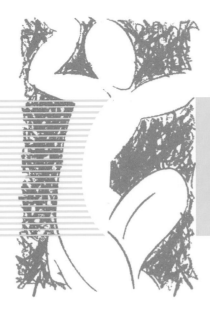

# 8

# POSTEROLATERAL THORACIC AND THORACOLUMBAR PROCEDURES

# Costotransversectomy

Costotransversectomy was developed primarily for drainage of tuberculous abscesses prior to the development of the direct transthoracic procedures in the 1950s. Quite often there was a gibbous deformity resulting from the destruction of the vertebral bodies due to the tuberculous infection and then either bony fragments or more likely abscess contents would press on the spinal cord causing a paraparesis. Surgeons learned to drain these abscesses via Capener's costotransversectomy approach, thus alleviating the paralysis in many cases. This procedure was a very significant advance in spinal surgery although currently seldom used. Nevertheless, it still has application for unique circumstances.

Costotransversectomy involves resection of ribs and transverse processes from a posterolateral approach, allowing access to the vertebral body area in the front of the spinal canal without entering the thorax and without doing a laminectomy.

## Exposure

Most patients requiring this procedure have some element of gibbus deformity (sharp, angular kyphosis). A straight incision is made parallel to the midline but just lateral to the main muscle mass of the long paraspinal muscles, that is, at about the tip of the transverse process area in the thoracic spine (Fig. 8–1A). Depending on the length of spine to be exposed, 3 to 5 ribs and transverse processes are exposed (Fig. 8–1B). Dissection is carried along the dorsal surface of the transverse processes exposing them to their bases and laterally on the ribs approximately 2 to 3 cm beyond the tip of the transverse process (Fig. 8–1C). The transverse process is resected using a bone rongeur. With careful subperiosteal dissection, the ribs are exposed and cut distally. Closer to the spine, the ribs curve anteriorly where they join the vertebral body; the soft tis-

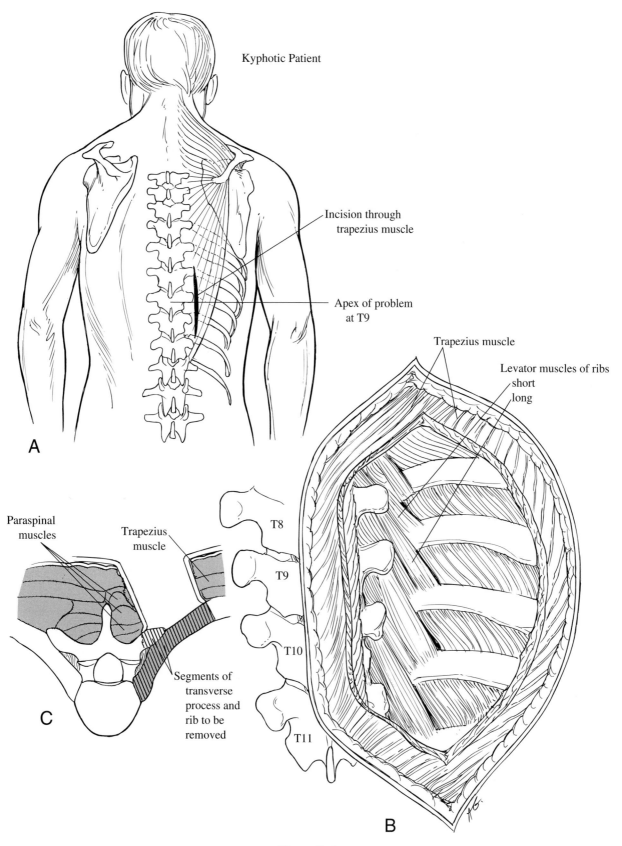

Kyphotic Patient

Incision through
trapezius muscle

Apex of problem
at T9

A

Trapezius muscle

Levator muscles of ribs
short
long

Paraspinal
muscles

Trapezius
muscle

T8

T9

Segments of
transverse
process and
rib to be
removed

T10

C

T11

B

*Figure 8–1*

337

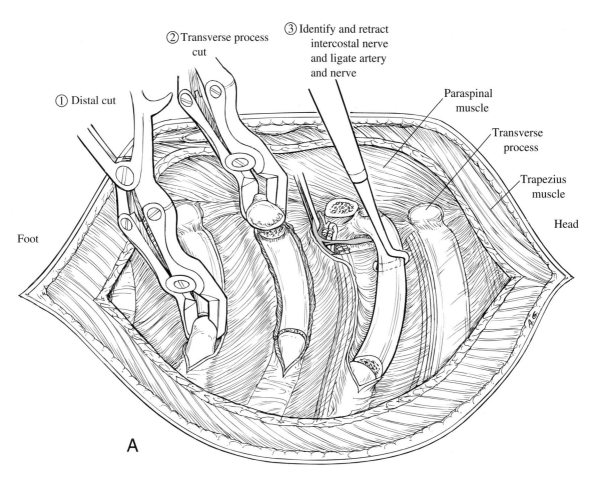

① Distal cut

② Transverse process cut

③ Identify and retract intercostal nerve and ligate artery and nerve

Paraspinal muscle

Transverse process

Trapezius muscle

Head

Foot

A

*Figure 8–2*

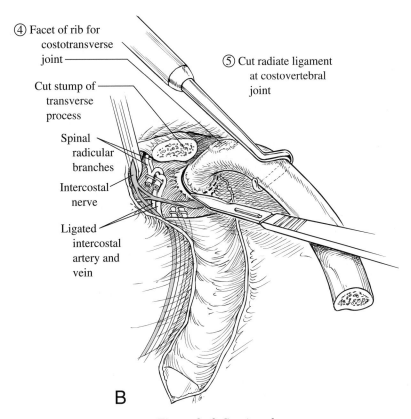

④ Facet of rib for costotransverse joint

⑤ Cut radiate ligament at costovertebral joint

Cut stump of transverse process

Spinal radicular branches

Intercostal nerve

Ligated intercostal artery and vein

B

*Figure 8–2 Continued*

## Drainage of Abscess

The ribs are gradually nibbled away and usually can be disarticulated from the vertebral body to drain an abscess in the region of the vertebral body. This exposure allows adequate visualization for the drainage of abscesses and for biopsy of tissue in the vertebral body area, but it does not provide adequate exposure for good bone grafting. Drainage is instituted; curettage of the vertebral bone is carried out; and any sequestered material is removed. Cancellous bone can be inserted in this area, but the formal type of strut grafting that is possible through the transthoracic approach is not usually feasible (Fig. 8–3).

## Cord Decompression

The more gibbus deformity there is the easier the spinal cord decompression can become. Similar to the transthoracic approach for cord decompression, a bone cavity must be created anterior to the posterior cortex of the vertebral bodies at the apical vertebra and at least one vertebra above and below the apical vertebra. The vertebral body excision is carried across to the deep side cortex, taking care to leave the posterior cortex of the vertebral body intact. After this cavity has been created in the vertebral bodies, the cortex is removed distally or proximally or both to the apex and then gradually into the apical area. Since the intercostal nerves have been identified in the rib resection, follow these nerves inward toward the dural sac and gradually identify the cord in that area. As in the transthoracic approach, dissect and remove bone on the deep side first working toward yourself rather than working away, which allows the cord to rotate the empty cavity and leave a ledge of bone behind it, which is very difficult to remove.

## Arthrodesis

Arthrodesis in a sense can be obtained by the insertion of cancellous bone into the cavity after the removal of the vertebral bodies. However, it should be understood that these bone grafts are not anterior enough to deal with an angular kyphosis and may have to be augmented later using a transthoracic approach. When there is no significant kyphotic deformity, then the grafting may be adequate, but the circumstances for this are relatively rare.

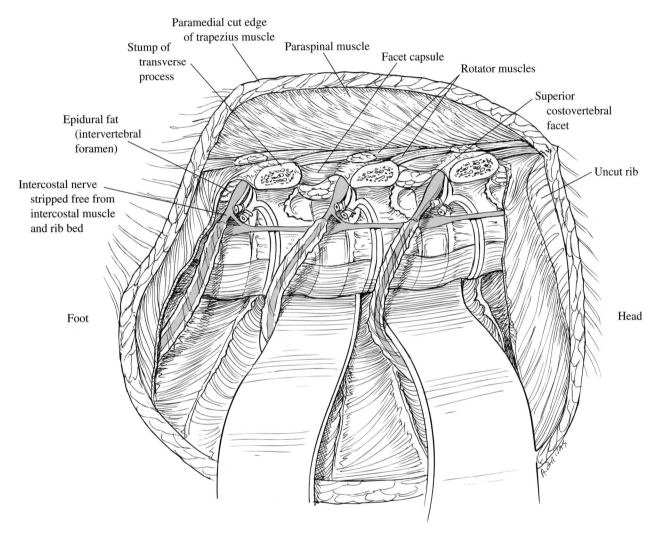

Paramedial cut edge
of trapezius muscle

Paraspinal muscle

Facet capsule

Rotator muscles

Stump of
transverse
process

Superior
costovertebral
facet

Epidural fat
(intervertebral
foramen)

Uncut rib

Intercostal nerve
stripped free from
intercostal muscle
and rib bed

Foot

Head

*Figure 8–3*

# Intrathoracic Extrapleural Approach to the Thoracolumbar Spine

This approach is not new and has been used extensively; for example, by Kaneda for the insertion of his instrumentation, by Bohlman for decompression of late burst fractures in the thoracolumbar junction region, and in general surgery for the removal of renal tumors and other surgical problems.

The skin incision is along the 11th rib beginning at the lateral margin of the sacrospinalis muscle and continuing to the tip of the rib or to the abdominal wall if necessary (Fig. 8–4). The rib is carefully stripped so that the pleura is not penetrated. With blunt instruments, the surgeon dissects the parietal pleura off the inside of the chest wall moving upward to the point of exposure of the 10th rib and intercostal muscle between the 9th and 10th ribs and downward until the diaphragm is reached (Fig. 8–5). This extrapleural dissection is carried out to the diaphragm for a space of about 3 cm and to the lateral border of the vertebral bodies (Fig. 8–6). Once this space is developed, the diaphragm can be divided beginning at its vertebral body attachment and moving laterally along the chest wall (much in the same manner as done for the transthoracic approach). Posteriorly, as the diaphragm is detached, the retroperitoneal space is entered, which then can be developed with gauze sponges on the surgeon's fingertip milking the undersurface of the diaphragm (Fig. 8–7). The upper lumbar vertebrae are approached by division of the three layers of the abdominal muscles just beyond the tip of the rib, taking care not to penetrate the peritoneum, and then dissecting the peritoneum off the inner surface of the abdominal muscles until the retroperitoneal space is developed. All of the retroperitoneal structures are swept medially in order to continue dissecting the diaphragm off the chest wall. At this point the lateral border of the vertebral bodies can be identified, the psoas muscle lying over the lateral portion (Fig. 8–8). Any segmental vessels that need to be divided are ligated at the midvertebral body. From this point on the exposure for the procedure is identical to that in the transthoracic retroperitoneal approach described in Chapter 6.

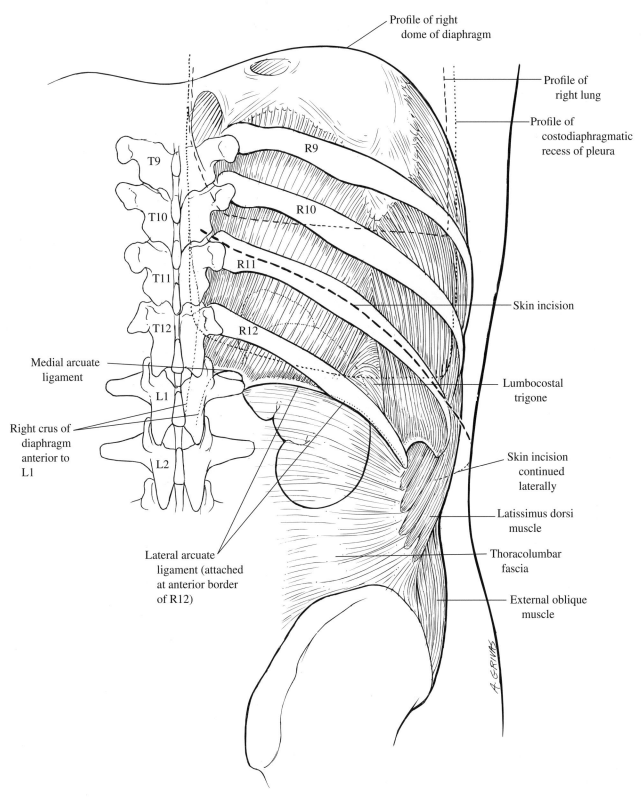

Profile of right
dome of diaphragm

Profile of
right lung

Profile of
costodiaphragmatic
recess of pleura

R9

R10

T9

T10

T11

R11

T12

R12

Skin incision

Medial arcuate
ligament

Lumbocostal
trigone

L1

Right crus of
diaphragm
anterior to
L1

L2

Skin incision
continued
laterally

Latissimus dorsi
muscle

Thoracolumbar
fascia

External oblique
muscle

Lateral arcuate
ligament (attached
at anterior border
of R12)

A. GRIVAS

*Figure 8–4*

343

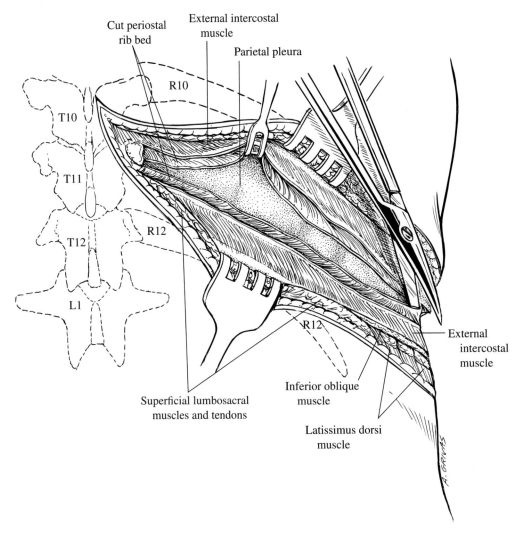

Cut periostal rib bed

External intercostal muscle

Parietal pleura

R10

T10

T11

T12

R12

L1

R12

External intercostal muscle

Superficial lumbosacral muscles and tendons

Inferior oblique muscle

Latissimus dorsi muscle

*Figure 8–5*

344

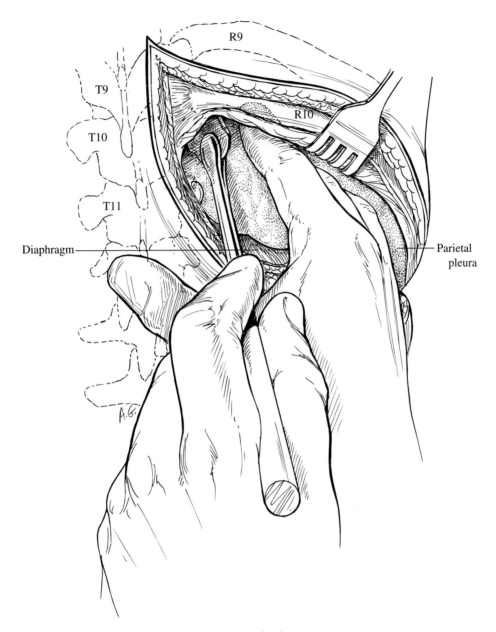

R9

T9

T10

R10

T11

Diaphragm

Parietal
pleura

*Figure 8–6*

345

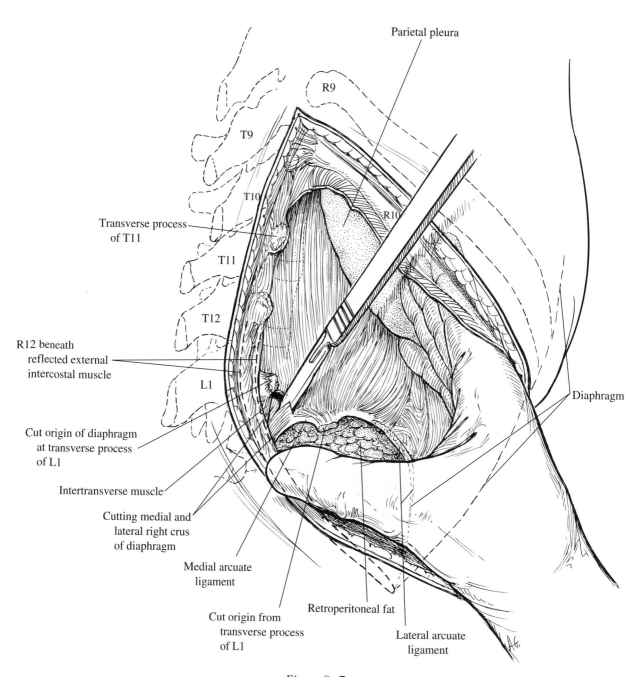

Parietal pleura

R9

T9

T10

R10

Transverse process
of T11

T11

T12

R12 beneath
reflected external
intercostal muscle

L1

Diaphragm

Cut origin of diaphragm
at transverse process
of L1

Intertransverse muscle

Cutting medial and
lateral right crus
of diaphragm

Medial arcuate
ligament

Cut origin from
transverse process
of L1

Retroperitoneal fat

Lateral arcuate
ligament

*Figure 8–7*

346

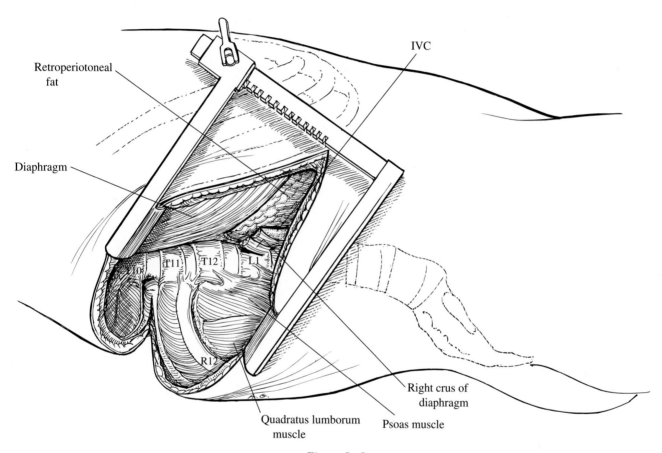

Retroperiotoneal
fat

IVC

Diaphragm

T11 T12 L1

R12

Quadratus lumborum
muscle

Right crus of
diaphragm

Psoas muscle

*Figure 8–8*

347

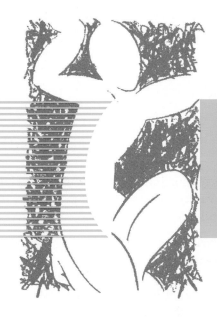

# 9

# COMBINATION ANTERIOR AND POSTERIOR THORACIC AND THORACOLUMBAR PROCEDURES

# Anterior Diskectomy
# and Hemivertebra Excision

The hemivertebra is first identified either by direct visualization, which usually can be done by subperiosteal exposure of the curvature and hemivertebra area, or by an x-ray, which can be obtained in the operating room.

If the hemivertebra is being excised in the thoracic spine, the rib leading directly to the hemivertebra is usually removed. The rib head at the level of the hemivertebra must be removed (Fig. 9–1). The periosteum is dissected subperiosteally exposing the white disks. The disks are excised back to the posterior annulus. It is important to carry the dissection across the spine to the opposite side leaving only the most lateral annulus as a stabilizing structure. Hemivertebrae often stop in the midline and ineffective closure will occur if the wedge is not carried to the opposite side (Fig. 9–2). Once the disk above and below the hemivertebra have been removed back to the posterior annulus, the exposed hemivertebral body is quickly removed back to the posterior cortex using rongeurs followed by curettes in a transverse, rotating motion so the hard, white bone of the posterior cortex is exposed but not penetrated (Fig. 9–3).

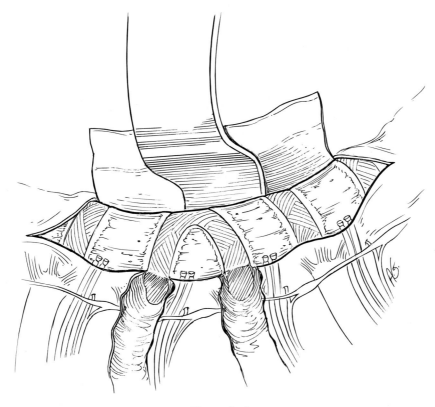

*Figure 9–1*

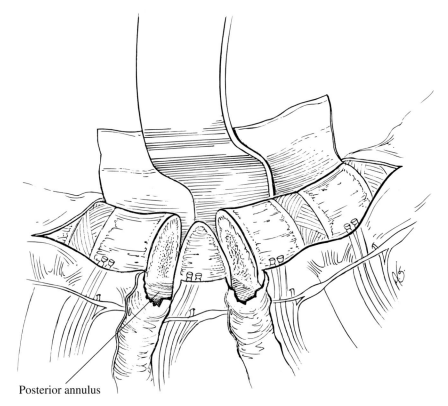

Posterior annulus

*Figure 9–2*

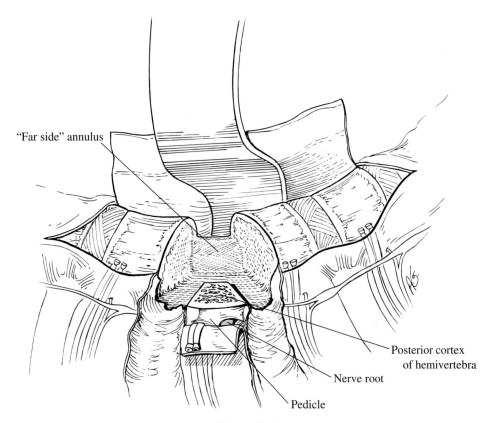

"Far side" annulus

Posterior cortex
of hemivertebra

Nerve root

Pedicle

*Figure 9–3*

351

At this point, the two posterior annuli and the firm, white bone of the posterior cortex are exposed, and the spinal canal must be entered. The authors have found that it is easier to enter the canal through the posterior cortex of the bone than through the soft annular tissue. Some surgeons prefer to use a diamond-tipped burr to enter the canal (Fig. 9–4), while others use very fine gouges or curettes. Once an opening is made, it is gradually enlarged with curettes and/or rongeurs (Fig. 9–5). The problem usually is not the removal of the bone, but bleeding from the epidural veins lying just beneath the cortical bone. Thrombin-soaked Gelfoam pledgets usually control this problem, but occasionally bipolar cautery may be necessary.

Once this initial window has been made, the dissection is carried upward and downward until the annular tissue is noted and removed. This is done in the midline and carried across to the far side leaving the near side bone to be removed last. The dissection is directed to the posterior bony cortex toward the foramen lying in the lower half of the hemivertebra. The bone is nibbled away until the foramen has been fully opened and the exiting nerve root can be seen.

The final remaining structure is the pedicle, located in the superior half of the hemivertebra. The posterior cortical bone is gradually nibbled upward from the foramen and laterally from the midline until just the pedicle remains (Fig. 9–6A). Dissection must include the annulus above the pedicle, leaving the pedicle as an isolated structure. The base of the pedicle should be nibbled off anteriorly until the waist of the pedicle is reached (Fig. 9–6B). The remainder of the pedicle is removed from the posterior approach. Bone chips are placed in the bone space along with pledgets of thrombin-soaked Gelfoam or a fat graft against the dura.

If the procedure is being done in the lumbar spine or lumbosacral area, the exposure is easier, since there is no rib head to be removed and the disk spaces are usually wider. At the lumbosacral area the greatest problem is the large arteries and veins, which must be carefully exposed and retracted to adequately remove a hemivertebra.

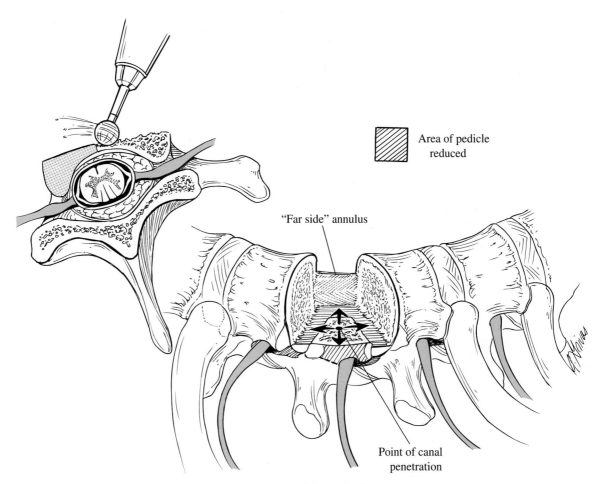

Area of pedicle reduced

"Far side" annulus

Point of canal penetration

*Figure 9–4*

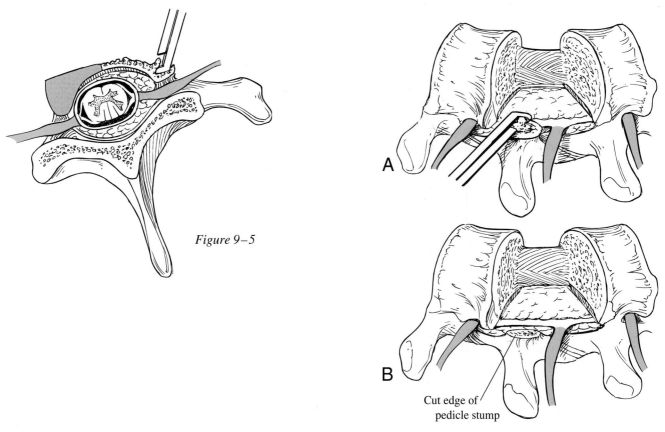

*Figure 9–5*

A

B

Cut edge of pedicle stump

*Figure 9–6*

# Posterior Hemivertebra Excision

For removal of the posterior portion of the hemivertebra, the patient is placed in a direct prone position. The spine is exposed in the area to be fused and the proper level identified, preferably by x-ray in the operating room. Once the proper level is identified, the ligamentum flavum above and below the hemivertebra is removed, much the same as for a Luque procedure (Fig. 9–7A). The hemilamina is removed using a standard laminectomy-type approach from midline to lateral aspect (Fig. 9–7B). As the intervertebral foramen is approached, the inferior and superior facets are removed and the nerve root can be seen to exit at the foraminal level. The ligamentous material is excised superiorly to the pedicle, leaving the transverse process and the pedicle as the only remaining structures (Fig. 9–7C). In the lumbar spine the transverse process can be transected at its base with a neurorongeur or Kerrison rongeur and the lateral parts left in place. In the thoracic spine it is easier to excise the whole transverse process posteriorly. With a Kerrison rongeur, the laminar bone is nibbled away medially, inferiorly, superiorly, and then laterally so only the pedicle itself remains (Fig. 9–8A). If the pedicle has been properly prepared anteriorly by adequate bone removal, it can be grasped with a fine-tipped rongeur with one jaw inside the pedicle and the other jaw laterally outside the pedicle (Fig. 9–8B). The pedicle is then gently twisted and rotated and will come out as a single piece (Fig. 9–8C). If this does not occur, it can be removed by progressive bites with a fine-tipped rongeur or with a curette. At the conclusion of the hemivertebra resection, the nerve roots that exit above and below the pedicle can be seen. Depending on the individual case, it may be necessary to do additional fusion surgery above and below this area.

The method for closure of the wedge depends on the individual situation. In very young children, for instance under age 2, the bone stock is usually inadequate for any type of internal fixation and casting is the desired method of correction of the deformity. In children a little older where there is an adequate bone stock, the wedge can be carefully compressed into a partially closed alignment by using a rod with two small hooks. Another alternative, if the pedicles are large enough, is to insert two pedicle screws above and below the pedicle and a small rod is placed between the two screw heads. In the pediatric CD system, a screw can be used at one site and a hook in the other.

The most likely cause of trouble with hemivertebra excision is the downcoming pedicle. It may impinge on the exiting nerve root since there are two nerve roots exiting a common foramen. The downcoming pedicle must be carefully watched during the procedure; and if there is too much pressure on the nerve root, the correction must be stopped or the pedicle partially or completely removed. This may hamper the internal fixation capabilities, but protection of this nerve root is of extreme importance. Finally, adequate bone chips are applied to the area to give a good fusion. All too often, the surgeon becomes entranced with the hemivertebra excision and forgets that the purpose of the operation is to do a spine fusion and the hemivertebra removal is merely an apical wedge osteotomy for such a fusion operation.

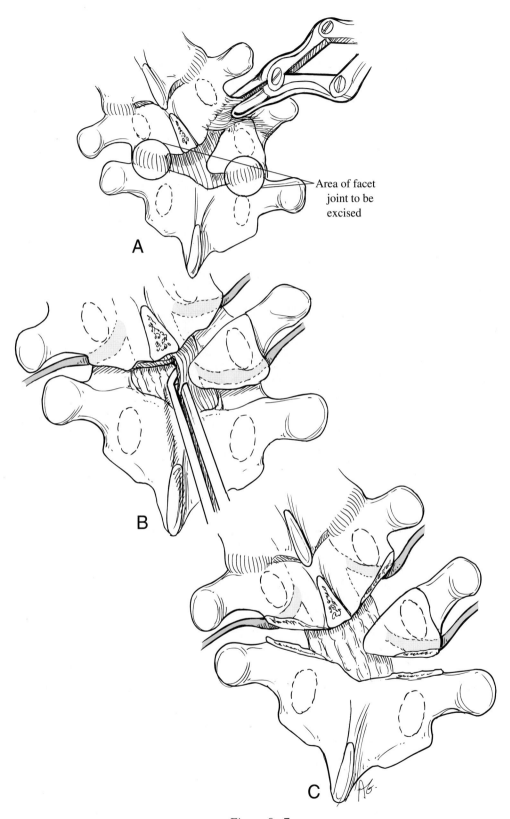

Area of facet
joint to be
excised

A

B

C

*Figure 9–7*

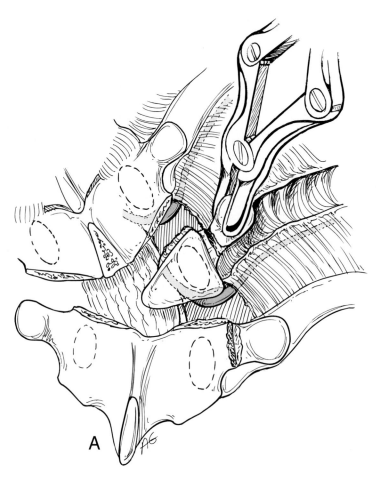

Figure 9–8

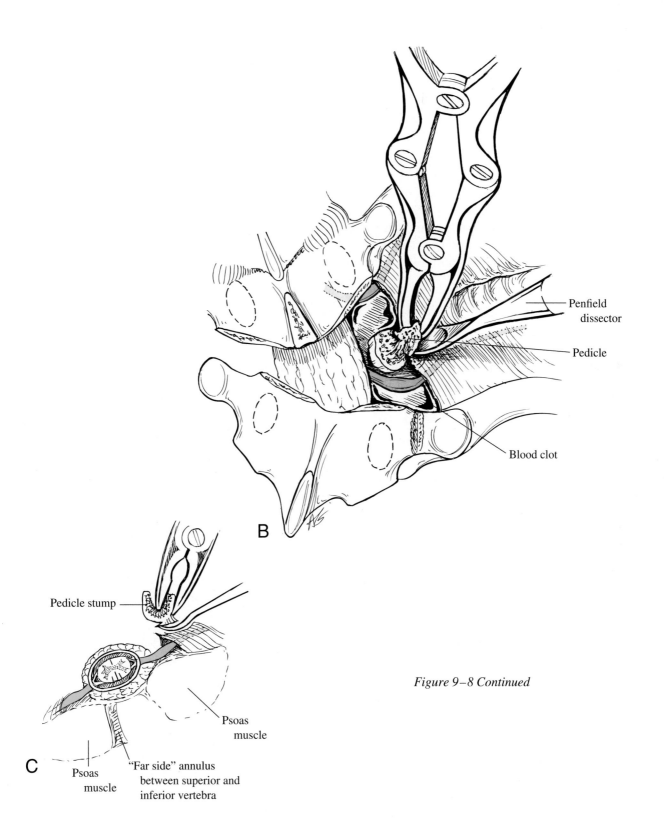

Penfield
dissector

Pedicle

Blood clot

B

Pedicle stump

Psoas
muscle

C

Psoas
muscle

"Far side" annulus
between superior and
inferior vertebra

*Figure 9–8 Continued*

# Convex Epiphysiodesis of the Spine

The purpose of the operation is to completely arrest growth on the convex side of a scoliosis. This is usually a congenital problem but might be a difficult infantile idiopathic or juvenile curvature. It is useless if there is no growth capability in the concavity of the scoliosis, for example, a unilateral unsegmented bar.

TECHNIQUE

The patient is placed on the operating table in the direct lateral position. Both the anterior and posterior areas are appropriately prepped and draped. Two incisions are made: anterior and posterior exposures. The anterior exposure can be transthoracic, transthoracic-retroperitoneal, or retroperitoneal, depending on the surgical area. The posterior exposure is *only* of the convexity of the curve.

Markers are inserted in the front and back and the upper and lower ends of the surgical area. Proper area identification of front and back is critical.

Once the correct levels have been identified, the anterior area is subperiosteally exposed from just anterior to the foramen to the lateral margin of the anterior longitudinal ligament (Fig. 9–9). The lateral one-half of the disk is removed, along with the lateral one-half of the adjacent growth plates (Fig. 9–10).

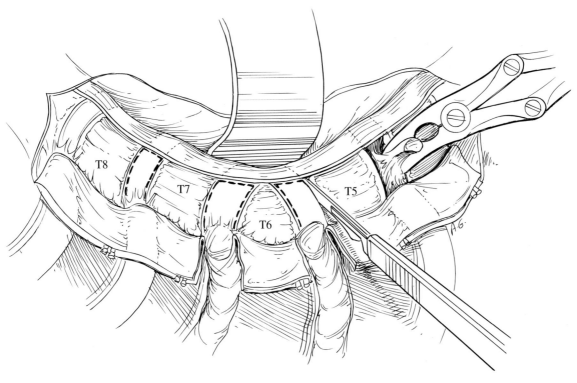

*Figure 9–9*

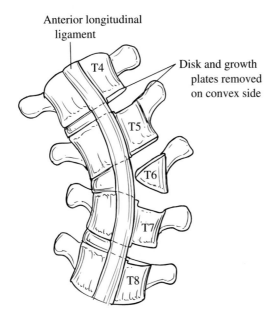

Anterior longitudinal
ligament

Disk and growth
plates removed
on convex side

T4

T5

T6

T7

T8

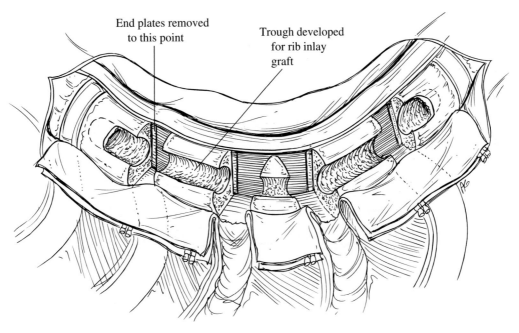

End plates removed
to this point

Trough developed
for rib inlay
graft

*Figure 9–10*

# COMBINATION THORACIC AND THORACOLUMBAR PROCEDURES

A trough is created in the vertebral bodies and bone graft is inserted in the lateral half of the disk space (Fig. 9–11A). Additional bone chips are added (Fig. 9–11B). The periosteum is reapproximated and the anterior incision closed.

Posteriorly, the convexity of the curve is exposed subperiosteally, the facet joints excised, the lamina decorticated, and bone graft applied (Fig. 9–12). The concavity must never be exposed. The posterior incision is then closed.

It is easiest to apply the corrective plaster cast while the patient is still anesthetized. If a chest tube has been inserted, it is brought out anterolaterally through the chest window of the cast. It can then be removed without disturbing the cast.

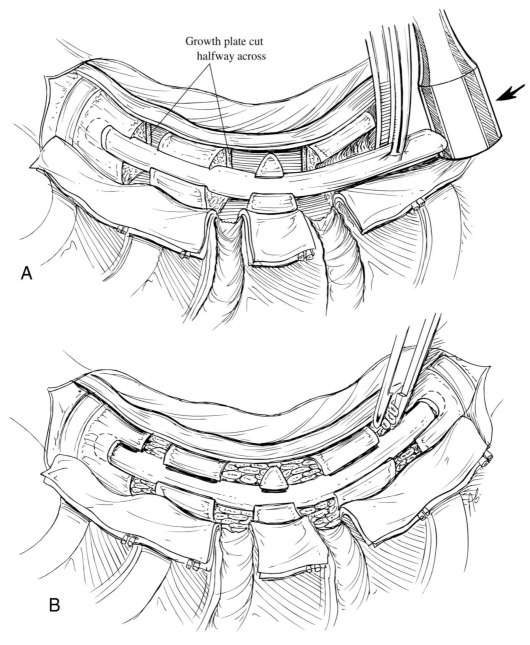

Growth plate cut
halfway across

A

B

*Figure 9–11*

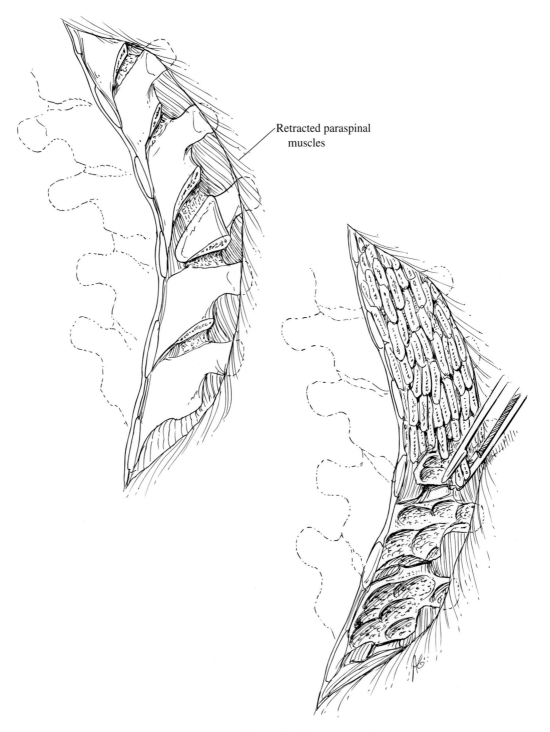

Retracted paraspinal muscles

*Figure 9–12*

361

# Correction of Fixed Thoracic Lordosis

Correction of fixed thoracic lordosis is a complex procedure requiring both anterior and posterior surgery. It is highly desirable that these be done under the same anesthetic if at all possible. The purpose of operation is to restore the spine to either a straight or preferably kyphotic alignment from a lordotic alignment in the chest. This is usually necessary because of progressive respiratory insufficiency owing to the spine's encroachment into the thoracic cavity (Fig. 9–13).

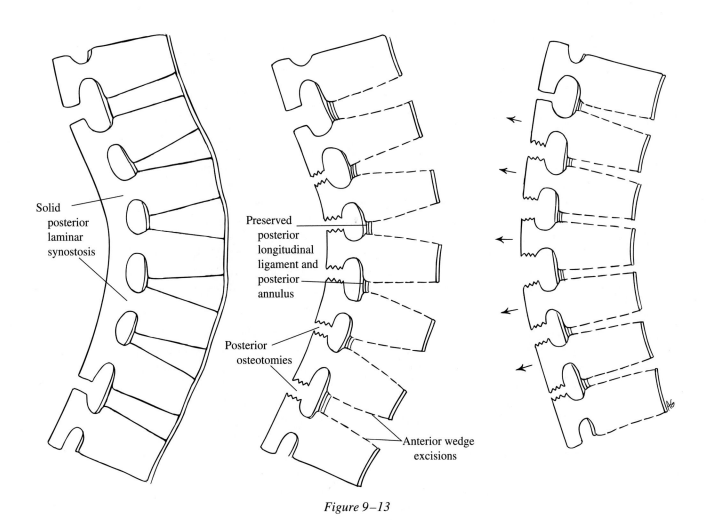

Solid posterior laminar synostosis

Preserved posterior longitudinal ligament and posterior annulus

Posterior osteotomies

Anterior wedge excisions

*Figure 9–13*

363

# COMBINATION THORACIC AND THORACOLUMBAR PROCEDURES

The spine is approached anteriorly. The amount of vertebra exposed is determined by the preoperative evaluation from the clinical and x-ray findings. Disks are thoroughly removed in this area along with wedges of bone on each side, the wedges facing anteriorly because of the lordosis rather than laterally, as previously described for scoliosis. Because of the intrusion of the spine into the mediastinum, this exposure usually is not easy. The key is to obtain gaping wedges anteriorly and not packing the wedges with bone, since the purpose is to close the wedges with the posterior instrumentation (Fig. 9–14). Once the wedges have been created they are simply left open and the chest closed (Fig. 9–15). Depending on whether the deformity is stiff or flexible, resection of the convex ribs may be necessary. To accomplish this, an incision is made in the periosteum just posterior to the rib head and out for about 3 cm, subperiosteally exposing the ribs; then segments of bone are removed and saved for later bone grafts.

Double chest tubes are inserted and the chest is closed. The patient is placed prone. A posterior midline incision is made and the dissection carried down to expose the spine, and, if necessary, the ribs on the opposite side of the thoracotomy. This is a difficult exposure because the spine is down inside the chest, and it is often difficult to move the muscles laterally. Occasionally, it is necessary to excise the paraspinal muscles. Because of the fusion, these muscles are nonfunctional. Once the spine is thoroughly exposed posteriorly, the ligamenta flava between the vertebrae are excised, as for a Luque procedure. This would be true of an idiopathic lordoscoliosis or lordosis due to some disease such as Marfan's or neurologic problem.

If the problem is a congenital thoracic lordosis, a plaque of bone will be found posteriorly representing spontaneously fused or nonsegmented laminae, and osteotomies have to be created opposite the levels that were osteotomized anteriorly. For this, precise x-ray identification is necessary. These osteotomies are done with a burr and/or Kerrison rongeur. In a lordotic spine, the spinal cord is displaced up against the laminae and is more easily injured than in a kyphosis. Once the ligamenta flava are removed and/or osteotomies completed, double loops of wire, preferably 0.12 mm, are passed on each side, giving four strands of wire under each lamina. Two metal rods are prepared. These must be very strong, 6 mm-diameter, hard rods. The ends of the rods are flattened to prevent intrusion into the canal. The wires are brought up around the rods and loosely twisted in position. The correction begins to take place by sequentially tightening the wires, starting at the ends and working gradually toward the middle. It usually takes three and sometimes four passes up and down the rods before the laminae are aligned against the arched rods. For flexible curves, one rod can be inserted, the spine is brought into the corrected alignment, and then the second rod is added as a stabilizing device. For ridged deformities, it may be necessary to osteotomize and resect ribs on both sides of the spine. The authors have corrected flexible, idiopathic-type lordosis without rib resections and without an anterior procedure, but in most cases, it is necessary to use an anterior release and one- or both-side rib resections. Thorough bone grafts should be applied and often the amount of rib removed provides adequate bone for grafting. The length of fusion is determined by the length of the pathologic lordosis, which is usually longer than any coexisting scoliosis.

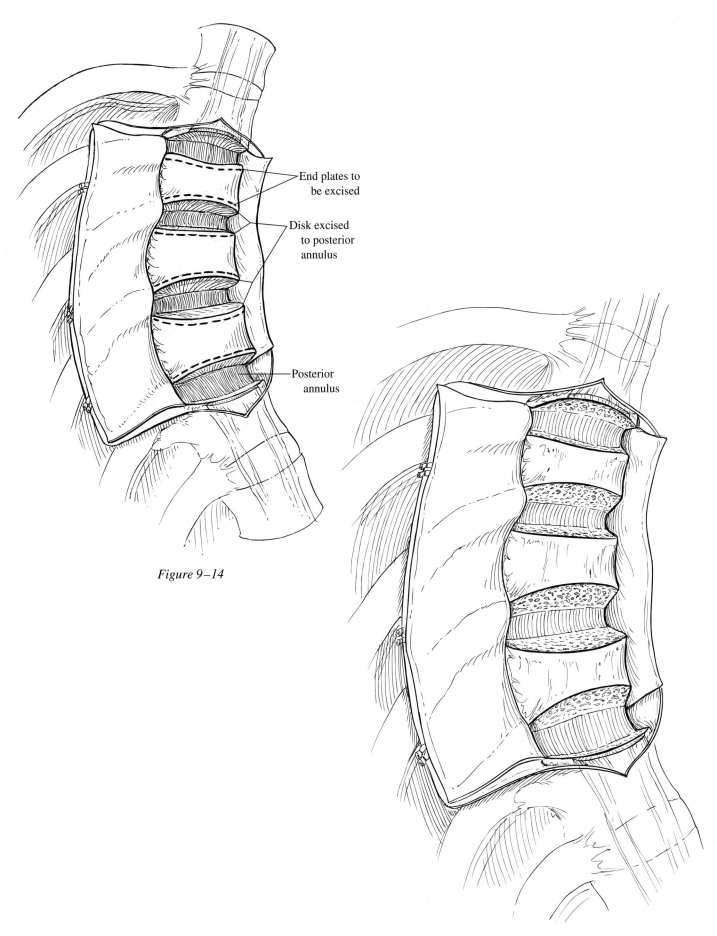

End plates to
be excised

Disk excised
to posterior
annulus

Posterior
annulus

*Figure 9–14*

*Figure 9–15*

365

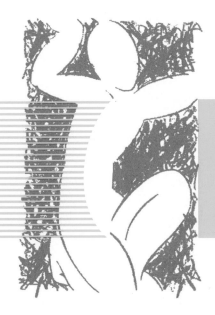

# 10

# ANTERIOR LUMBOSACRAL PROCEDURES

# Anterolateral Flank Approach, Retroperitoneal L2–S1, without and with 12th Rib Resection

The patient is placed in the lateral decubitus position, tilted about 45 degrees posteriorly, with the convexity of the spine uppermost. If there is no scoliosis, approach from either side is possible with equal facility. The left side, dealing with the aorta rather than the vena cava, is generally preferred. The kidney rest is elevated and the feet dropped for more exposure. A curvilinear incision is made from the midinguinal ligament or ipsilateral pubic tubercle to the tip of the 12th rib curving around the iliac spine (Fig. 10–1). This is carried through the subcutaneous fat, the external and internal oblique and transverse abdominal muscles, and lumbocostal fascia laterally (Fig. 10–2). The length and orientation of the lumbotomy incision are modified, depending on the level of exposure needed. For the L4–5 and L5–S1 levels, the incision is more anterior and the rectus sheath is divided. For the higher levels, L2–3 and L3–4, the incision is carried into the flank and the lumbodorsal fascia is divided as necessary.

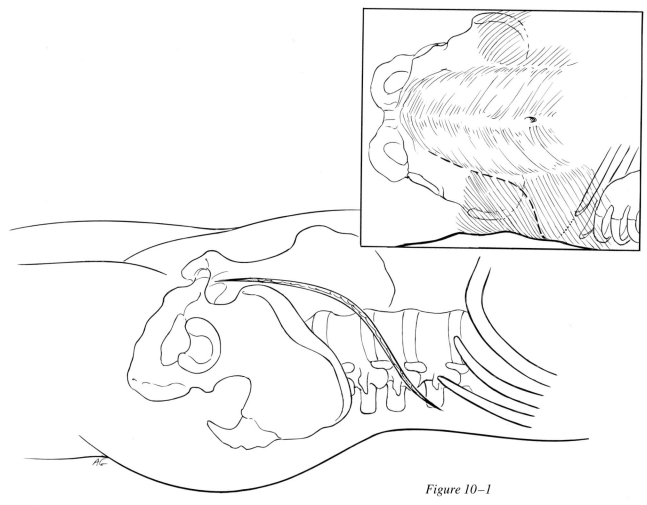

*Figure 10–1*

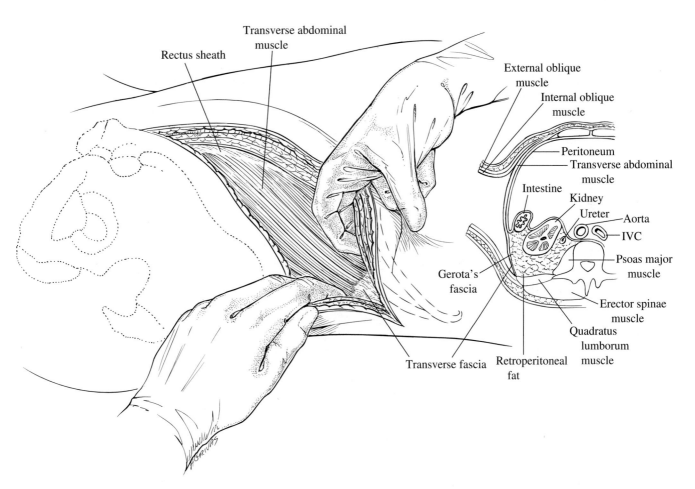

*Figure 10–2*

369

# ANTERIOR LUMBOSACRAL PROCEDURES

The extraperitoneal space is entered and manual, blunt, and gauze dissection is carried medially and anteriorly to the edge of the rectus sheath and inferiorly to the inguinal ligament or pubic tubercle, separating the anterior abdominal muscles from the peritoneum and peritoneal contents (Fig. 10–3). The peritoneum and the abdominal muscles should be generously separated on the cephalad side to leave a good margin of muscle or fascia free of peritoneum to facilitate the closure of the incision.

The oblique muscles and then the transverse abdominal muscle are divided further in the line of the skin incision to the lateral edge of the rectus sheath (Fig. 10–4). Often for wider exposure, the anterior sheath of the rectus is divided in line with the incision and the tethering tissues are divided in line with the semilunar line. The inferior epigastric vessels may be exposed.

The peritoneum is then freed laterally and posteriorly entering the retroperitoneal space (plane) bounded posteriorly by the quadratus lumborum and psoas muscles.

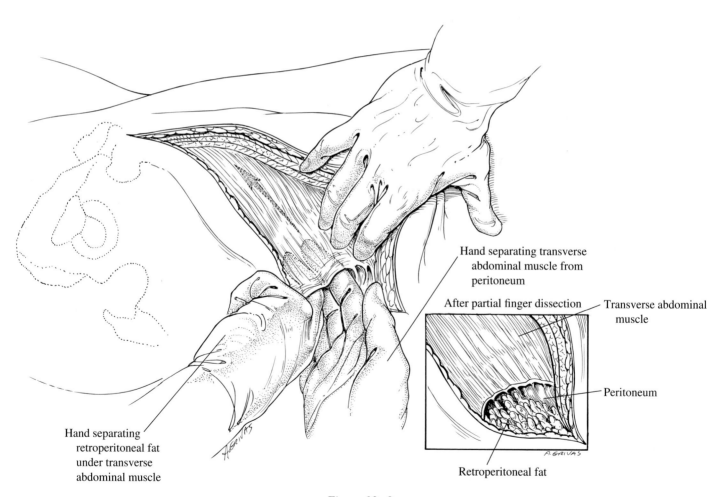

Hand separating transverse abdominal muscle from peritoneum

After partial finger dissection

Transverse abdominal muscle

Peritoneum

Hand separating retroperitoneal fat under transverse abdominal muscle

Retroperitoneal fat

*Figure 10–3*

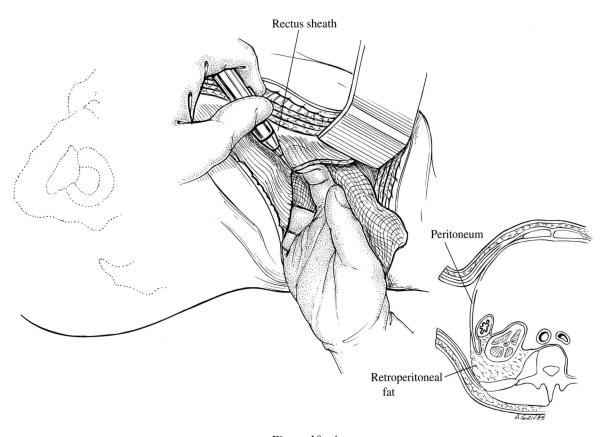

Rectus sheath

Peritoneum

Retroperitoneal
fat

*Figure 10–4*

371

# ANTERIOR LUMBOSACRAL PROCEDURES

At the higher L2 and L3 levels, Gerota's fascia is encountered. Gerota's fascia is continuous with the peritoneum and surrounds the kidney, ureter, adrenal gland, and peritoneal fat and is loosely applied to the quadratus lumborum and psoas muscles. The layer blends loosely with the psoas fascia and is attached to the vertebral column anterior to the medial margin of the psoas. In this plane, by manual and blunt dissection, the peritoneal contents are pushed anteriorly and medially across the quadratus lumborum and psoas muscles (Fig. 10–5).

The wound margins are padded with moist sponges and a self-retaining, Burford or Balfour, retractor is inserted. Exposure of the spine from L2 to the iliac vessels is achieved (Fig. 10–6).

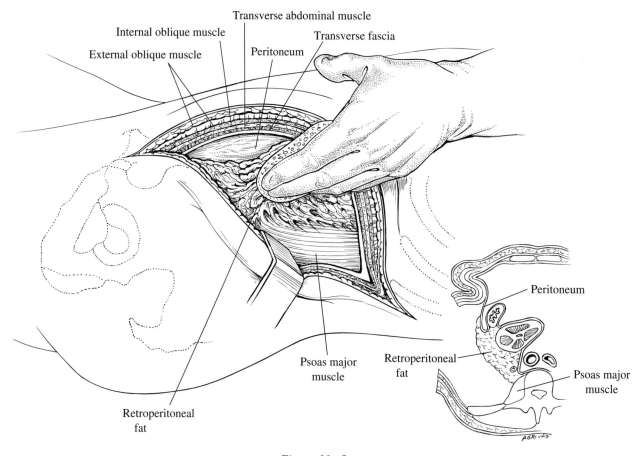

*Figure 10–5*

372

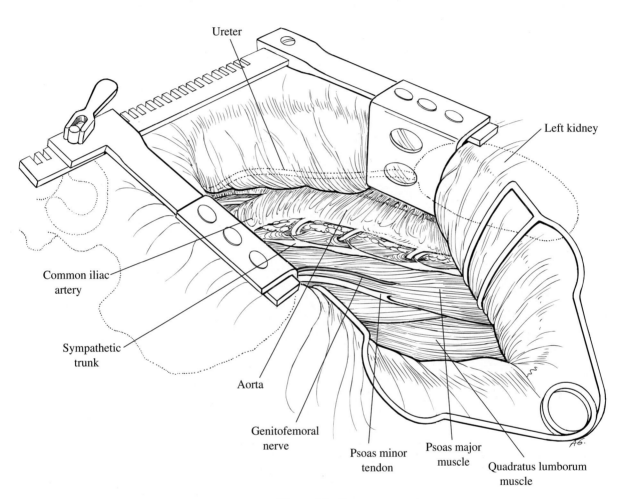

Ureter

Left kidney

Common iliac
artery

Sympathetic
trunk

Aorta

Genitofemoral
nerve

Psoas minor
tendon

Psoas major
muscle

Quadratus lumborum
muscle

*Figure 10–6*

Slips of the psoas muscle are elevated off the spine. The prevertebral arteries and veins are exposed, dissected free, doubly clipped and ligated or divided, and then peeled medially and laterally as previously described (Fig. 10–7).

For wider exposure of the L4–L5 disk space cephalad to the iliac vessels, the left iliac artery may need to be mobilized and retracted with a Penrose drain. The iliac vein also may need mobilization and retraction. The iliolumbar vein, when encountered, is exposed, doubly clipped and divided or ligated, stitch-tied and divided. As previously noted, if this vessel is large, it may need to be divided using vascular clamps and oversewn. The iliac veins, iliolumbar veins, and tributaries are shown in Figure 10–8.

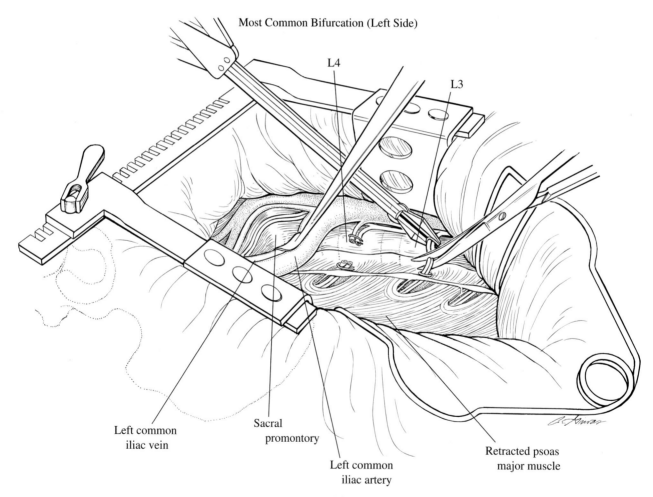

*Figure 10–7*

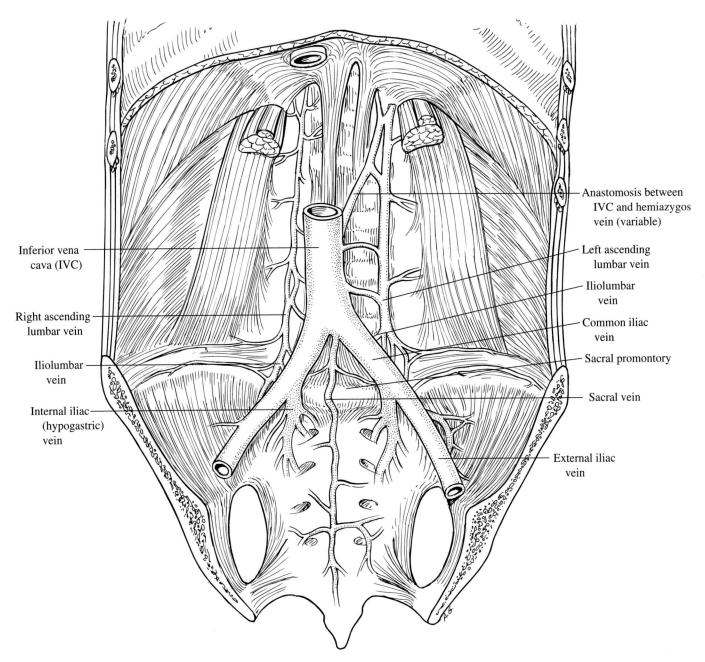

Inferior vena
cava (IVC)

Right ascending
lumbar vein

Iliolumbar
vein

Internal iliac
(hypogastric)
vein

Anastomosis between
IVC and hemiazygos
vein (variable)

Left ascending
lumbar vein

Iliolumbar
vein

Common iliac
vein

Sacral promontory

Sacral vein

External iliac
vein

*Figure 10–8*

375

The L5–S1 disk space is best exposed caudad to the iliac vessels, but staying retroperitoneally, using digital and gauze dissection. The peritoneal contents are pushed anteriorly to the dependent side and retracted. The sacral promontory is palpated and exposed. Presacral arteries, veins, and nerves are visualized. The vessels are occluded with Ligaclips quadruply and divided. The nerves are pushed medially and laterally without division, if exposure is not compromised. If the aortocaval bifurcations are low, the L5–S1 disk may need to be exposed cephalad to the iliac artery and vein (Fig. 10–9). Retract the iliac artery with a Penrose drain. Carefully dissect the iliac vein off the spine looking for the *iliolumbar* vein and *venous anomalies*. This is a more difficult exposure and requires added precautions in dealing with the blood vessels. Variations in the aortocaval bifurcations, although uncommon, may modify the approach to the L4–5 and L5–S1 disks.

After the orthopedic procedure is completed, hemostasis is secured. Peritoneal contents are allowed to fall into place. No drains are left. Before the wound is closed, the kidney rest is lowered, the extension of the table is removed, and the table is placed in favor of mild flexion to reduce muscular tension.

The abdominal muscles are then approximated anatomically with a continuous strong suture of PDS 0, the first layer incorporating the transverse and internal oblique muscles. As the transverse muscle becomes well developed, it is approximated separately. The abdominal wall muscles are then pushed in, reducing tension on the suture line and avoiding tearing of the muscle. The external oblique muscle is similarly closed. The subcutaneous tissue is approximated with 2-0 suture and 3-0 is used as a subcuticular suture.

Although the L2–S1 exposure is achieved by the anterolateral, retroperitoneal, flank approach, as described, oftentimes this exposure is less than optimal, making the orthopedic procedure more difficult and time-consuming. For these reasons, the anterolateral flank approach for this level is combined with resection of the 12th rib.

Removal of the 12th rib frees the insertions of the diaphragm and the transverse muscle and fascia at the tip and releases the lumbocostal ligament, an extension of the lumbodorsal fascia, attached to the 12th rib and the first two lumbar vertebrae. Cephalad retraction is made easier and better exposure of the spine is obtained.

The flank incision is tailored in length, appropriate to the lower level desired, and extended overlying the 12th rib. The 12th rib is removed subperiosteally, taking special precautions to avoid injury to the pleura. The flank incision is extended posteriorly through the lumbodorsal fascia, the posterior, inferior serratus muscle, and lumbocostal ligament.

Should the pleura be opened, it may be repaired if the pleural tissue holds sutures well. If the pleura is thin and friable, it is best to insert a chest tube in the posterior gutter and establish conventional continuous suction.

The wound closure is carried out as previously described for the flank incision. The extended segment of the incision is closed in a similar manner approximating the divided lumbodorsal fascia, posterior, inferior serratus muscle, latissimus dorsi muscle, subcutaneous tissues, and skin.

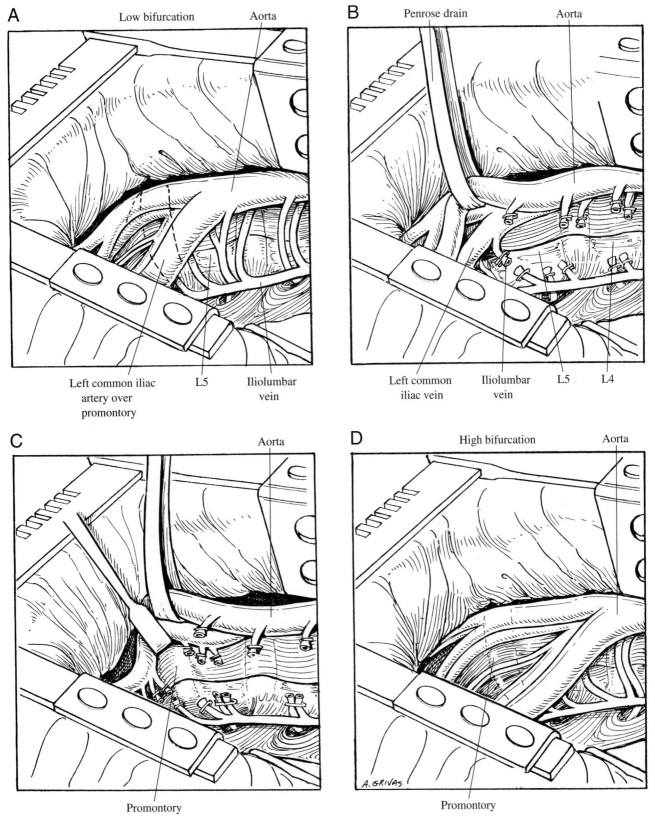

A     Low bifurcation     Aorta

Left common iliac    L5    Iliolumbar
artery over                vein
promontory

B    Penrose drain      Aorta

Left common    Iliolumbar    L5    L4
iliac vein      vein

C                Aorta

Promontory

D    High bifurcation     Aorta

Promontory

A. GRIVAS

*Figure 10–9*

377

# Transperitoneal Approach

This approach may be used for correction of spondylolisthesis. The patient is positioned supine on the operating table. The hips are hyperextended. The abdomen is entered through a Pfannenstiel incision extending from one lateral edge of the rectus sheath to the other (Fig. 10–10). The rectus muscles are divided with electrocautery. The inferior epigastric arteries are doubly ligated and divided. The peritoneum is entered.

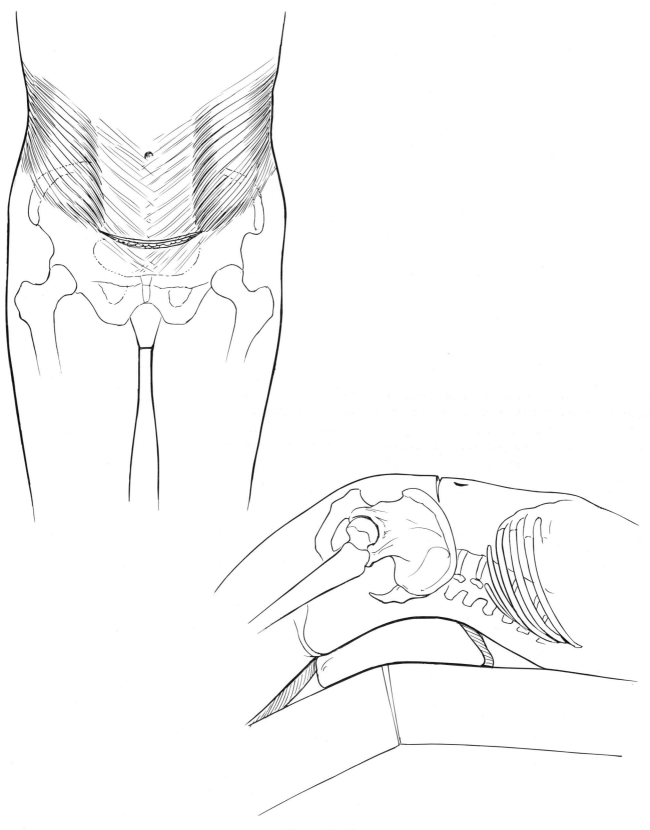

*Figure 10–10*

At this point, the patient is put in the Trendelenburg position and the bowel contents of the peritoneal cavity are pushed cephalad and kept in place with moist sponges and an abdominal retractor. The presacral hollow is exposed. The presacral peritoneum may be elevated with saline injection. A midline longitudinal incision is made in the retroperitoneum in front of the sacrum. The presacral arteries, veins, and nerves are exposed (Fig. 10–11). The nerves are peeled medially and laterally, preserving them, if exposure is not compromised. The arteries and veins are doubly ligated and divided. The promontory, L5–S1, and L4–5 levels are then exposed below the bifurcation of the aorta.

After the corrective orthopedic procedure, the retroperitoneum is closed with 3-0 running chromic catgut. Abdominal muscles and the anterior rectus sheath are approximated with #1 running chromic catgut. The subcutaneous tissue is closed with 2-0 generic Vicryl as a running stitch. The skin is approximated with 3-0 generic Vicryl as a subcuticular suture.

NOTE: Although L3–4 and L4–5 spaces may be exposed anteriorly between the inferior vena cava and aorta, the anterolateral, extraperitoneal flank approach for these levels, as well as the lower lumbar spine, is preferred because of better exposure. Thus, the anterior, transperitoneal approach to the lower lumbar spine is less often utilized now.

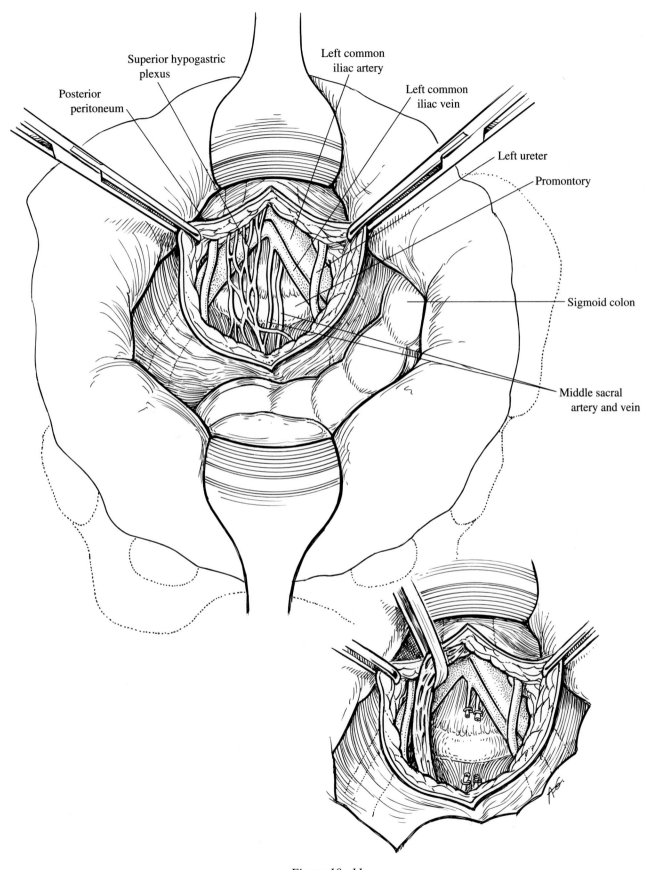

Posterior peritoneum

Superior hypogastric plexus

Left common iliac artery

Left common iliac vein

Left ureter

Promontory

Sigmoid colon

Middle sacral artery and vein

*Figure 10–11*

381

# Retroperitoneal Approach

## BASIC DISKECTOMY L4–5 AND L5–S1

Multiple techniques have been described for anterior lumbar interbody fusions with variations in both graft type and construct and recipient site preparation. The specific technique selected should be based on the goals of the surgery, which include not only solid arthrodesis, but also in many cases structural stabilization and distraction. Common to all anterior lumbar interbody fusions is a safe and thorough diskectomy with preparation of the interbody space for bone graft insertion. The approach to the disk can be directly anterior or anterolateral depending on the goal and technique of the surgery, patient positioning on the table, and the anterior exposure chosen.

Most commonly used are retroperitoneal approaches where the patient is positioned in one of two basic positions: (1) a lateral decubitus position or posteriorly reclined to varying degrees from this position (Fig. 10–12A) or (2) supine for a more anterior approach to the spine (Fig. 10–12B). The lateral decubitus approach or one of its variations provides a more anterolateral approach to the spine, if this is the goal, and gravity helps with exposure since the viscera will fall away from the site of surgery. The advantage of the supine position is that it allows for procedures more easily carried out by a direct anterior approach and the disk space is opened up in the anteroposterior plane to theoretically permit more even compression across multiple, cortical-type graft constructs. The disadvantage is that retraction may be more difficult since gravity does not pull the viscera from the site of surgery. Whichever approach is chosen, it is important to position the patient appropriately so that high-quality surgery can be achieved through an adequate exposure.

After the anterior abdominal exposure is accomplished, the key structure for identification of spinal structures is the psoas muscle. This is particularly true in the retroperitoneal approach, but also in the transperitoneal approach. The spine is immediately medial to the psoas muscle and usually partially covered by it. The psoas muscle, the intervertebral disks, vertebral bodies, and vascular structures can be easily palpated. The paravertebral sympathetic plexus lies immediately medial to the psoas muscle and should be appropriately respected during the exposure of the anterior surface of the lumbar spine.

Adequate retraction is necessary for a safe and efficient anterior diskectomy. Several approaches for retraction can be used, but important to all of them is the protection of vascular structures and surrounding soft tissue at risk from instruments used in the procedure. Retraction can be achieved with hand-held retractors only, with hand-held retractors in combination with Steinmann pins that are placed in a rectangular construct surrounding the disk to be operated on at the lateral extents of the exposure both above and below the disk space, or with a self-retaining systems. Regardless of the particular system selected, adequate and safe exposure and retraction is the key to prevent any intraoperative complications from injury to vascular, visceral, urologic, and neural structures.

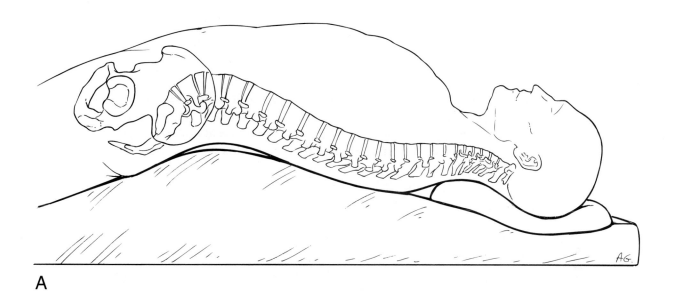

A

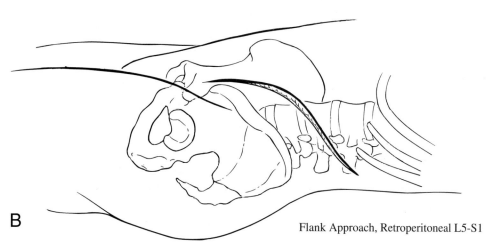

B

Flank Approach, Retroperitoneal L5-S1

*Figure 10–12*

The L4–5 level can present difficulties with retraction because of the great vessels present at this level and the individual anatomic variation in their position. Exposure of the L4–5 level is done by blunt dissection with mobilization of the distal aorta and the left common iliac vessels to the right. It is usually necessary to divide small lateral branches off of the left common iliac vessels to obtain optimum exposure. Occasionally the ascending lumbar vein, the first major branch off of the common iliac vein, requires transection after first securing it with double ligatures on each side. Additional exposure can be obtained by ligating the segmental vessels that usually cross the midportion of the vertebral bodies beginning with L4. The sympathetic trunk is mobilized and retracted laterally. The ureter and vascular structures are retracted medially.

After isolating the anterior surface of L4–5, retroperitoneal soft tissue is removed from the annulus from medial to lateral with coagulation as needed and care taken to protect the sympathetic plexus located more laterally during the exposure. The annular window to be removed is then outlined using electrocautery with a straight tip mounted on an extension handle. An annular rectangular window is then made in the disk utilizing a #15 blade mounted on a long handle. The transverse incisions are made adjacent to the end plates above and below the disk, cutting away from the great vessels at all times (Fig. 10–13). The lateral extensions of these incisions are based on both exposure and the extent of annulus to be removed as determined by the surgical goal and individual anatomic variation. The goal usually is not to remove all of the annular structures as they contribute significantly to stability, but rather an appropriate amount to safely and efficiently remove the disk and allow easy insertion of the graft. From a practical perspective, the removal tends to be approximately 3 cm in width. A Cobb elevator can then be used to separate the cartilage end plate from the bony end plates prior to its removal (Fig. 10–14). A major portion of the anterior annulus and the bulk of the disk can then be removed with a large pituitary rongeur or, sometimes more easily, with a long-handle Leksell rongeur (Fig. 10–15). A combination of straight, angled, and ring curettes as well as pituitary rongeurs can be used to remove the remainder of the intervertebral disk up to but not including the remainder of the annulus fibrosis laterally and posteriorly (Fig. 10–16). A nerve hook or small angled curette can be used to palpate the posterior margin of the vertebral body to help determine the depth of the diskectomy, proceeding with greater caution the more posterior. The goal of the diskectomy is usually to remove as much of the disk as safely as possible to obtain the maximum area for fusion. Up to this point in the procedure, it is important not to violate the bony end plates, since this will lead to unnecessary blood loss and poor visualization.

The end plates are then decorticated to expose bleeding subchondral bone by a number of methods utilizing curettes, high speed burrs, chisels, or osteotomes. The techniques used are dependent on the surgeon's experience and preference, the patient's normal and abnormal anatomy, and the surgical procedure chosen. If the anterior interbody fusion is going to consist of either autologous or allograft morselized cancellous bone, then meticulous carpentry is not necessary to decorticate the end plates. Consequently, osteotomes or a high speed burr can

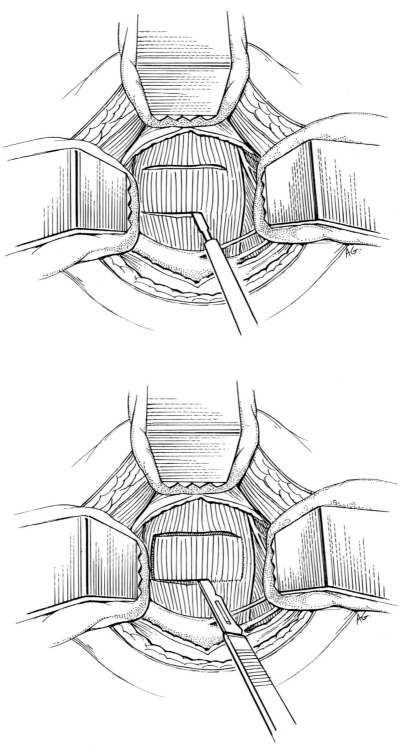

*Figure 10–13*

rapidly accomplish decortication. However, when distraction and structural stability are to be achieved, usually some type of cortical construct, it is of paramount importance to maintain the integrity of the subchondral plates to allow for graft impaction and distraction and still have bleeding surfaces of subchondral bone to encourage graft incorporation and fusion. In this situation, meticulous carpentry with the use of chisels, osteotomes, or a high speed burr is necessary to create the correct surfaces to prevent graft dislodgement and maintain the structural integrity of the subchondral end plate.

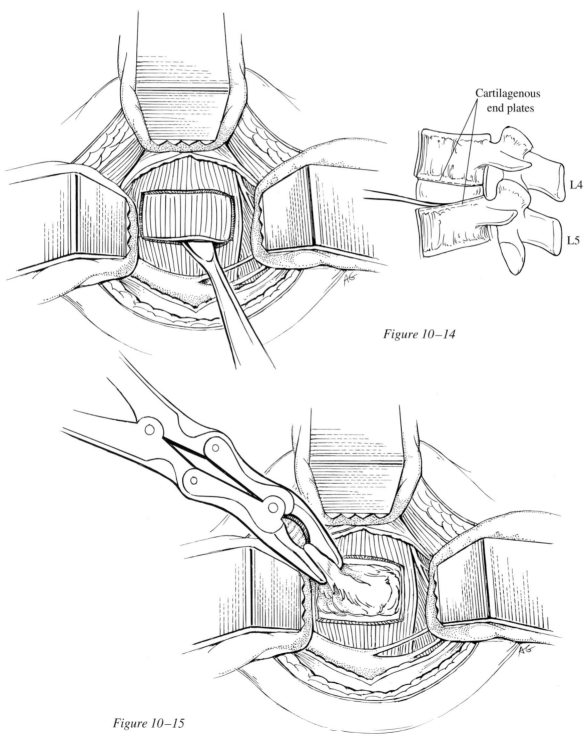

Cartilagenous
end plates

L4

L5

*Figure 10–14*

*Figure 10–15*

The L5–S1 level can be deeply seated in the pelvis and require different approaches to exposure and retraction. Usually adequate exposure is obtained by mobilizing the common iliac vessels *cephalad* and laterally with careful division of the presacral vessels. It is very important to use blunt dissection in this area to avoid injuring the branches of the sympathetic plexus and vascular structures. Appropriate retraction is obtained and must be carefully observed and maintained at this level because of the vascular anatomy. The diskectomy is completed as previously described with constant vigilance of the structures at risk. The level of inclination at L5–S1 is obviously different from that at the L4–5 and should be correlated with the preoperative and intraoperative x-rays to guide the procedure. Generally speaking, suction drains are not necessary.

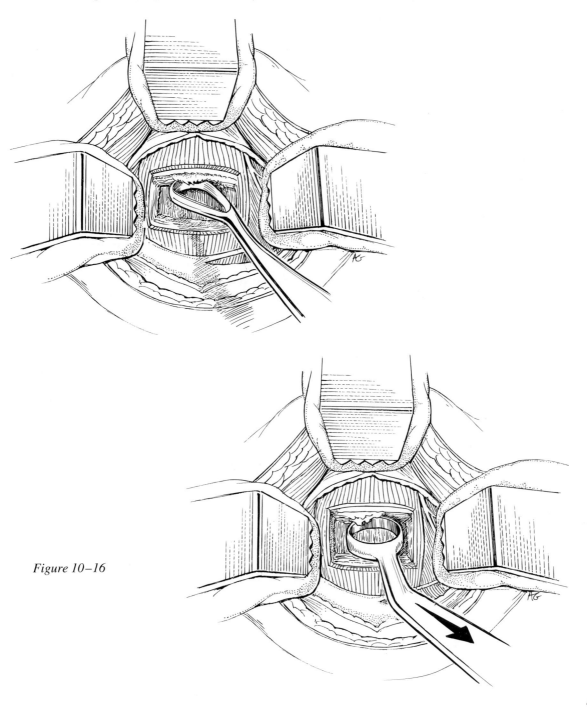

*Figure 10–16*

387

# Basic Fusion L4–5 and L5–S1 with Cancellous Graft

Autologous and/or allograft cancellous bone can be used for an anterior interbody fusion in the lumbar spine. However, this has obvious limitations with regard to structural stability and distraction and should only be undertaken if structural stability will not represent a real or potential problem. For example, if correction of the deformity is the goal and the dimensions of the intervertebral disk space will change after the posterior procedure, cancellous grafting is usually chosen. One can anticipate settling with this type of fusion and consideration must be given to posterior neural structures at risk when this occurs.

Depending on the surgeon's preference, the L5–S1 disk is exposed and retracted. The diskectomy is carried out and the cartilagenous end plates removed with decortication to bleeding subchondral bone. The cancellous graft is morselized prior to insertion. The source of this graft can be an autologous iliac graft obtained through the same abdominal incision from the side exposed, through a separate incision over the opposite iliac crest, or multiple types of allograft. If a posterior procedure is carried out first, a posterior iliac graft can be harvested to be used anteriorly.

The next step is the careful insertion of the cancellous bone graft, beginning posteriorly, filling the disk space with gentle impaction of the graft layer by layer with a suitably sized impactor (Fig. 10–17A,B). The cancellous bone graft is carried out to the anterior edge of the vertebral bodies. This bone should not be over-impacted, since this can potentially lead to posterior structure injury or iatrogenic stenosis. Gelfoam impregnated with thrombin solution is placed over the intervertebral level to help with hemostasis and perhaps assist in forming a layer or membrane to isolate the cancellous graft to the interspace, although some of the anterior portion of the graft often migrates.

The retractors are removed and the L4–5 disk space is then exposed. After exposure and retraction are obtained at the L4–5 level, the same procedure used at L5–S1 is repeated (Fig. 10–17C). Both levels are then evaluated to be certain adequate hemostasis has been achieved. The wound is irrigated and closed in anatomic layers. In most cases a deep drain is not necessary.

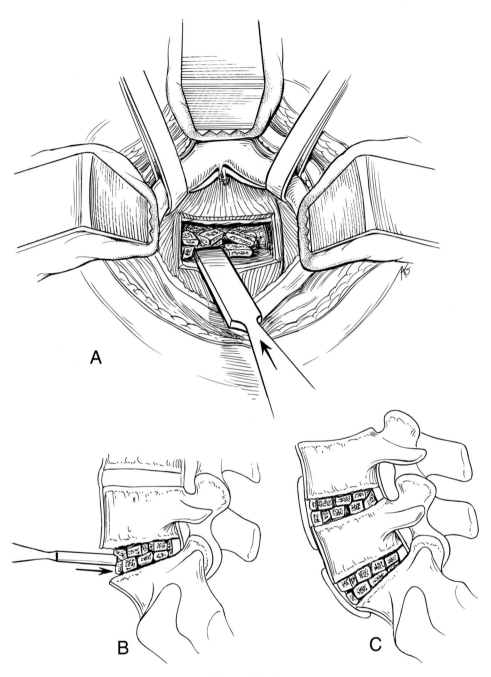

*Figure 10–17*

# BASIC FUSION L4–5 AND L5–S1 WITH TRICORTICAL ILIAC GRAFT

A basic technique, when indicated, utilizes tricortical iliac allograft. These grafts come in various sizes and shapes and can be contoured for appropriate fit. Autologous iliac grafts harvested through the same abdominal incision can be used if preferred or indicated. This technique has many modifications, all of which provide structural stability and often distraction of the interspace to some extent. It should be apparent that other sources for grafts can be used for this procedure, such as fibula, femur, or tibia, and the surgical approach can be directly anterior or anterolateral. Unlike the fusion technique utilizing cancellous graft, meticulous carpentry is of paramount importance to safely achieve the goal of a solid interbody fusion.

Patient preparation, positioning, and exposure are carried out as previously described. Unless there are mitigating factors in favor of approaching L4–5 first, the procedure is begun at L5–S1. This can sometimes be quite difficult because of the inclination of the L5–S1 interspace as well as its deep location in the pelvis. If it is not possible to carry out the procedure at this level, the technique can be modified by preparing the interspace and inserting the grafts in a plane that is somewhat less than parallel to the end plates as allowed by the anatomic constraints or cancellous grafting can be undertaken as previously described. This is a decision that occasionally needs to be made intraoperatively and the surgeon should be prepared to take alternative approaches when confronted with restrictive anatomy.

The diskectomy at L5–S1 is carried out to the point of decortication. A high speed burr may be used for decortication, but anatomic constraints may require the use of straight or curved osteotomes. Regardless of the approach taken, the end plates are carefully decorticated avoiding violation of integrity of the subchondral plate, which is necessary for structural support. Beginning posteriorly and on the S1 side of the interspace, decortication is meticulously carried creating a ridge or lip of bone both posteriorly and anteriorly to help prevent graft dislodgement in these directions. The same procedure is carried out on the L5 side. The subsequent dimensions of the prepared interspace are measured for appropriate graft selection (a caliper is particularly helpful). The interspace is packed with Gelfoam and a sponge while the grafts are being prepared (Fig. 10–18).

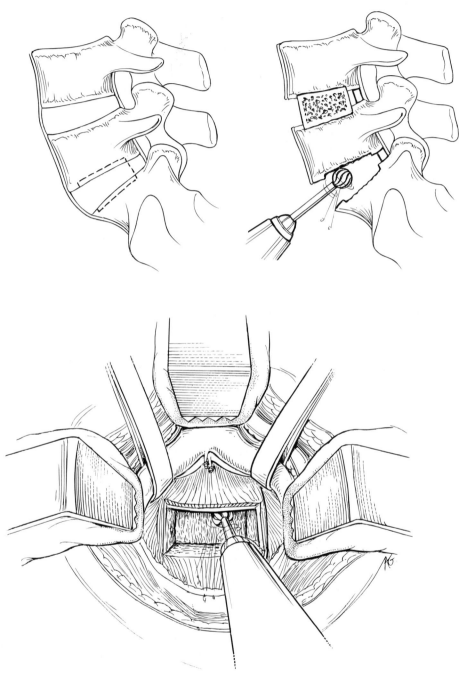

*Figure 10–18*

Generally, an attempt is made to fill as much of the interspace with bone grafts as possible. This usually requires two tricortical iliac grafts, but in some cases, three are possible for larger interspaces and one larger graft supplemented with cancellous graft as needed to fill the interspace for very small interspaces (Fig. 10–19A–E). The tricortical iliac grafts selected are contoured using a burr and/or rongeur to create grafts with smooth edges that are slightly larger than the measured interspace height so that they are securely locked in place after impaction and the operating table flexion is removed. The two grafts are contoured as similarly as possible with regard to their top and bottom surfaces as well as their anteroposterior diameter. The top and bottom surfaces are contoured to match the inclination of the decorticated end plates, which are often not entirely parallel. It is sometimes helpful to taper the leading edge of the graft to allow for insertion and impaction.

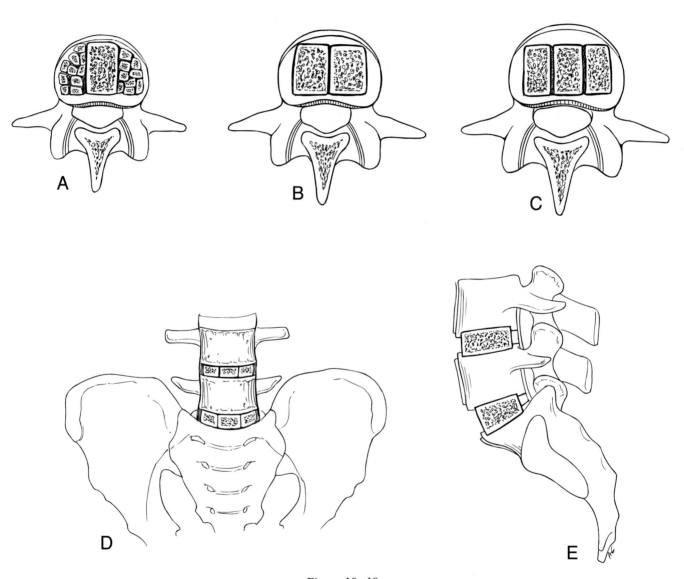

*Figure 10–19*

393

The Gelfoam and sponge are removed from the interspace. Some surgeons prefer to use laminar spreaders to further distract the interspace prior to graft insertion. The two grafts are lined up next to each other at the entrance to the interspace to make a final evaluation for placement and fit. The first graft is carefully inserted and impacted into one side of the interspace past the anterior lip created by the burr, avoiding injury to nearby vascular structures during its insertion. The remaining graft is similarly impacted (Fig. 10–20).

Both grafts should fit very snugly and are evaluated for stability with a small Cobb elevator or Kocher clamp, keeping in mind that additional stability will be achieved when the flexion is removed from the operating table. Sometimes one of the grafts may appear slightly loose compared to its counterpart. If such is the case, the flexion should be removed from the table to re-evaluate graft stability, which is oftentimes achieved by this maneuver. If not, it is sometimes necessary to create a new graft construct rather than take the chance of graft expulsion.

Should any interspace remain that has the potential for fusion, additional allograft or autograft chips from the graft preparation are inserted and impacted to complete the grafting at this level. Hemostasis is evaluated and Gelfoam is placed over the interspace. The retraction is removed, allowing the soft tissues to return to their normal position over the interspace.

Retraction is then repositioned to expose the L4–5 level and the same procedure is repeated at this level. The flexion is removed from the operating table and both levels are evaluated one last time for graft stability and hemostasis. If any questions remain about graft position, intraoperative x-rays should be taken. Otherwise, the wound is closed in anatomic layers. Deep suction drains generally are not necessary after this procedure.

If the authors plan to perform a posterior stabilization procedure, they generally proceed with the patient under the same anesthetic unless there are mitigating factors requiring staging the anterior and posterior procedures.

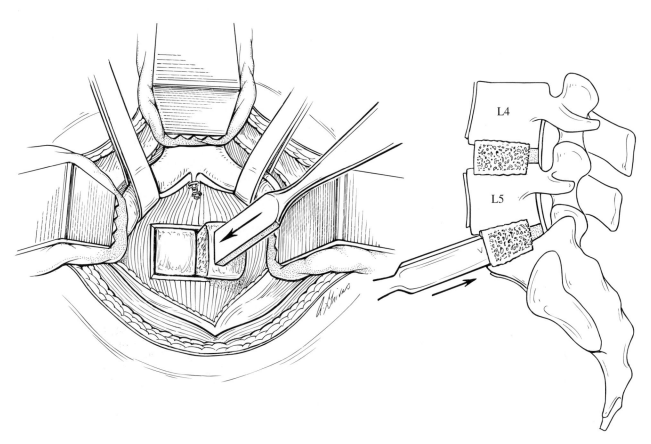

*Figure 10–20*

# ANTERIOR INTERBODY FUSION L4–5 WITH THE SELBY TECHNIQUE

An alternative technique to anterior interbody fusion using a tricortical construct and instrumentation for recipient site preparation has been described by David K. Selby and coworkers with original referencing of the technique to Henry V. Crock. This is a retroperitoneal approach with the patient on the operating table in the supine position. The exposure is carried down to the anterior lumbosacral spine and, for purposes of this discussion, the procedure will be described for an L4–5 interbody fusion. This technique is applicable at other levels of the lumbar spine. It requires a direct anterior approach once the lumbosacral spine has been exposed.

With the exposure completed and adequate retraction obtained, the appropriate disk level is identified. A complete diskectomy is carried out with curetting of disk material from the end plate down to subchondral bone. A depth gauge is used to determine the depth of the vertebra and this is compared to marking lines on an appropriately sized dowel cutter. A circular cutting chisel is used to make two starting cuts to seat the teeth of the dowel cutter (Fig. 10–21). The circular chisel used comes in sizes graded from 0 to 3 equivalent to the dowel cutters and is used to measure which cutter will be used in the intervertebral space. Selby recommends using the smallest size that provides distinct cuts on both sides of the interspace.

The dowel cutter is used to ream out two circular cuts across the intervertebral space parallel to the end plates (Fig. 10–22). A Hudson brace on a T ratchet handle or an air-powered drill is recommended to carry out this step. The depth of the vertebra is measured with a depth gauge and is compared to the marking lines on the dowel cutter so that the posterior circular cut is not carried too far, which could result in potential neural injury.

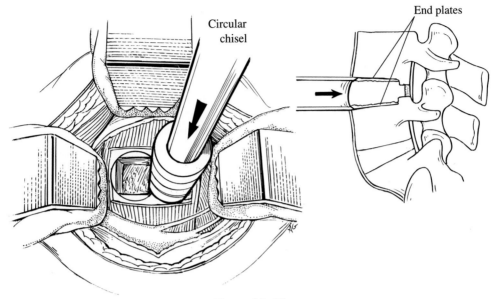

Circular
chisel

End plates

*Figure 10–21*

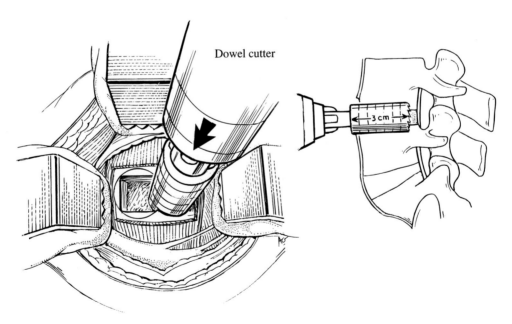

Dowel cutter

3 cm

*Figure 10–22*

397

A core evacuation gouge can is used to remove the remaining bone fragments (Fig. 10–23). Selby leaves a portion of the most posterior rim of the circular cuts to provide a buttress for seating of the grafts and prevent potential posterior extrusion of the graft into the neural tissues.

The grafts are harvested for insertion. Dowel cutters are graded in size from 0 through 4 so that the higher number, which is larger, is used to take a graft for the number below it, such as using a #4 dowel cutter to obtain graft for the recipient site that has been cut with a #3 dowel cutter. The graft is harvested with the dowel cutters from the patient's anterior iliac crest or allogeneic grafts can be taken with the dowel cutters. Dr. Selby has precut plugs from a bone bank, which has a set of the dowel cutters for this system to save on intraoperative time. Regardless of the source, two such cylindrical appropriately sized grafts are obtained.

The operating room table is flexed to help open up the interspace and the two grafts are inserted concurrently and tapped in place with alternating taps from an impactor (Fig. 10–24). After the grafts are inserted, the flexion of the operating table is removed to firmly lock the grafts in place. It should be noted that the grafts are fashioned slightly larger than the precut holes, which allows for maximum compression. In order to avoid graft extrusion, Dr. Selby recommends a 2–3 mm recess both anteriorly and posteriorly. If there is any question of improper graft placement, an intraoperative x-ray should be taken at the time.

After the graft has been appropriately seated and hemostasis assured, Surgicel is placed over the interspace and the wound is closed. Deep suction drains are generally not necessary.

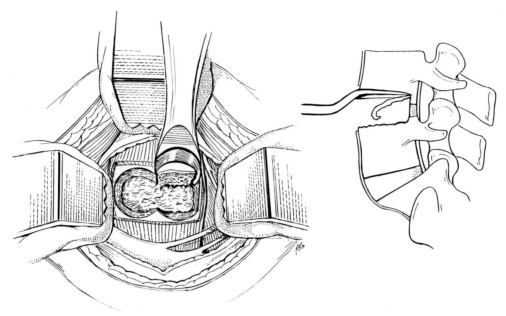

*Figure 10–23*

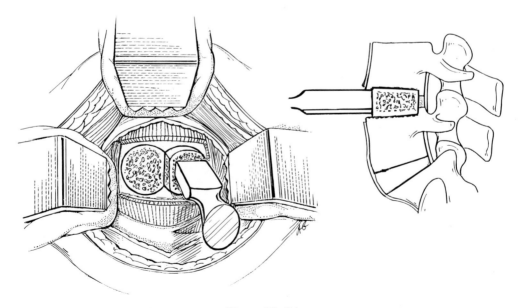

*Figure 10–24*

399

Some surgeons have chosen to modify this technique and use the circular cutting chisels with or without the cutting dowels to make the two parallel cuts in the intervertebral space with removal of the intervening ridge with a high speed burr. This results in a rectangular cut in the interbody space (Fig. 10–25A,B). Various types of tricortical constructs can then be inserted into the space. Some surgeons utilize a femoral ring (harvested from allogeneic femoral shaft) with the middle of the femoral ring filled with either cancellous allograft chips or portions of bone removed from the vertebral bodies during the formation of the recipient graft site (Fig. 10–25C,D). Some bone banks will supply this graft with multiple small fenestrations to theoretically allow for increased graft incorporation. Otherwise, multiple fenestrations can be drilled into the femoral ring with a small drill bit with care being taken not to compromise the structural integrity of the graft. It has been proposed that the cortical femoral ring construct allows for immediate distraction and structural stability with increased incorporation of grafts by the cancellous central portion, which does not have to go through the creeping substitution phase of fusion that a cortical construct does.

The Selby technique is relatively easy at the L4–5 interspace, but the lumbosacral junction can sometimes provide great difficulty in utilizing this instrumentation for an interbody fusion. In some cases with a deeply seated lumbosacral junction, it may not be possible to use these instruments or a modification in the angulation of the instruments and cuts are made with a subsequent construct that does not lie parallel to the vertebral body end plates after insertion. However, if patients are appropriately selected for this technique and the exposure is done correctly, as described by Selby and coworkers, this is not usually a problem.

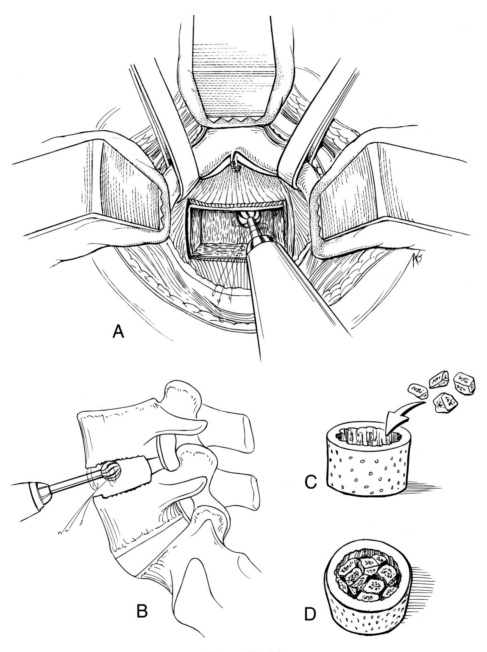

*Figure 10–25*

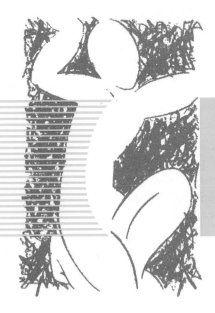

# POSTERIOR LUMBAR AND LUMBOSACRAL PROCEDURES

# Positioning the Patient

The proper positioning of the patient on a frame should allow for full chest excursion, the abdomen to hang completely free of pressure to decrease venous bleeding, and the safety of the neck. Many frames also allow for adjustment in the amount of lumbar curvature in the sagittal plane to facilitate the procedure (Fig. 11–1). The basic cross-sectional anatomy is seen in Figure 11–2.

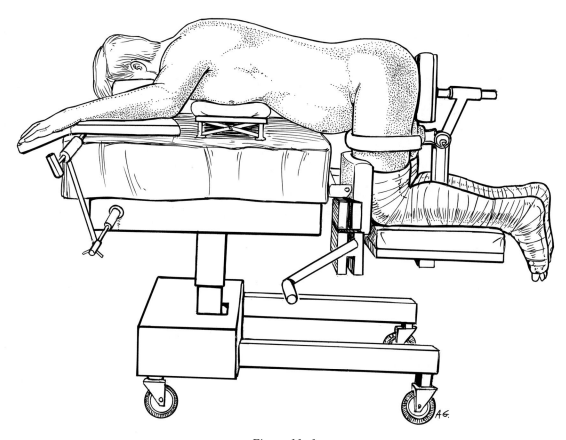

*Figure 11–1*

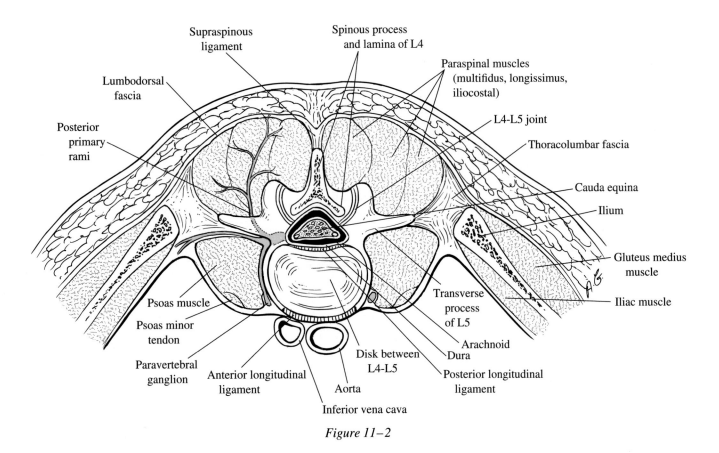

*Figure 11–2*

405

# *Exposures*

## MIDLINE APPROACH

The posterior midline approach to the lumbar spine is a time-honored, traditional approach that has its greatest utility in decompressive procedures and osteotomies but also is used widely for posterior and posterolateral fusions with and without spinal instrumentation. The incision is centered over the spinous processes.

The dissection is carried down to the spinous processes utilizing the full extent of the skin incision. Self-retaining retractors are used to hold back the skin margins. Depending on the quality of the tissues and other factors such as a previous surgery, the fascia overlying the spinous processes is divided with a sharp scalpel or electrocautery. A Cobb elevator is used to separate the fascia from the spinous processes bilaterally. The paraspinal muscles are reflected subperiosteally from the posterior structures with the Cobb elevator taking care to stay on the bone and out of the muscles. Initially the Cobb elevator is faced inward (Fig. 11–3A) along the lateral border of the spinous processes down to where it unites with the lamina. The Cobb elevator is then reversed to allow subperiosteal stripping of the paraspinal muscles from the posterior elements to the facet joints bilaterally (Fig. 11–3B). This dissection can be facilitated by using the Cobb elevator with a sponge to pack the wound and provide further hemostasis. Depending on the surgical procedure to be undertaken and the surgeon's preference, retractors are inserted to reflect both margins of the wound for further exposure and soft tissue removal from the posterior elements (Fig. 11–3C). Using various sized rongeurs and curettes, meticulous removal of soft tissue is undertaken to delineate all posterior osseous elements of interest. Avoid violating the facet capsules.

If a decompressive procedure such as a laminectomy is being undertaken, then the exposure is complete. However, if a posterolateral fusion is being undertaken, then the exposure is continued bilaterally over the facet joints onto the transverse processes and further laterally to the tips of the transverse processes to be fused. For this additional exposure, the self-retaining retractors are removed and hand-held retractors, such as a Hibbs retractor or a Myerding retractor, are used to expose the soft tissue attachments of the paraspinal muscles to the lateral structures. Using a scalpel, or electrocautery, the soft tissue attachments are cut from the lateral structures (Fig. 11–3C). A Cobb elevator is used to dissect down the lateral face of the superior facet of the vertebral body onto the transverse process at that level and to carefully reflect laterally the paraspinal muscles dorsal to the intertransverse membrane (Fig. 11–3D). Large rongeurs and electrocautery with an extension tip can be used to further denude the transverse processes, lateral face of the superior facet, and the pars interarticularis to completely expose the osseous structures. In the course of doing this, significant bleeding from vessels immediately lateral to the pars interarticularis is encountered. These vessels usually can be adequately controlled with electrocautery or, in some cases, more safely with a bipolar coagulator. It is helpful to coagulate those vessels before tearing them with the Cobb elevator.

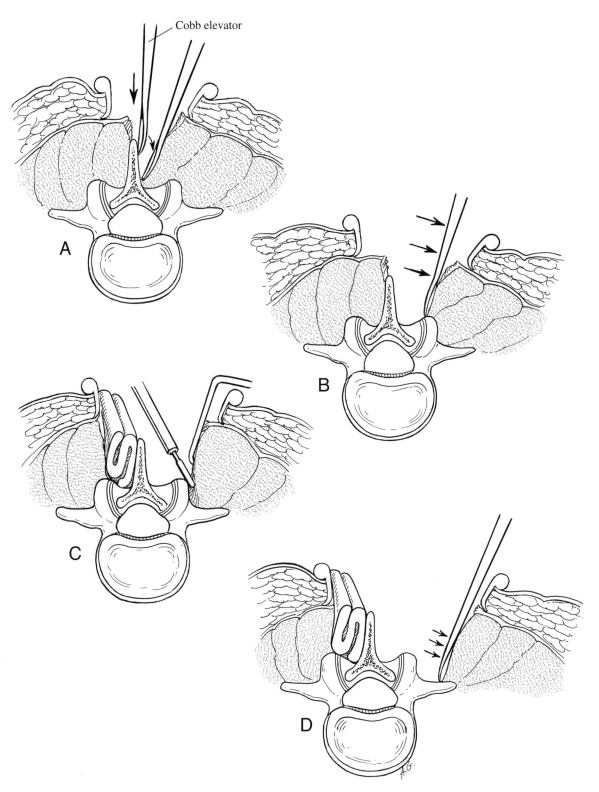

Cobb elevator

A

B

C

D

*Figure 11–3*

407

For an L4–S1 posterolateral fusion, the dissection is completed. The critical components of this exposure are adequate visualization and retraction, hemostasis, and meticulous removal of soft tissue from the posterolateral osseous elements if a fusion is to be undertaken (Fig. 11–4). For a decompressive laminectomy, it is very important to see the lateral border of the pars interarticularis at both levels in order not to remove too much bone. The correct level of exposure is of paramount importance and intraoperative x-rays should be taken for confirmation if there is doubt.

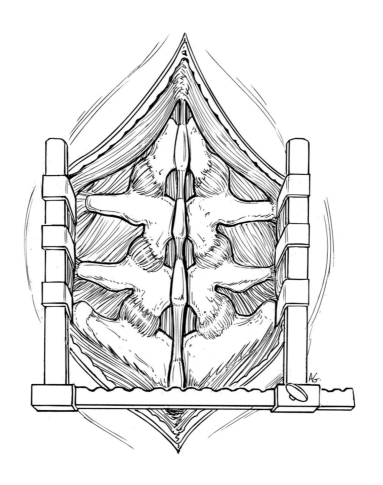

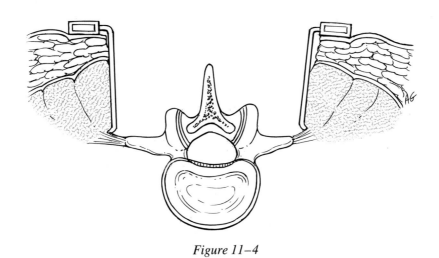

*Figure 11–4*

# PARASPINAL APPROACH L4–S1

The paraspinal approach to the lumbar spine presented here is attributed to Wiltse and coworkers as first described in 1968, with new uses and refinements described by Wiltse in 1988. This is a posterolateral approach to the lumbar spine through the paraspinal muscles that allows surgical procedures to be carried out on the posterior and lateral structures of the lumbar spine. This approach was initially developed for posterolateral in situ fusions. However, it has also been advocated by Wiltse for removal of herniated "far lateral" disks and pedicle screw placement.

The lower back is prepared and draped in the usual sterile fashion. A midline incision is made centered over the appropriate area of pathology and via sharp dissection or electrocautery carried down to the level of the deep fascia (Fig. 11–5A). Short, deep self-retaining retractors are placed to reflect the wound margins. A Cobb elevator or similar instrument is used to dissect the subcutaneous tissue from the deep fascia layer laterally on both sides. This is done in such a way as to allow bilateral deep fascial incisions to be made approximately two fingerbreadths or 2 cm lateral to the midline on either side (Fig. 11–5B). A scalpel or electrocautery is then used to split the lumbodorsal fascia. The fascial layer immediately below (fascia of the erector spinae) that envelops the muscle is also split (Fig. 11–5C). A natural cleavage plane can then be found between the multifidus and longissimus muscles. This can be identified by placing a finger for blunt dissection between these muscles at or above the L4 level as the fibers of the multifidus move laterally below this level and require splitting with either a scalpel or cautery. After the cleavage plane above L4 is identified and extended with a finger or a Cobb elevator, the depths of the wound should be over the facet joint of L4–5, which is easily palpable (Fig. 11–6). The scalpel or electrocautery is used to split the decussating paraspinal fibers below the L4 level to osseous structures, which are usually the sacral ala and the L5–S1 facet (Fig. 11–7). Deep, long-handle, self-retaining retractors are placed between the two exposed muscles groups for retraction (Fig. 11–8). Soft tissue in the depths of the wound is removed with a large rongeur. A Cobb elevator is used to expose the lamina of the vertebra and the transverse processes. Care should be exercised during this portion of the exposure as the nerve roots traverse just below the intertransverse membrane (Fig. 11–9). Extreme caution should be used with dissection of the loose posterior element as in spondylolisthesis. The remainder of the exposure is consistent with the intended surgical goal as described elsewhere.

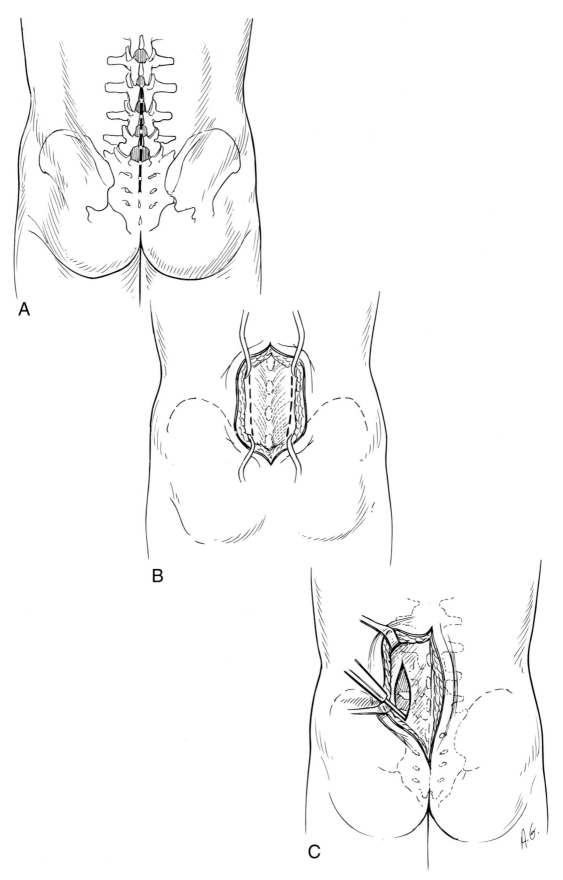

A

B

C

*Figure 11–5*

411

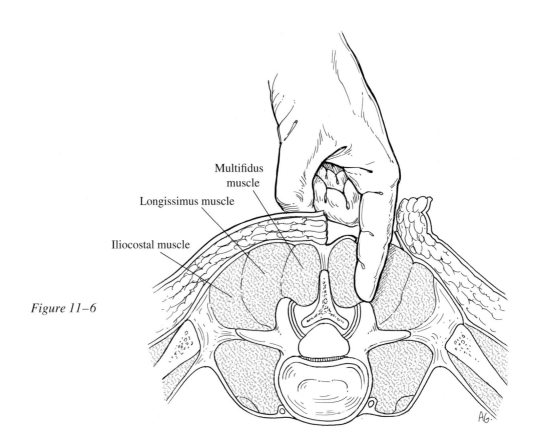

Multifidus
muscle

Longissimus muscle

Iliocostal muscle

*Figure 11–6*

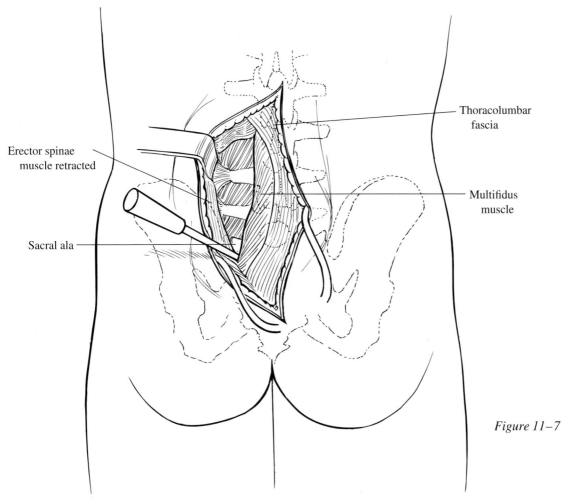

Erector spinae
muscle retracted

Sacral ala

Thoracolumbar
fascia

Multifidus
muscle

*Figure 11–7*

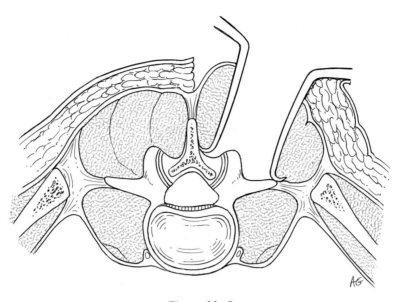

*Figure 11–8*

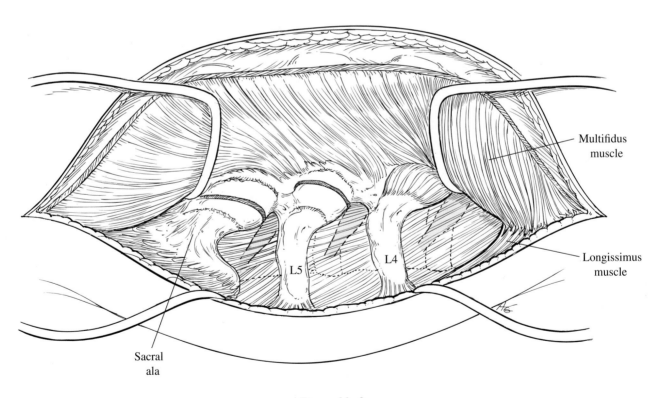

Multifidus
muscle

Longissimus
muscle

Sacral
ala

L5

L4

*Figure 11–9*

413

# Basic Disk Surgery

## STANDARD HEMILAMINOTOMY
## AND DISKECTOMY (L4–5 DISK)

For a routine or "traditional" diskectomy, the approach is midline centered over the level or levels of pathology. Identifying the appropriate level for the skin incision can be done in several ways. When a limited incision is used as in a microdiskectomy, prior to draping the level of incision is identified by placing one or two 20 gauge spinal needles perpendicular to the skin and lateral to the spinous processes of the presumed level by palpation (Fig. 11–10). An antiseptic solution is used to cover the skin at the site of this insertion. A cross-table, lateral x-ray can be taken to confirm the correct level. The second approach is a similar positioning of these needles after the routine prepping and draping of the lower back. A third approach would be that after an initial incision, an instrument is placed in the interlaminar space to mark the level over the presumed lamina or marking a spinous process with a clamp. Ultimately, an x-ray of a metallic probe placed in the disk provides the most accurate determination of level.

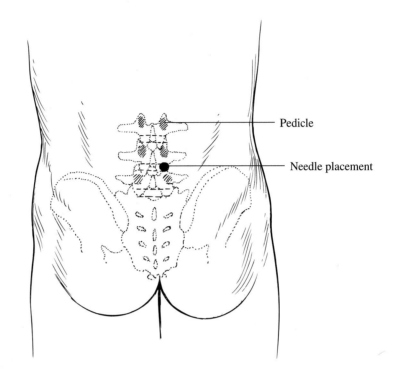

Pedicle

Needle placement

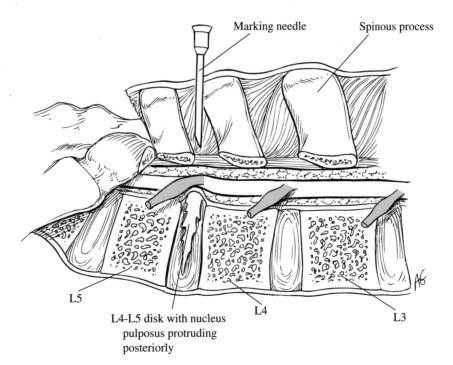

Marking needle

Spinous process

L5

L4-L5 disk with nucleus
pulposus protruding
posteriorly

L4

L3

*Figure 11–10*

An initial skin incision is made consistent with the operative approach. To facilitate hemostasis, the subdermal and subcutaneous tissues down to a level dorsal to the lamina may be infiltrated with 25 to 50 cc of a 1 : 500,000 epinephrine solution. The dermal incision is completed with a scalpel and carried down to the lumbodorsal fascia overlying the spinous processes of L4 and L5. The lumbodorsal fascial attachments to the spinous process and the interspinous and supraspinous ligaments should be maintained. Some surgeons believe that maintaining the lumbodorsal fascial attachment to the spinous process on closure of the wound contributes to spinal stability. Consequently, a slightly paraspinous incision is made into the lumbodorsal fascia just lateral to the bulbous tips of the spinous processes (Fig. 11–11). The length of the incision is based on the extent of exposure. A Cobb elevator with the sharp edge facing medially is inserted in the spinous process of L4 just under its bulbous tip to begin the subperiosteal dissection, which is carried down to the junction of the lamina and the base of the spinous process of L4 and repeated at L5 (Fig. 11–11). With the Cobb elevator reversed so that the flat side faces laterally, the subperiosteal dissection is continued over the L4 lamina, the L4–5 interlaminar area, and the L5 lamina to move the soft tissues laterally to the facet joint capsule of L4–5 (Fig. 11–12A). Avoid injuring the facet capsule. Further removal of soft tissue from the L4–5 interlaminar area is done with a straight curette and/or rongeur.

Once the L4–5 interlaminar area is identified and exposed, a self-retaining retractor is inserted, such as the Williams self-retaining retractor with the blade placed laterally over the facet joint capsule and the pointed tip placed medially, two deep angled Gelpi retractors at both ends of the wound if the exposure is large enough, a Taylor retractor with the point locked under the outer side of the L4–5 facet joint (Fig. 11–12B), or a Selby lateral mass retractor placed under the lateral edge of the L4–5 facet joint after a Cobb elevator or scalpel is used to release the soft tissue attachments to the outer face of the facet. The Williams and deep Gelpi retractors are easily adjustable and require no additional mechanism to maintain their position. The Taylor and Selby retractors can be hand held by an assistant or a gauze pack can be used to create a loop with one end attached to the retractor and the other end attached to a weight that drops lateral to the patient on the operating table, to the foot of the surgeon to maintain the correct amount of tension and retraction, or it can be tied to the operating table out of the sterile field. If a bilateral exposure is being done at the same level, a larger self-retaining retractor, such as the Watanabi retractor, Colles retractor, or Karlin crankshaft retractor, can be used to expose both sides simultaneously.

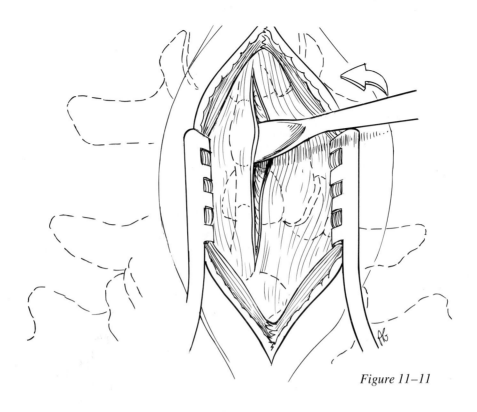

*Figure 11–11*

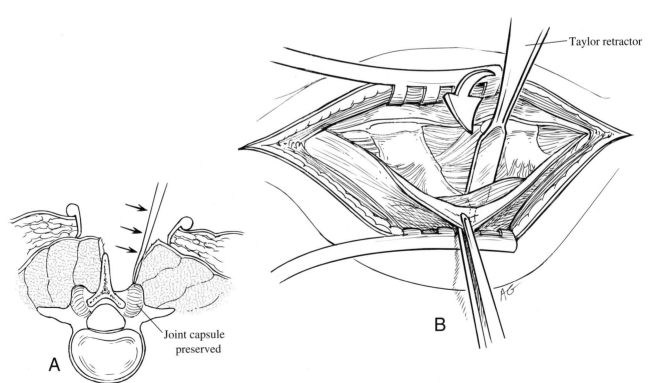

Taylor retractor

Joint capsule
preserved

A

B

*Figure 11–12*

417

After meticulous dissection of the soft tissue in the interlaminar area is carried out, the superficial layer of the ligamentum flavum is identified in the interlaminar space. To gain access to the intraspinal canal, the ligamentum flavum must be transgressed. Depending on the philosophy of the surgeon, the ligamentum flavum can be removed entirely, a portion removed, or it can be split and retracted for later repair. Removal of the lateral half of the ligamentum flavum will best facilitate the exposure. This is done by initially defining the attachment of the ligamentum flavum to the undersurface of the caudal edge of the L4 lamina with an angled curette and to the cephalad edge of L5 using a straight or angled curette. A #15 blade scalpel or a curette is used to create an incision in the superficial layer of the ligamentum flavum located in the lateral third of the interlaminar area. If a scalpel is chosen, feather the blade in such a fashion so the cutting edge is always seen (Fig. 11–13). A curette or #4 Penfield elevator is used to raise from lateral to medial the superficial layer of the ligamentum flavum from the deep portion. An angled Kerrison or pituitary rongeur is used to remove the superficial ligamentum flavum. The deep layer of the ligamentum flavum is now exposed.

The deep layer of the ligamentum flavum is incised in the same fashion as the superficial layer, but greater caution must be exercised because of the proximity of the dura to the undersurface of the deep layer. Consequently, a #4 Penfield elevator will be safer in creating a vertical vent in line with the vertical striations of the deep layer of the ligamentum flavum from lamina to lamina (Fig. 11–14A). Upon traversing this layer, a layer of epidural fat over the dura is often encountered. This cannot be relied on as a protective layer since a large, space-occupying lesion in the spinal canal, such as a herniated disk, may cause the dura to be immediately adjacent to the undersurface of the ligamentum flavum. A Freer-Davis or Penfield #4 elevator can be used to retract the dura medially away from the ligamentum flavum. An angled Kerrison rongeur is used to remove the lateral leaf of the ligamentum flavum (Fig. 11–14B). If more exposure is needed, the angled Kerrison rongeur can be used to remove a portion of the medial leaf of the ligamentum flavum.

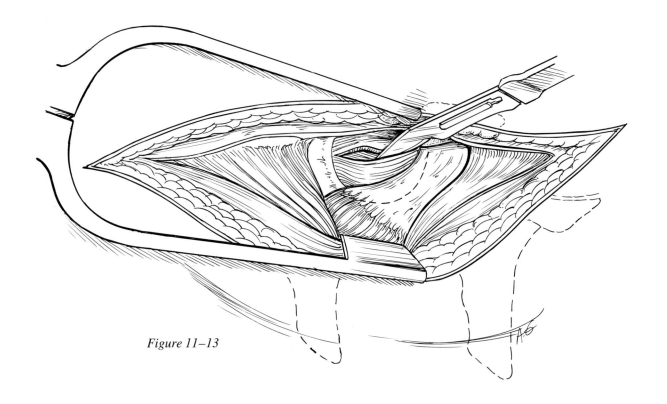

Figure 11–13

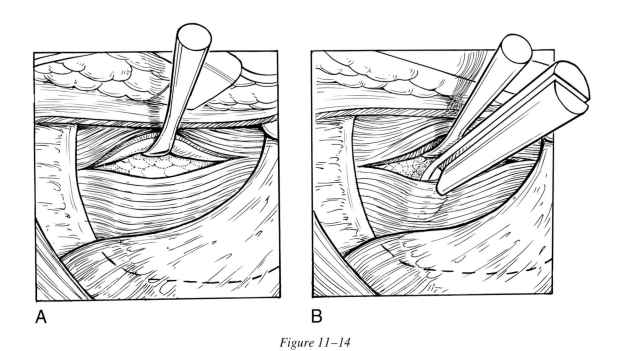

A                                B

Figure 11–14

At this point, the epidural fat, dura, nerve root, and longitudinal blood vessels in the lateral recess are identified. Should this exposure be inadequate, a laminotomy is carried out, removing as much of the inferior edge of the cephalad lamina, superior edge of the caudad lamina, and a portion of the lateral wall as needed. Bone removal may not be necessary at the L5–S1 level, but moving cephalad in the lumbar spine more bone removal is needed, with up to a centimeter of the cephalad lamina requiring resection at the L3–4 level. The facet capsule should not be disturbed (Fig. 11–15).

It is imperative to identify the nerve root prior to exposing the disk (Fig. 11–16). If this is not readily apparent, the constant landmark that represents the key to localizing the nerve roots and the disk is the pedicle. The pedicle can be palpated with a nerve hook or a Murphy hook as well as feeling the neuroforamen at the level of exposure.

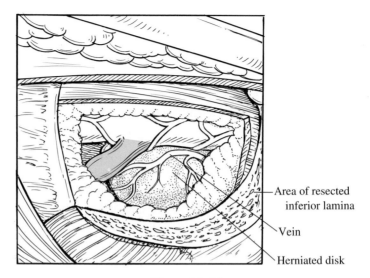

Area of resected
inferior lamina

Vein

Herniated disk

*Figure 11–15*

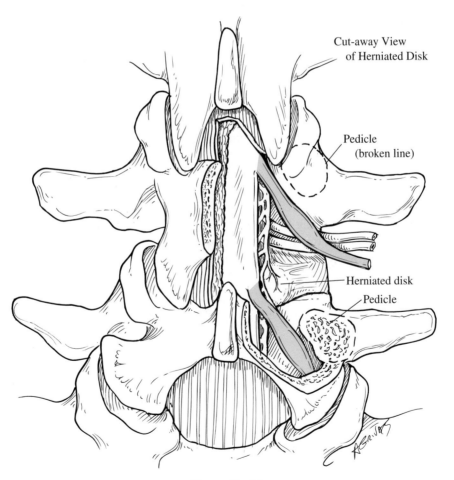

Cut-away View
of Herniated Disk

Pedicle
(broken line)

Herniated disk

Pedicle

*Figure 11–16*

421

A #4 Penfield elevator is used to facilitate exposure of the nerve root by blunt dissection. If soft tissue is not abundant, a nerve root retractor is used to carefully retract the nerve root medially as well as slightly elevating it (Fig. 11–17). No undue tension should be placed on the nerve root. Any bleeding encountered from violation of the epidural veins can be controlled with Surgicel or Gelfoam and Cottonoids placed in the canal above and below the disk or with *bipolar* coagulation. Care should be taken to minimize violation of the epidural veins as this can contribute to increased scar formation and may theoretically contribute to devascularization of intracanal structures.

A second nerve root retractor may be used to retract the thecal sac medially over the disk. A #4 Penfield elevator is used to palpate the disk and bluntly dissect its margins medially, laterally, caudally, and cephalically. However, if an extruded herniated nucleus pulposus is present, it may be immediately identified under the nerve root or in the canal. Epidural bleeding encountered directly over the disk is best controlled with bipolar coagulation. A nerve hook is used to explore the area under the dura and over the disk for extruded fragments of herniated nucleus pulposus that can be pulled out from under the dura or nerve root. Removal of such a fragment may relieve some of the tension on the nerve root and decrease bleeding as well as allowing better visualization. When the herniated nucleus pulposus is encountered, its boundaries are palpated with the nerve hook and an attempt is made to identify a defect in the annulus. If a defect is encountered, the nerve hook is used to sweep the free fragments from the defect to permit insertion of pituitary rongeurs for disk removal. If this defect is located too medially for adequate disk removal, enlarge the defect laterally to gain better exposure.

If no extruded fragments are encountered, the annulus is incised to allow for disk removal with a pituitary rongeur. A minimal annular window can be made with a #4 Penfield rongeur or a slightly larger window can be created with a linear or cruciate incision using a #15 scalpel (Fig. 11–18). If a more thorough diskectomy is intended, a rectangular annular window can be made with a #15 scalpel. Great care should be exercised not to injure the dura and nerve root. This can be facilitated by making the cephalad and caudad incisions separately from medial to lateral away from the dura and completing the rectangle with the scalpel blade facing away from the nerve root.

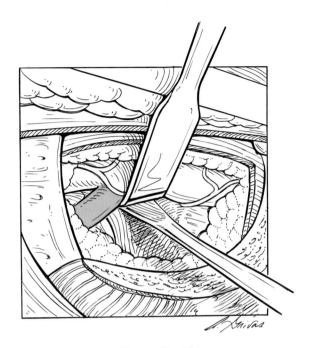

*Figure 11–17*

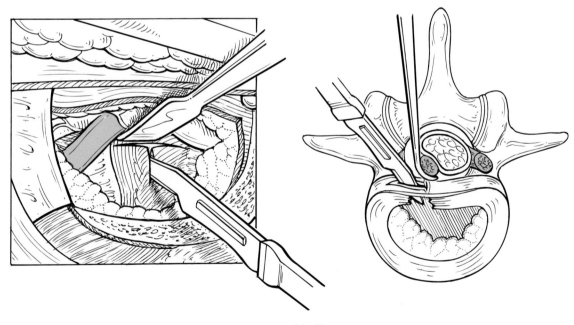

*Figure 11–18*

423

An appropriately sized pituitary rongeur is inserted through the window into the disk to remove any free fragments (Fig. 11–19). The extent of disk material removed is dependent on the surgeon's philosophy and the goals of the procedure. This can range from removal of only the herniated fragment, a so-called "minimal diskectomy"; removal of the herniated portion of the disk and all loose fragments intradiskally; to radical removal of the disk, even bilaterally, in addition to curetting the end plates. Regardless of the extent of disk removal, caution should be exercised in the extent to which the pituitary rongeur is manipulated into the depths of the disk to avoid catastrophic vascular injury anteriorly. This can be avoided by sounding the bottom of the disk and the annulus anteriorly and noting how deep this is on the rongeur or by marking the rongeur relative to the size of the given disk (Fig. 11–20A).

If a more radical diskectomy is to be carried out after the initial removal of free fragments and disk material, a down-pushing curette is used to remove disk material in the midline under the dura as well as disk more laterally located relative to the annulus window (Fig. 11–20B,C). An up and down biting pituitary rongeur can be used to remove the curetted disk material. A straight curette is used to remove more midline and deeper disk material followed by a pituitary rongeur to remove the freed fragments.

Regardless of the amount of disk removed, optimal control of the pituitary rongeur and curette is obtained by placing both hands on the instruments and stabilizing them on the patient to prevent their tips from slipping and injuring anterior structures, the dura, or the nerve root. If an assistant is not available to handle the retraction of the neural structures for exposure, the two-handed technique with the nerve root retractor in the left hand and the pituitary rongeur in the right hand can be undertaken with care. However, there are several self-retaining devices available for neural retraction to allow a surgeon to use both hands when surgical instruments are placed in the depth of the wound near vital structures.

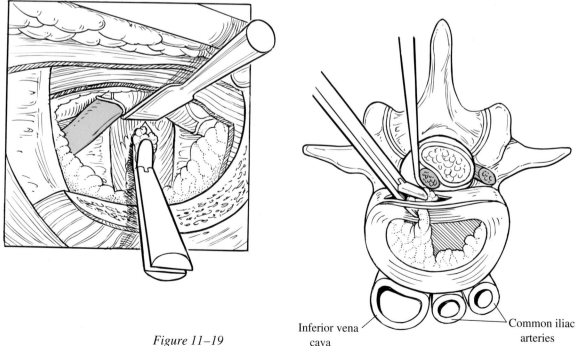

*Figure 11–19*

Inferior vena cava

Common iliac arteries

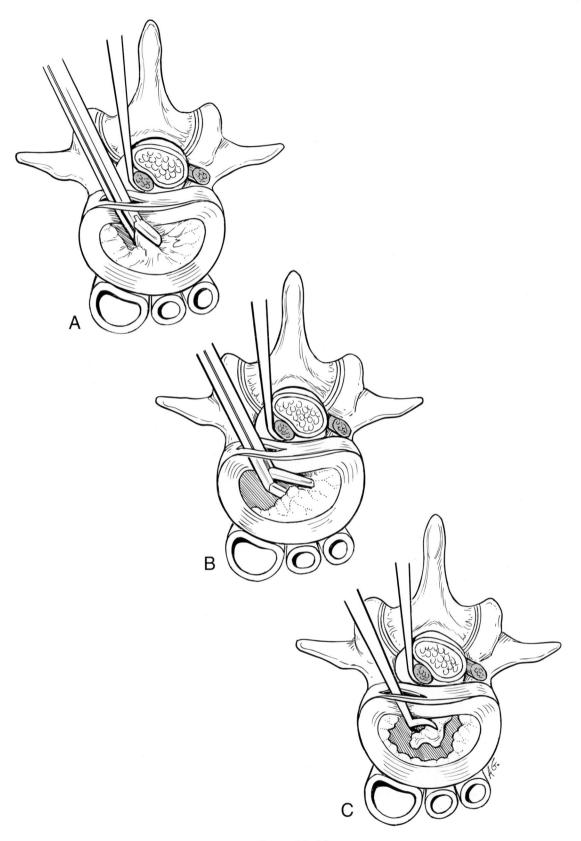

*Figure 11–20*

On completion of the diskectomy, it is important to ascertain that no free fragments remain in the intradiskal space, under the dura or nerve root, or in the neuroforamen. The canal is carefully evaluated with a nerve hook or #4 Penfield rongeur for any missed fragments.

If meticulous hemostasis has been maintained throughout the procedure, the wound should be dry. The wound is profusely irrigated prior to closure. If postoperative epidural narcotics are used for analgesia, a catheter can be placed intraoperatively. Depending on the surgeon's preference and the degree of hemostasis, a deep suction drain can be placed. The wound is closed in layers. If the deep fascial layer has been maintained, it can be reapproximated to the medial portion attached to the spinous process.

# Decompression in Spinal Stenosis (A 3 Level Laminectomy)

A total laminectomy can be indicated for a number of reasons, but its primary purpose is for decompression in central spinal stenosis. A midline approach is recommended.

After dissection and exposure of the laminae with meticulous soft tissue removal from the interlaminar areas above and below the laminae and out to the facet joints, appropriate retractors are inserted. It is important to completely expose the pars interarticularis at the level of the laminectomy as this structure will determine the extent of bone removal. Violating or compromising this structure can lead to postoperative fracture and/or instability.

An intraoperative survey x-ray should be taken if there is any question as to the correct level prior to completion of the exposure or beginning of the laminectomy.

There are a number of techniques to perform a total laminectomy and depending on the pathology encountered, a combination of these techniques can be used. Hand-held instruments such as a Leksell rongeur and angled or 90 degree Kerrison rongeur traditionally have been used.

A box cutter or other large bone cutter is used to remove the spinous process down to the lamina and the interspinous ligaments above and below the spinous process (Fig. 11–21A). If hand-held instruments are preferred, a Leksell rongeur can be used to remove the dorsal portion of the lamina to decrease its thickness, which allows for easier removal with subsequent instruments. Or, the lamina can be thinned with a high-speed burr (Fig. 11–21B). An angled curette is used to expose or dissect the caudal edge of the lamina from the ligamentum flavum. The Leksell rongeur can be used to remove the majority of the lamina if, to create a safe plane, an angled curette or #3 or #4 Penfield elevator is used to release the ligamentum flavum from underneath the lamina and the tip of the Leksell is carefully positioned to prevent dural injury (Fig. 11–22A). Sliding a Cottonoid underneath the lamina provides further protection for the dura. Another alternative for removing the lamina is with an appropriately sized straight or angled Kerrison rongeur (Fig. 11–22B).

426

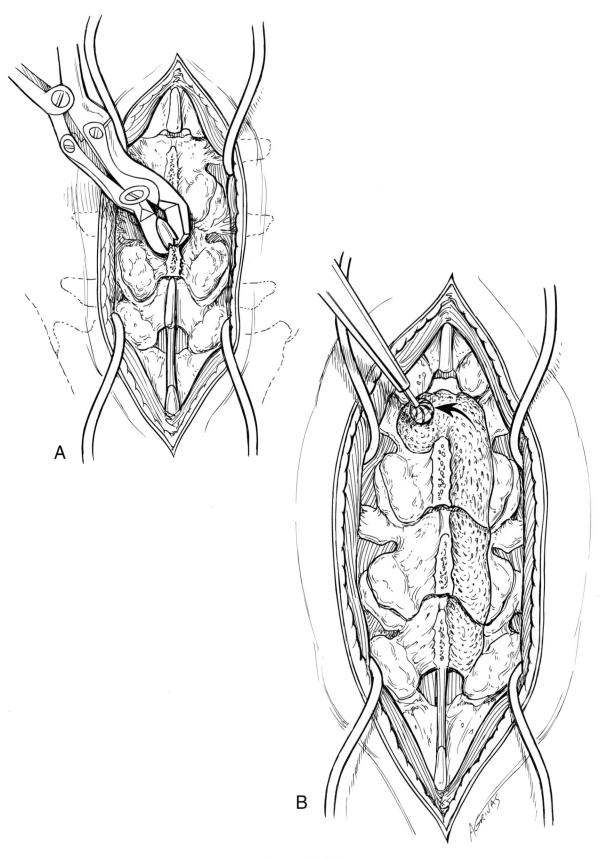

A

B

*Figure 11–21*

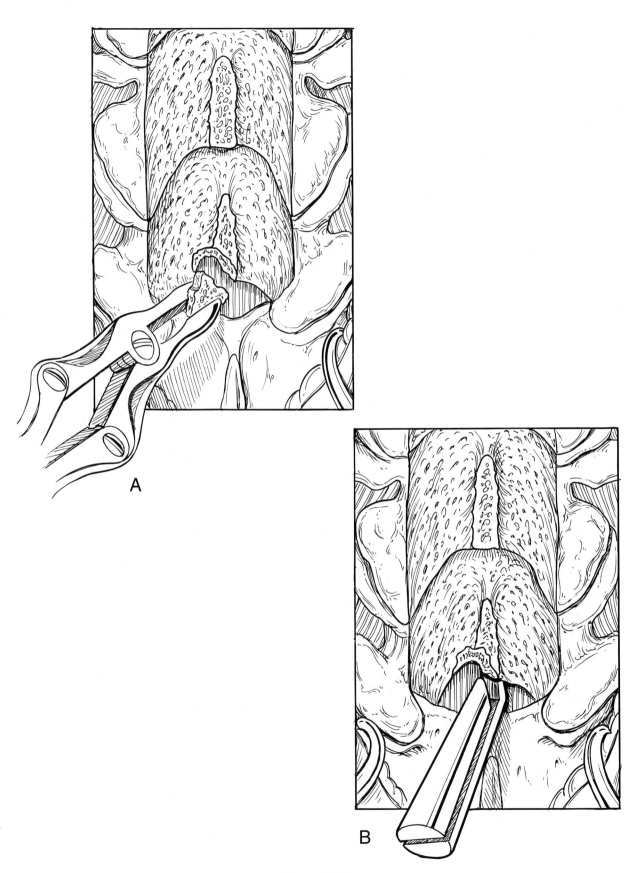

*Figure 11–22*

Once the lamina is removed in its midline, the remaining ligamentum flavum is removed with a scalpel (Fig. 11–23A) or an angled Kerrison rongeur (Fig. 11–23B). The ligamentum flavum is separated from the dura using a #3 or #4 Penfield elevator to depress the dura and resect the ligamentum flavum with the tips of the angled Kerrison rongeur.

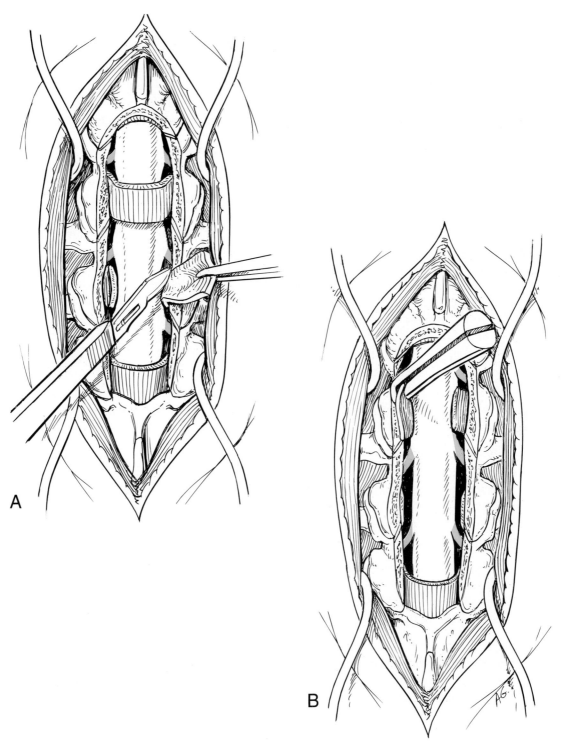

*Figure 11–23*

The remaining lamina at its lateral boundaries is then removed. If the ligamentum flavum is not to be retained, a #4 Penfield elevator is used to separate the dura from the lateral spinal canal wall and an angled Kerrison rongeur is used to remove the remaining lamina up to the medial wall of the pedicle. When hand-held instruments are used, such as an angled Kerrison rongeur, it is helpful to use a Cottonoid to separate the dura and exposed nerve roots from the instruments. Some surgeons prefer to use a 90 degree Kerrison rongeur, which they believe is less likely to result in dural injury. In removing the remaining lateral extent of the lamina and the lateral wall up to the medial edge of the pedicle, it is of paramount importance to expose the pars interarticularis bilaterally so not too much of the pars is removed with resultant fracture. The medial edge of the superior facet is removed during this procedure. It is also important to identify the pedicle and its medial edge, the nerve root, and the extent of osseous resection. The facet capsule and superior and inferior facets (except for undercutting) must be preserved if fusion is not done.

Any other decompressive procedures, such as foraminotomy, uncinate spur removal, and diskectomy, can be carried out through the midline decompression. The exposed dura is covered. Although there is no convincing evidence that any one particular technique is superior in protecting the dura and decreasing scar formation, there are proponents for covering the dura with fat grafts harvested from the midline incision or the buttocks. This does carry a small risk of a cauda equina syndrome which has been documented. Thrombin-soaked Gelfoam, muscle, or synthetic materials have been placed over the dura. Some surgeons, however, choose not to place any material over the dura prior to wound closure. In most cases a deep subfascial drain is placed in the wound.

# LATERAL STENOSIS

A multitude of pathologic conditions can result in lateral or neuroforaminal stenosis. A thorough preoperative assessment utilizing CT scans can clarify the pathoanatomy involved in the stenosis.

Although various approaches to the neuroforamen exist, the most widely used and optimal exposure is a midline approach and a laminectomy. If the pathology is unilateral, a hemilaminectomy is performed. In some circumstances, a laminotomy can be done, but this often makes the decompression difficult depending on the normal anatomy of the lumbar spine of the individual and the pathoanatomy present.

The structures in the lateral wall that can contribute to lateral stenosis are the inferior facet, superior facet, pedicles, herniated disks and uncinate spurs. The goal of the procedure is to resect those offending structures causing compressive phenomena of the nerve root.

A total laminectomy will provide an optimum and safe exposure for visualization and decompression, for dural and nerve root retraction, and for efficient and safe placement of the instruments. Consequently, a midline approach with a total laminectomy is the procedure used for neuroforaminal decompression in this discussion.

The medial portion of the lateral wall is removed as described previously for total laminectomy. It is imperative to maintain the pars interarticularis in adequate dimensions for its integrity and stability. The nerve roots are identified with the key anatomic structure being the pedicle. The medial wall of the pedicle and its inferior border into the neuroforamen are palpated with a nerve hook or Murphy hook (Fig. 11–24). The amount of stenosis in the neuroforamen can be determined by using a Murphy hook in the up-down (cephalad-caudad) and the front-back (anterior-posterior) directions as stenosis in both planes is important. Alternatively, a dural separator or "hockey stick" or gallbladder probes up to a diameter of 5 mm can be used to determine the dimensions of the neuroforamen. These maneuvers serve only to confirm the stenosis and indicate where bony resection needs to take place. Consequently, the preoperative imaging, such as CT scanning with reformatting, is very important.

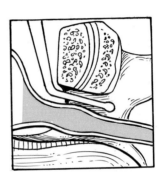

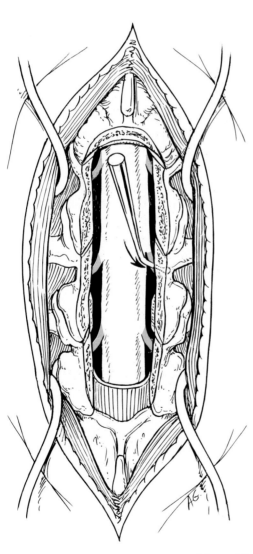

*Figure 11–24*

At this point in the procedure any lateral recess stenosis is resected and herniated disk material removed to optimize exposure and visualization. After the lateral wall has been removed up to the medial margin of the pedicle surrounding the neuroforamen, an appropriate-sized, angled Kerrison rongeur is used to enlarge the opening of the neuroforamen, protecting the nerve root at all times (Fig. 11–25A,B). From small to large Kerrison rongeurs are progressively used to enlarge this opening and reach laterally as far as safely possible without compromising the pars interarticularis. The Kerrison tips are directed dorsally, cephalad, and caudad and can be used to remove a portion of the pedicle if contributing to tension on the nerve root. The remainder of the foraminotomy, to remove the most lateral osseous structures, is best achieved with a series of curved, angled Kerrison rongeurs, which involves following the contour of the curvature underneath the roof of the neuroforamen and hooking the lateral aspect of the opening with the jaws to prevent any neural injury. These curved, angled Kerrison rongeurs can be oriented in the dorsal, cephalad, and caudad directions to complete the osseous decompression (Fig. 11–25C). If the pedicle is causing tethering or increased tension on the nerve root, a portion of the pedicle can be removed with an angled Kerrison. However, this is more easily carried out by careful neural retraction and utilizing small chisels or osteotomes.

Sometimes overlooked contributing pathoanatomy to lateral stenosis is represented by uncinate spurs, which arise from the caudal vertebral body, L5 in this case, and are located cephalad to the L5 pedicle and caudal to the edge of the L4–5 disk space. These can be best seen by CT scans with reformatting. If strategically located and large enough, they can be contributing to nerve root tension with tethering of the nerve root laterally by a foraminal ligament. If this situation exists, a foraminotomy alone is inadequate since there will still be impingement and tension on the nerve root. These spurs can be removed from a caudad to cephalad direction using various types of small chisels placed under the root. The disk below the spur is exposed and a portion adjacent to the spur is removed. The uncinate spur can be removed with a chisel or use a curette to remove the bone underneath the spur and then impact the spur or resect it with an osteotome (Fig. 11–25D).

The nerve root is carefully examined to see that all tension has been removed, and the neuroforamen is probed to identify adequate osseous resection. If multiple foraminotomies are to be performed, the remaining levels are carried out in the same fashion, placing small pledgets of Gelfoam with or without Cottonoids at the completed levels to assist with hemostasis.

The nerve root and dura can be covered with several materials. Some surgeons prefer to place steroid-impregnated Gelfoam over the nerve root to decrease inflammation and postoperative leg pain from a nerve root that is irritated by both stenosis and an inflammatory process. Otherwise, the wound is closed over a suction drain.

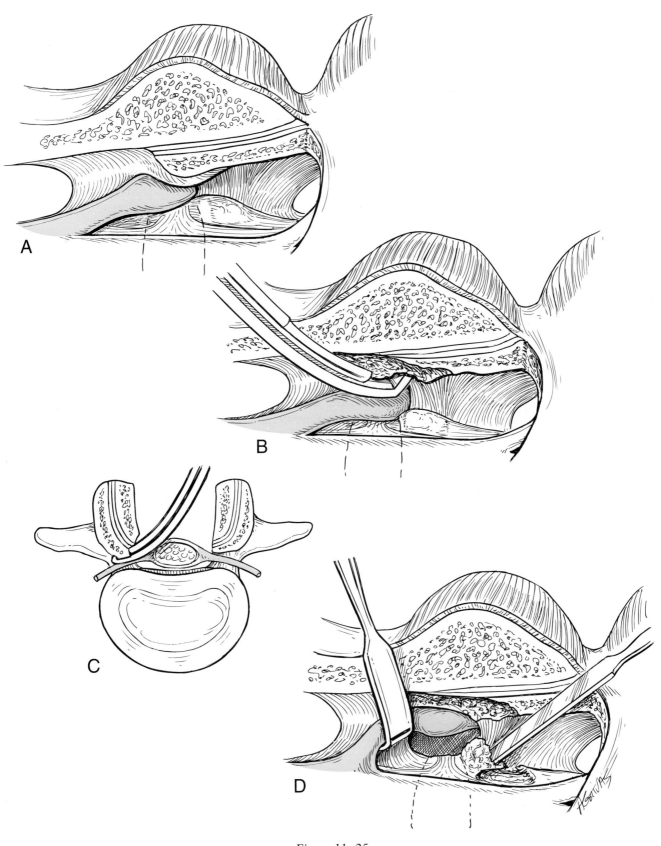

*Figure 11–25*

# *Arthrodesis*

The indications for lumbar fusions are beyond the scope of this atlas. However, the type of fusion selected should be consistent with the surgical goals and consistent with the surgeon's experience and ability.

The key to all posterior fusions is adequate exposure of the structures to be fused with meticulous soft tissue removal and decortication utilizing the full extent of the posterolateral structures available. Autologous bone graft is preferred for posterior and posterolateral fusions in the lumbar spine. For the procedures to be described, the graft source is the posterior iliac crest and is usually harvested through the same midline incision.

## POSTEROLATERAL FUSION L4–S1 THROUGH A MIDLINE APPROACH WITHOUT INSTRUMENTATION

Following induction of anesthesia, intubation, and placement of appropriate monitors and a Foley catheter, the patient is transferred to the operating table in the prone position with a spine frame to maintain normal lumbar lordosis. The lumbar spine is prepared and draped in the usual sterile fashion after which a midline approach is utilized to expose the posterolateral structures of L4 and L5 out to the tips of the transverse processes (Fig. 11–26). If there is any question as to the correct levels, an intraoperative x-ray should be taken prior to the exposure. The type of retraction used for optimal exposure is dependent on what is available and surgeon preference. Various types of hand-held and self-retaining retractors have been previously described. During the exposure, it is often necessary to excise some of the paraspinal muscles over the intertransverse membrane and transverse processes not only for exposure but to create a space for the bone graft. Too much muscle removal increases the dead space and too little removal can put undue stress and tension on the paraspinal muscles.

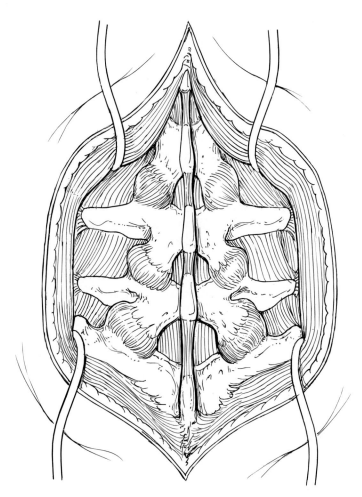

*Figure 11–26*

After meticulous removal of all soft tissues from all posterolateral structures of L4, L5, and S1, an incision with a scalpel or electrocautery is made at the tips of the transverse processes of L4 and L5 on one side. Wiltse transverse process retractors are placed with their blunt ends under the tips of the transverse processes (Fig. 11–27). This allows for adequate exposure to further remove the soft tissue from the transverse processes as well as the paraspinal musculature overlying the intertransverse membrane. Great care is taken to retain this limiting membrane as it is the structural support where the bone graft will lie and its integrity protects the underlying nerve root at that level. The paraspinal musculature over the transverse membrane can be removed by sweeping over the intertransverse membrane with a Cobb elevator or can be removed with a Leksell rongeur or a large pituitary rongeur if it is at all adherent to this membrane. Various curettes can then be used to remove soft tissue from the lateral wall including the outer face of the superior facet of L4 and L5 as well as the pars interarticularis and the L4–5 and L5–S1 facets. The capsules from the facets are removed and the posterior three quarters of the facet joint is denuded of its cartilaginous surfaces with osteotomes, rongeurs, or a burr (Fig. 11–28). This side of the wound is then packed off with sponges.

The same procedure is repeated on the opposite side. The wound is profusely irrigated and packed off with sponges bilaterally. The posterior iliac graft is harvested from either the right or left side at the surgeon's discretion. The procedure for harvesting of posterior iliac crest graft is described elsewhere (see page 522). After the graft has been harvested, the iliac donor site is profusely irrigated and packed with a lap sponge (the use of smaller sponges is discouraged as they can be overlooked at the time of closure). Some surgeons prefer to apply bone wax or Gelfoam to the iliac donor site to aid hemostasis. The harvested bone graft is given to the nurse or surgical assistant for preparation prior to its insertion.

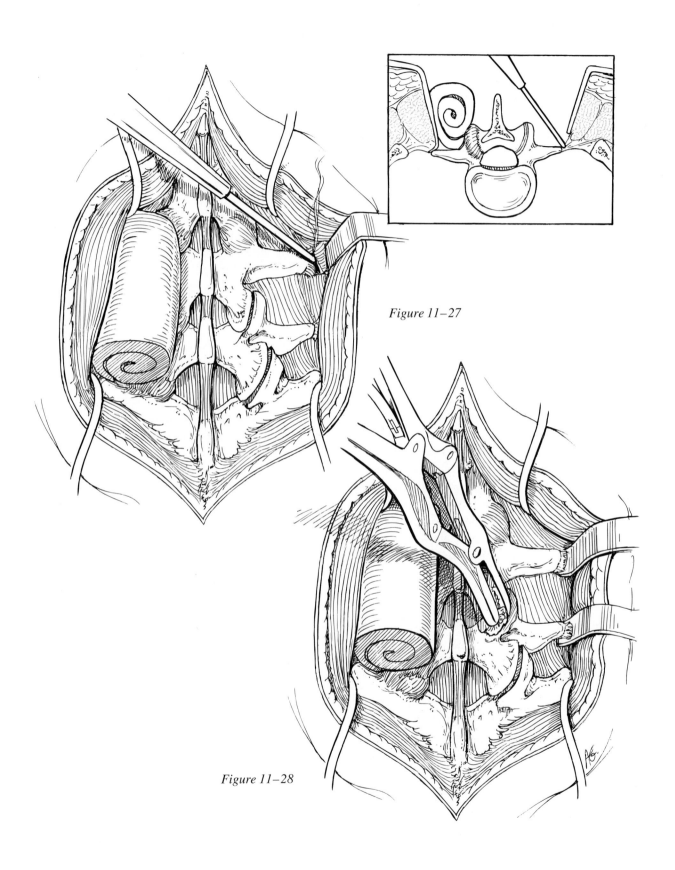

*Figure 11–27*

*Figure 11–28*

437

Next, decortication of the exposed posterolateral structures of L4, L5, and sacrum on one side only is carried out. High-speed burrs, various sized straight and angled curettes, rongeurs (with and without teeth), or various gouges can be used. Regardless of the technique chosen, decortication should be done systematically on one side at the outer face of the superior facet of L4 and then proceed down to the transverse process of L4. A rat-tooth or a needle-nosed Leksell rongeur can be used to carefully decorticate the transverse process of L4 and L5 to maintain integrity of the transverse process and create a bleeding recipient bed (Fig. 11–29). If the transverse processes are particularly fragile, a burr can be used with the least amount of trauma (Fig. 11–30). However, others have described the use of a curette to decorticate the transverse processes sweeping in a lateral to medial direction (Fig. 11–31). The pars intra-articularis of L4 and L5 and the outer face of the superior facet of L5 and S1 are similarly decorticated. If the facet joints were not decorticated as part of the cartilage removal, this is now completed using a needle-nosed Leksell rongeur, an osteotome as described by Moe (Fig. 11–32A), or a burr. An appropriately fashioned rectangular piece of cancellous graft is then carefully impacted into the L4–5 and L5–S1 facets (Fig. 11–32B).

With the decortication completed on one side, the next step is to complete the placement of cancellous and corticocancellous strips over the decorticated recipient site. The iliac graft should have been prepared prior to this step by morselizing a portion of the graft and preparing the corticocancellous strips with removal of any remnant soft tissues. A Cobb elevator is placed in the cephalad end of the wound to prevent migration of the graft in a cephalad direction. Wiltse transverse process retractors are placed under the tips of the L4 and L5 transverse processes. Grafting then begins in a systematic fashion at the outer face of the superior facet of L4 with placement of cancellous morselized grafts (Fig. 11–32C). Long strips of cancellous or corticocancellous grafts are then placed to span the gap over the intertransverse membrane from the L4 to L5 transverse processes and all of the sacrum (Fig. 11–33A). Some surgeons prefer to take a corticocancellous strip of allograft and wedge it underneath the transverse processes. However, this places the nerve root under the intertransverse membrane at risk. Morselized graft is then placed to fill voids and cover all remaining decorticated structures (Fig. 11–33B). If laminae are present, they should also be decorticated and grafted. The Cobb elevator and the Wiltse transverse process retractors are carefully removed in order not to displace any of the bone graft. Decortication and placement of graft is then carried out on the opposite side in the same systematic fashion.

All retractors are carefully removed in order not to displace the graft. The paraspinal muscles are carefully retracted over the graft to secure its position. Any devitalized paraspinal muscle is resected. One or two suction drains can be placed deep to the fascial layer or above the fascial layer dependent on the surgeon's philosophy and the needs of the individual case. The wound is closed in anatomic layers as previously described with the closure of the posterior iliac donor site over a deep suction drain, making certain that no sponges have been left in the donor site or midline area.

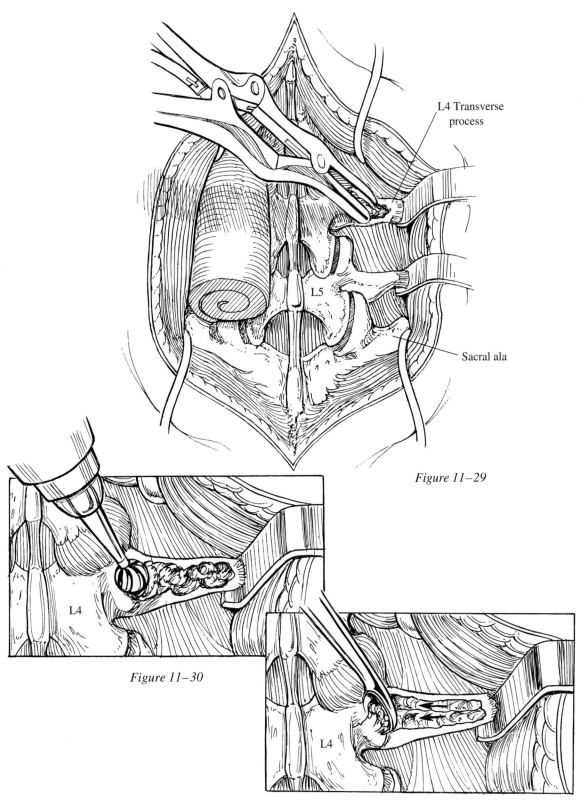

L4 Transverse process

Sacral ala

L5

*Figure 11–29*

L4

*Figure 11–30*

L4

*Figure 11–31*

439

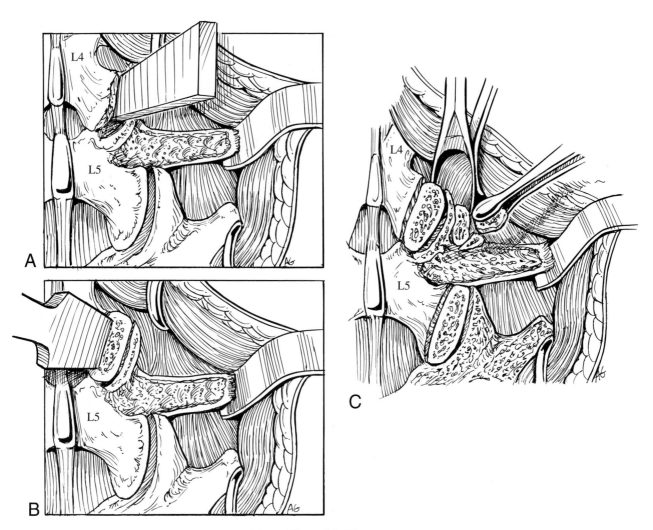

*Figure 11–32*

440

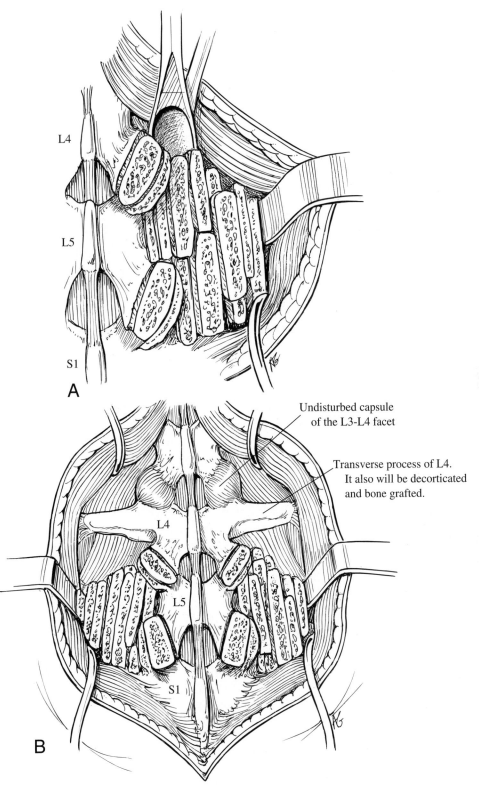

A

Undisturbed capsule
of the L3-L4 facet

Transverse process of L4.
It also will be decorticated
and bone grafted.

B

*Figure 11–33*

441

It is important to approach all fusion procedures in a systematic fashion to increase surgical efficiency and accomplish the ultimate goal of a solid arthrodesis. Meticulous soft tissue removal from the structures to be fused and decortication using the maximum area available for fusion are of paramount importance. Hemostasis is to be emphasized throughout the procedure with vigilance for all bleeders and packing off the portions of the wound that are not being worked on. The importance of hemostasis in not only to provide for optimal visualization of the surgical site but to decrease the transfusion requirements and their attendant risks. Electrocautery (cutting and coagulation modes), Gelfoam or Surgicel, bone wax, and a bipolar cautery should be available in all fusion cases. Attention to these details will lead to a more optimum outcome for all involved.

The paraspinal approach of Wiltse has been previously described (see page 410). As in the posterolateral in situ fusion of L4–S1, bone graft can be harvested through the same midline incision from the posterior iliac crest.

After the paraspinal approach has exposed the posterolateral structures of L5 and S1, all soft tissue is removed from these structures with various sized straight and angled curettes (Fig. 11–34). Debulking of the paraspinal musculature both medially and laterally is generally necessary to create a space for the subsequent fusion mass. This is carried out bilaterally after which both paraspinal wounds are irrigated and packed off.

The bone graft is harvested from one of the posterior iliac crest sites as indicated. The iliac donor site is packed off and the retractors are repositioned to expose one side. Decortication of the posterolateral structures of L5 and S1 is done using curettes, gouges, rongeurs, or a high-speed burr. Decortication is done systematically beginning at the outer base of the superior facet of L5 and continues to the transverse process of L5 and to the sacral ala. The L5–S1 facet and its posterior three fourths is decorticated of cartilage using an osteotome, curettes, a needle-nosed Leksell rongeur, or a high-speed burr. An alternative to decorticating the sacral ala is to create a flap of bone in the sacral ala that is reflected on top of the intertransverse membrane up to the caudal edge of the L5 transverse process (Fig. 11–35). Some believe this is a form of a vascularized flap graft. The fusion is carried out by placing a Cobb elevator just cephalad to the outer face of the superior facet of L5 with placement of cancellous bone followed by placement of either morselized cancellous or corticocancellous graft over the posterolateral structures of L5 and S1, or creating matchstick grafts of cancellous and/or corticocancellous graft to span the area between the L5 transverse process and the sacral ala. An appropriately fashioned plug of cancellous bone is placed in the decorticated facet joint of L5–S1 (Fig. 11–36). The paraspinal musculature is then carefully pulled over the graft to prevent its displacement. The same procedure is then carried out on the opposite side (Fig. 11–37).

Hemostasis is achieved, any devitalized paraspinal muscle is resected, and the wound is closed in anatomic layers over suction drains deep to the paraspinal fascia or superficial to it, depending on the surgeon's philosophy. The posterior iliac crest donor site is also closed over a deep suction drain.

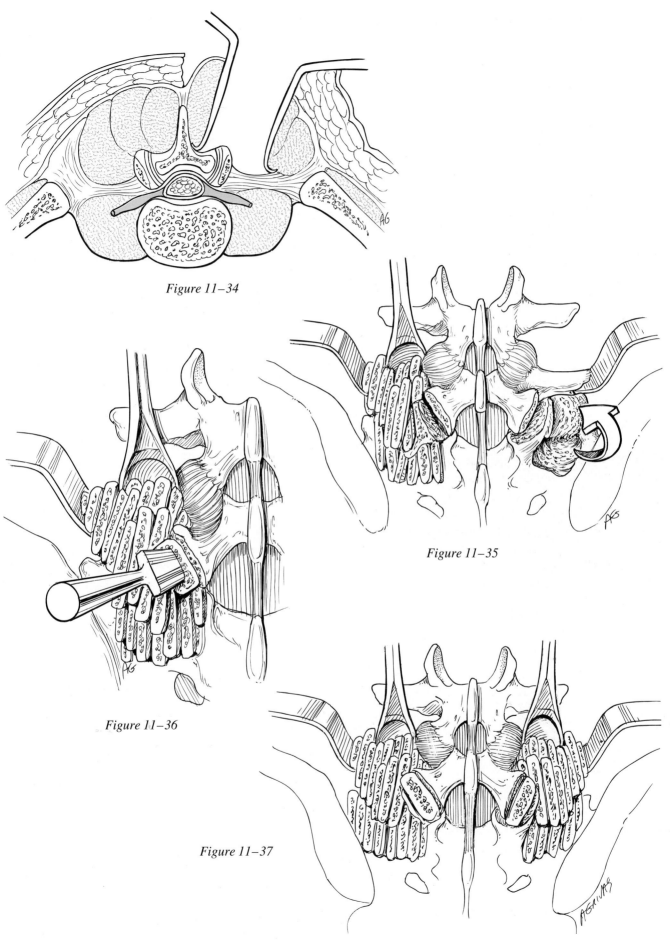

Figure 11–34

Figure 11–35

Figure 11–36

Figure 11–37

# Pedicle Procedures

After standard patient positioning and exposure, the most common exposure is the L4 to sacrum area (Fig. 11–38). Transverse processes and sacral ala should be well visualized and clean. The authors prefer the patient positioned in a more anatomic alignment with some lordosis rather than in the knee/chest flexion position, which eliminates lumbar lordosis. This latter position makes exposure of the intraspinal contents easier, but when internal fixation is used, it will tend to produce a position of fixation, which is not a normal lordosis for that patient.

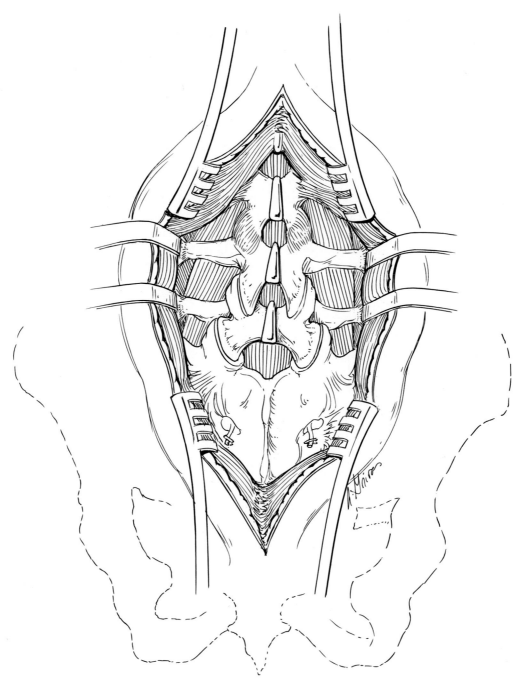

*Figure 11–38*

445

The optimal point of pedicle screw insertion is at the junction of the pars inter-articularis, the midpoint of the transverse process, and the inferior point of the superior articular facet (Fig. 11–39). It may be necessary to enter the pedicle slightly more laterally at the base of the transverse process just as it comes up into the superior articular process in order to have the fixation lateral enough to avoid any impingement on the intact facet joint and capsule at the first motion segment, L3–4. The sacral pedicle screw is located directly over the top of the sacral pedicle which is quite large, and the L5 pedicle screw should be on line between the L4 and the sacral pedicle screw to make insertion easy.

The small window made in the L5 pedicle screw insertion point can be made with a small burr, a curette, or an awl (Fig. 11–40). A blunt pedicle probe is inserted down the pathway of the pedicle. Thorough knowledge of pedicle anatomy is critical since the direction of the pedicle probe must match that particular vertebra. In the L4 and L5 region, the pedicle probe is angled inward about 15 degrees from vertical. The probe should be passed deep enough to enter the vertebral body but not so deep as to penetrate the anterior cortex. The authors prefer a depth gauge with centimeter markings (Fig. 11–41). Other surgeons prefer to use a #3–0 curette to make this passageway. The passing of the probe is done by feel of the surgeon as the canal of the pedicle is very cancellous bone, and its periphery is fairly firm cortical bone except in the very osteoporotic older individual. Not only is there the medial tilt of 15 degrees, but also there is a varying degree of cephalad or caudad tilt according to the alignment of that particular vertebra, which can best be determined by viewing lateral cross-table x-rays in the operating room.

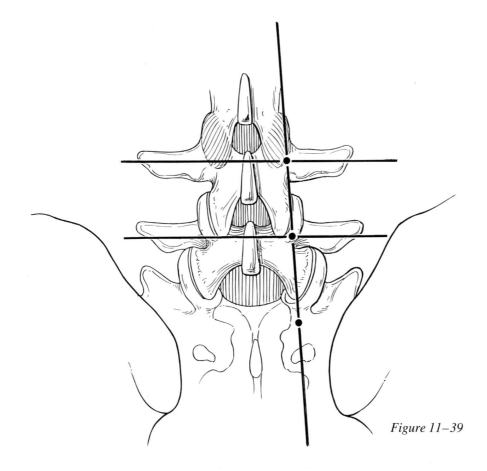

*Figure 11–39*

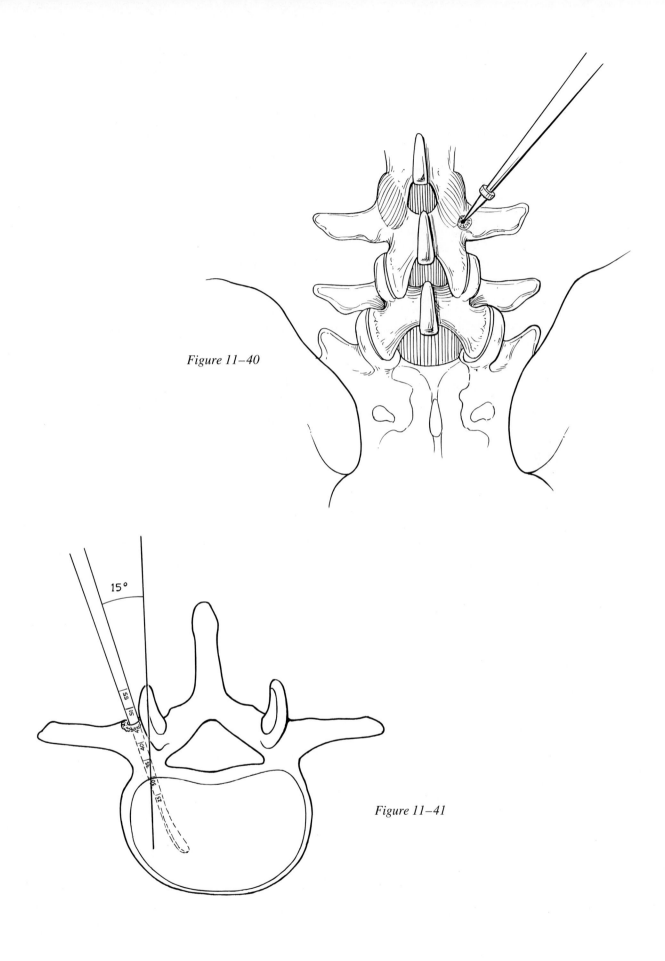

*Figure 11–40*

*Figure 11–41*

15°

On the sacrum, the same general angle of 15 degrees is usually optimal (Fig. 11–42). The bone of the sacrum is usually more osteopenic. Once the dorsal cortex is penetrated, it is very easy to pass down the cancellous bone until the hard cortical bone of the anterior cortex is reached, which can easily be felt or heard if the end of the pedicle probe is tapped with a mallet.

At this point, a depth gauge or other type of feeler should be passed down the passageway and all four quadrants should be palpated for bony integrity. This is a manual sensation in the fingertips of the surgeon and cannot be substituted with an x-ray or other device. For example, if no resistance along the medial wall of the pedicle is felt, then immediately redirect the probe and do not pursue the pathway.

If the spinal canal has been opened, for example, for decompression, then the nerve root is easily seen in this area; retract it gently in the area of the pedicle, and place a probe or blunt elevator along the medial wall of the pedicle to feel its position as well as any penetration of the medial wall.

Once all of the pedicle passages have been determined by vision and manual feel, the surgeon may place metallic markers in each pedicle and obtain a radiographic image, either a film or an image intensifier picture, to confirm position.

In extremely osteopenic bone where adequate purchase is not achieved, penetration of the anterior cortex of the sacrum is usually required. This should be done in the midportion of the sacral vertebral body and not in the alar area where there are nerves and other vital structures. Figure 11–43 shows a drill being passed through the anterior cortex. It is preferable to do this drilling by hand to gain the feel of passage through the cortex.

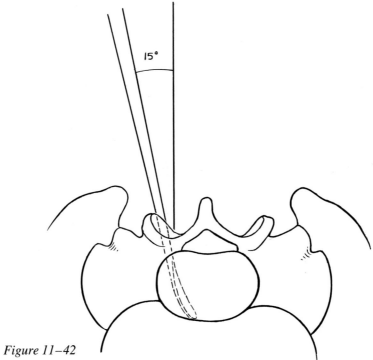

Figure 11–42

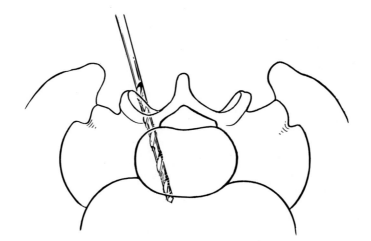

Figure 11–43

Some surgeons prefer to tap the pedicle with a tap the same size as the screw or one size smaller. In the patient with osteopenic bone this is seldom necessary, but it is necessary in the patient with very hard, firm bone. If the canal is open, palpate along the medial wall of the pedicle. If any of the threads of the tap come through, they can be immediately detected. Tapping should not be done until one is absolutely sure of the proper pathway of the pedicle (Fig. 11–44).

At this point, having confirmed the proper position and tapped if necessary, the screw is inserted. Figure 11–45A illustrates the insertion of a standard bone screw with a screwdriver.

The screw is inserted fully into the pedicle and about 2/3 to 3/4 into the vertebral body (Fig. 11–45B). It is not advisable to penetrate the anterior cortex as there are major blood vessels in this area, particularly at the L4 and L5 levels.

Figure 11–45C illustrates penetration of the anterior cortex of the sacrum with the pedicle screw when it is required.

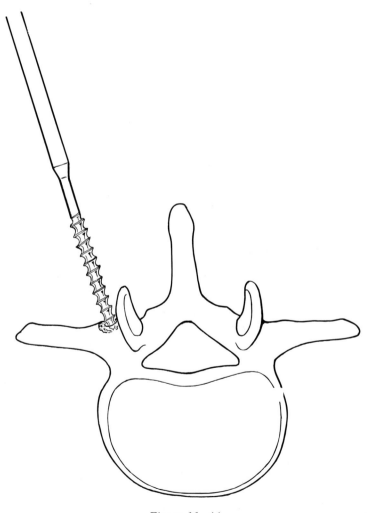

*Figure 11–44*

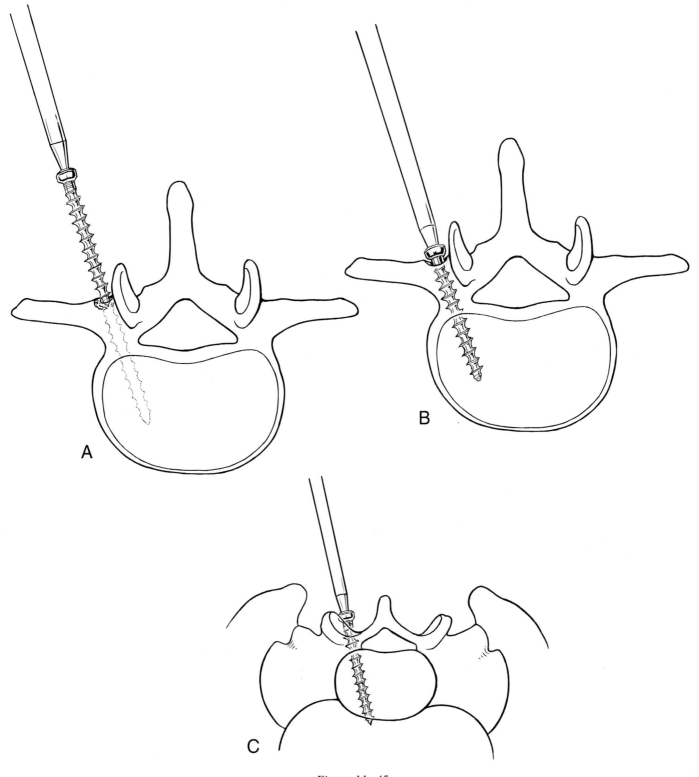

*Figure 11–45*

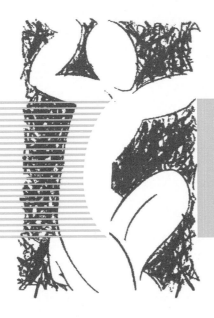

# SPONDYLOLISTHESIS AND OSTEOTOMY SURGERY

# Bohlman Technique

Smith and Bohlman have described a one-stage posterior decompression and posterolateral fusion combined with a lumbosacral interbody fusion through a posterior approach for L5–S1 severe spondylolisthesis. This procedure allows for adequate posterior decompression and an interbody fusion providing immediate stability of the lumbosacral junction with increased fusion potential in cases of spondylolisthesis that are grade III or greater in severity.

A midline exposure from the spinous processes of L3 down to S3 is executed and the posterolateral structures bilaterally from L4 to S3 are exposed (Fig. 12–1A). The loose posterior element of L5 is removed with complete decompression of the L5 nerve roots bilaterally and the lamina of S1 is removed. It may be necessary to remove a portion of the S2 lamina to allow for adequate dural and nerve root retraction as well as safe placement of the cannulated drill for the interbody graft placement. At this point in the procedure there should be complete visualization of the dura and nerve roots bilaterally from L4 to S3 (Fig. 12–1B).

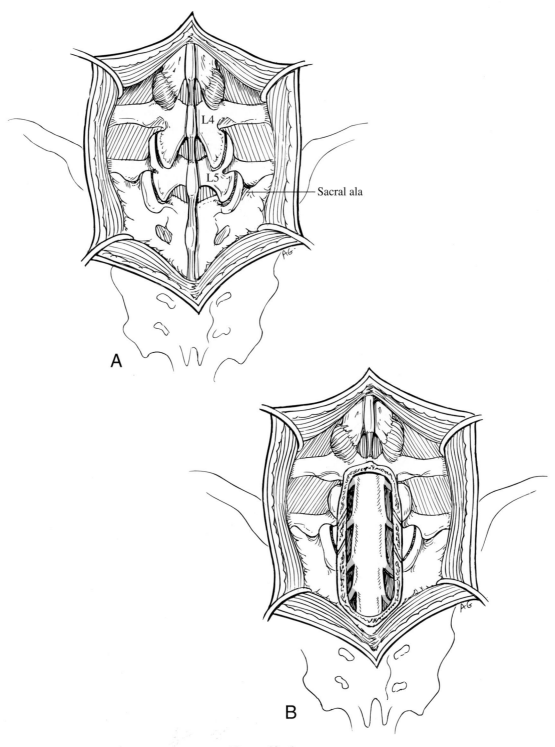

L4

L5

Sacral ala

A

B

*Figure 12–1*

# SPONDYLOLISTHESIS AND OSTEOTOMY SURGERY

The dura is then carefully retracted medially with no undue tension on the nerve roots from whichever side allows greater exposure to the posterior cortex of S1. The posterior cephalad portion of the sacral dome contributing to central stenosis is then carefully removed with an osteotome when preoperative myelography demonstrates a high-grade block owing to posterior sacral obstruction (Fig. 12–2A,B). The dura is retracted first to one side and then to the other so it is possible to work underneath the dura and completely remove the bump so that the dural sac is displaced forward. This decompresses the sacral roots; but, of course, it does not have any impact on the L5 roots, which are compressed more proximally (Fig. 12–2C). After removing the dome, it is possible to proceed forward to resect the disk (Fig. 12–2D, Pt. B) and the end plate of L5. This view is facilitated by removing the remainder of S1. The bone from the bump is returned to the bed as a cancellous bone graft. This is then coupled with a posterolateral L4 to sacrum fusion (Fig. 12–2E).

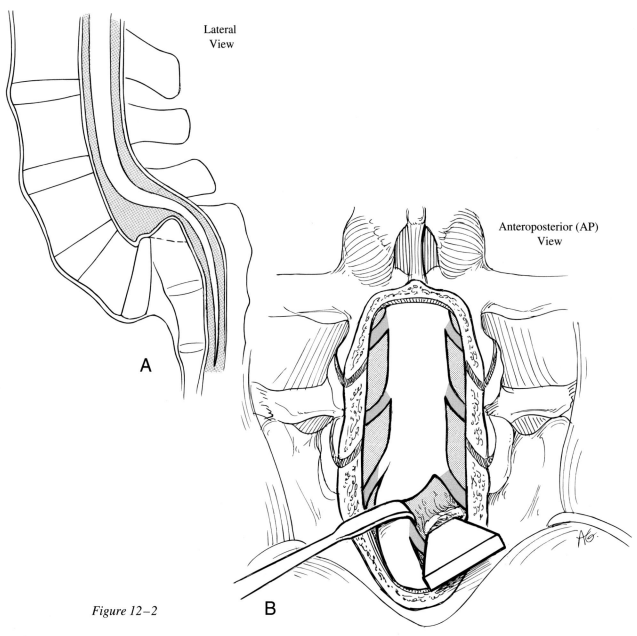

Lateral View

Anteroposterior (AP) View

A

B

*Figure 12–2*

456

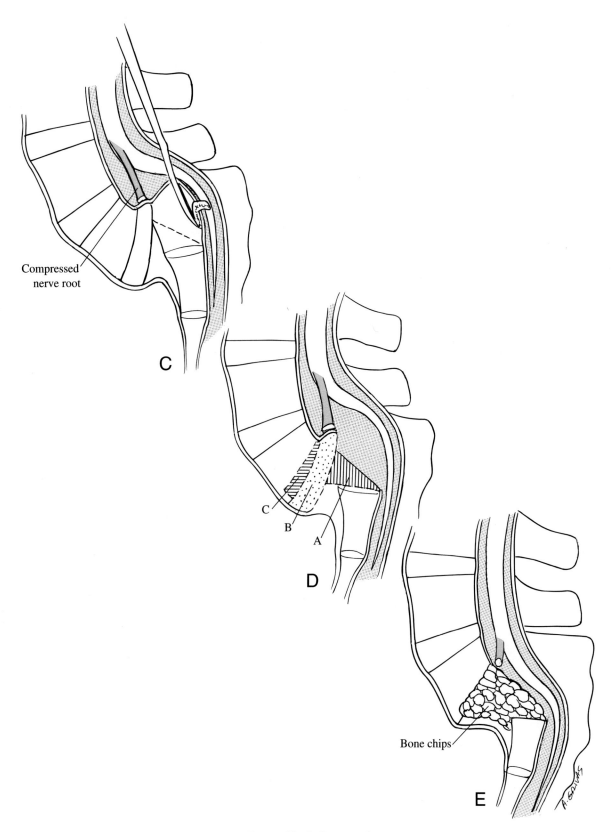

Compressed
nerve root

C

C
B
A

D

Bone chips

E

*Figure 12–2 Continued*

457

For the Bohlman technique an appropriately sized K-wire Steinmann pin for the cannulated drill is then placed through the posterior cortex of S1, through the S1 vertebral body, and through the L5–S1 interspace, and into the L5 vertebral body to its anterior cephalad cortex (Fig. 12–3). The cannulated drill is placed over this guide wire and attached to a hand-held apparatus. It is important to select the appropriately sized cannulated drill to accommodate the diameter of the fibular graft to be used to achieve a snug fit and prevent its migration. The drill is slowly and carefully turned to progress through the S1 vertebral body, the L5–S1 interspace, and up to the anterior cephalad cortex of the L5 vertebral body (Fig. 12–4).

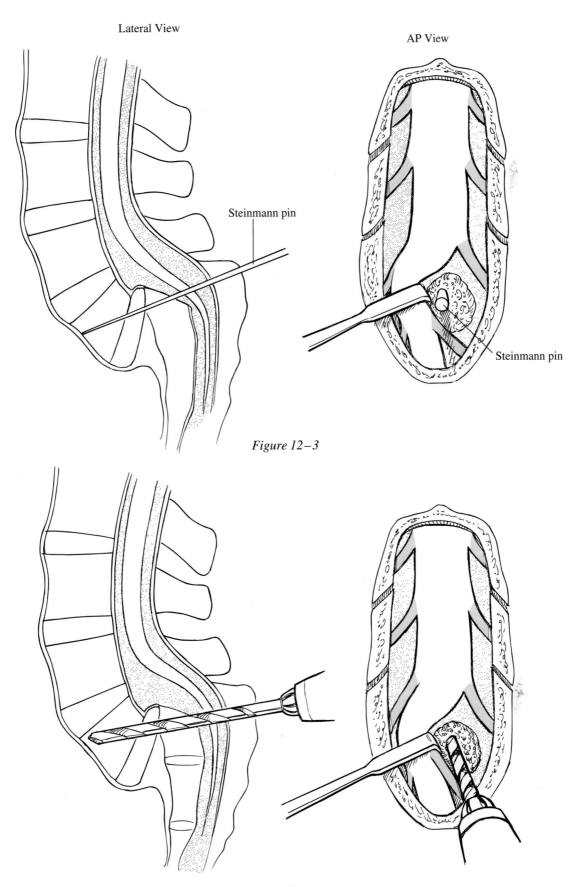

Lateral View

AP View

Steinmann pin

Steinmann pin

*Figure 12–3*

*Figure 12–4*

459

Portable cross-table, lateral x-rays are taken to confirm positioning of the guide wire and the depth of penetration of the cannulated drill to prevent any damage to the anterior structures. The fibular graft is placed into the hole created by the drill and carefully impacted anteriorly up to the cortical edge of the anterior cephalad surface of the L5 vertebral body (Fig. 12–5). Intraoperative x-rays are taken to confirm the placement of the graft. The remainder of the posterolateral fusion is carried out as described for L4–S1 (see page 434).

This procedure was initially described by Bohlman and Cook. However, others have modified the technique to include the use of C-arm image intensification for placement of the guide wire and cannulated drill as well as internal fixation. Smith and Bohlman do not believe internal fixation is necessary given the inherent stability of the fibular interbody construct.

This procedure can be relatively easy to perform; but great care should be taken with regard to retraction of the dura and nerve roots to prevent any neural injuries, which represents one of the more significant complications associated with this procedure. As well, the drill and subsequent fibular strut should be placed through the midline, if possible, and directed straight midline into the middle anterior cephalad portion of the L5 vertebral body.

Lateral View

AP View

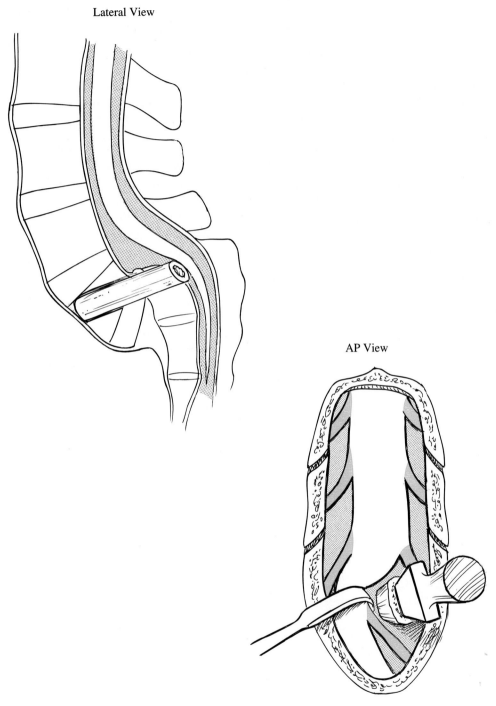

*Figure 12–5*

461

# Kellogg-Speed Technique

The Kellogg-Speed technique is used for an anterior interbody fusion of L5–S1 for spondylolisthesis generally greater than grade II in severity when an interbody fusion is deemed necessary and other techniques are not possible because of the pathoanatomic constraints involved. Although its use has been described as an isolated technique for anterior fusion alone, many spine surgeons would advocate its use only in conjunction with a posterior procedure (Fig. 12–6A).

The direct anterior approach to L5–S1 is performed through a transperitoneal approach with maximum anterior exposure (Fig. 12–6B,C). Depending on the degree of spondylolisthesis, this can be a difficult exposure with the L5 vertebral body placed deep in the pelvis. Also, this technique can be difficult depending on the positioning of the bifurcation of the aorta and vena cava. The disk space of L4–5 is identified intraoperatively. X-rays are taken if there is any question as to the correct level.

Based on preoperative and intraoperative x-rays, the appropriate angle and depth for a drill to be inserted and passed through the body of the L5 vertebra into S1 are determined. With the patient in the supine position, the direction is approximately perpendicular to the floor. It is of paramount importance to have adequate exposure with careful retraction of the vascular structures at risk.

Lateral View

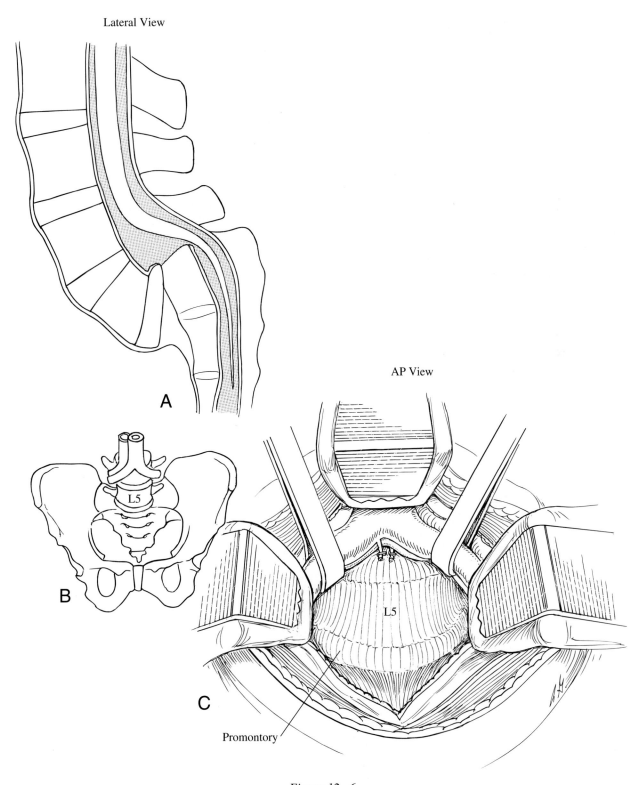

AP View

A

B

C

L5

L5

Promontory

Figure 12–6

463

Using a cannulated drill apparatus, generally one-half inch wide, the surgeon places an appropriately sized Steinmann pin or K-wire from the anterior cephalad portion of the L5 vertebral body just under the L4–5 disk through the L5 vertebral body, through the L5–S1 interspace, and into the S1 vertebral body up to but not through the posterior cortex of the S1 vertebral body (Fig. 12–7). This can be facilitated by using C-arm image intensification or portable cross-table, lateral x-rays with repositioning of the pin as indicated. The guide pin must be placed centrally in both the L5 and S1 vertebral bodies to avoid any injury to neural structures. The cannulated drill is placed over the guide pin. The drill can be attached to a power source or a hand-held device. The drill is carefully advanced down the guide wire and allowed to follow the course of the guide pin. The cannulated drill is advanced over the guide wire, through the vertebral body of L5, and through the L5–S1 interspace. Advancing the drill is easier until the body of the sacrum is reached, hereafter it can become more difficult. The goal is to carry the drill up to but not through the posterior cortex of the S1 vertebral body (Fig. 12–8). The drill is removed along with the guide pin. The depth can be determined from the guide pin, the C-arm, or with portable cross-table x-rays.

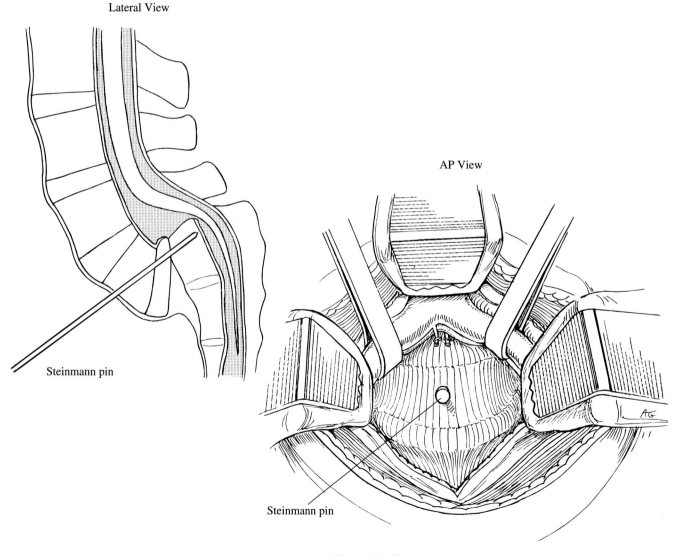

Lateral View

Steinmann pin

AP View

Steinmann pin

*Figure 12–7*

Lateral View

AP View

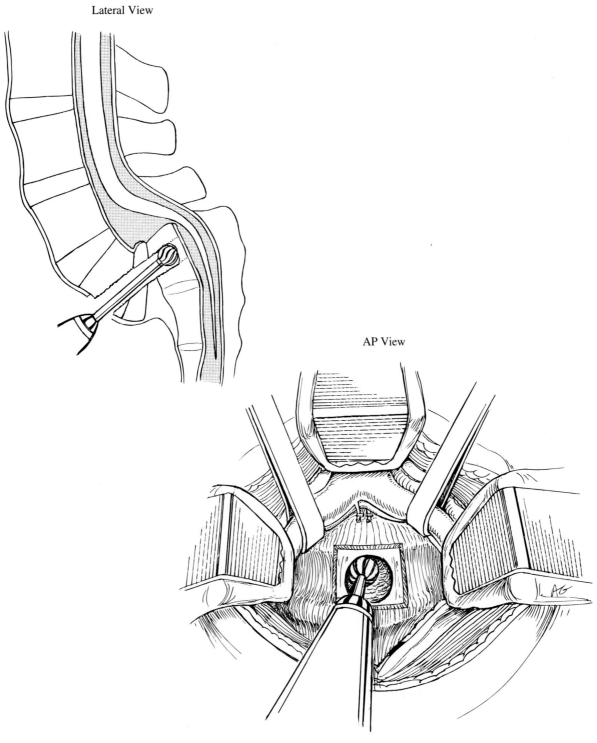

*Figure 12–8*

465

Either autologous iliac graft harvested through the same wound or fibular graft is used. The graft is fashioned to be slightly larger than the drill hole or the drill is selected in reference to the graft. The graft is then contoured to the width and length that the cannulated drill has progressed into the S1 vertebral body. The graft is then carefully inserted into the hole and impacted up to the posterior cortex of the S1 vertebral body, transfixing the L5 vertebra to the sacrum (Fig. 12–9).

Final x-rays are then taken in the posteroanterior and lateral planes to assure appropriate graft placement. Hemostasis is secured, and the wound is closed generally without a deep suction drain.

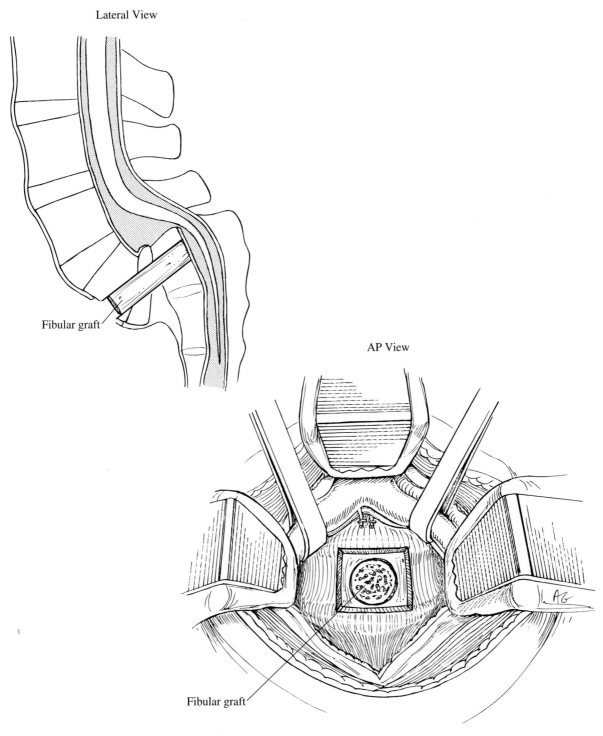

Lateral View

Fibular graft

AP View

Fibular graft

Figure 12–9

467

# Osteotomy

## MARIE-STRÜMPELL SPONDYLITIS (ANKYLOSING SPONDYLITIS)

### EXPOSURE

The soft tissues, namely the superspinous, interspinous ligament complex, ligamentum flavum, and facet joint capsules, are ossified, but the anatomy is retained. To correct the loss of lumbar lordosis (flatback) from ankylosing spondylitis, one or more osteotomies are performed in the upper lumbar area, usually L2–3, with a posterior closing wedge osteotomy used to obtain the correction of the flatback. Correction can be performed either through a posterior stage alone, breaking through the partially ossified disk anteriorly, or can be combined with an anterior release removing the disk and cutting the anterior longitudinal ligament (see disk removal, page 382). The latter technique is better for maintaining the correction obtained with osteotomy.

The amount of correction is determined by the amount of the loss of lordosis and the associated thoracic kyphosis. With careful preoperative planning using templates, it is possible to determine the amount of bone to be removed. In the preoperative planning, the wedge of bone to be removed has its apex at the posterior longitudinal ligament, which essentially shortens the spinal canal, while a wedge is opened anteriorly. If a large wedge of bone must be removed, it cannot be carried out at one site and more than a one-wedge osteotomy has to be performed. However, in the lumbar area because of the size of the vertebrae and the presence of cauda equina rather than cord, a large wedge of bone can be removed in most cases allowing correction through a single osteotomy.

The patient is positioned on a four-poster frame with supports under the thighs so the hips are extended as much as possible. When the patient's deformity (kyphosis and flatback) prevents this, the four-poster frame is positioned with its lower end at the break in the operating table. The table is flexed for patient positioning. The flex is reduced and the table straightened after the osteotomy is completed to help in the closure of the posterior wedge.

The posterior approach is via a midline incision in the upper lumbar area with subperiosteal dissection exposing the anatomy with fused ligament complexes. The correct vertebral level is confirmed with an intraoperative marker x-ray. The line of the osteotomy is through the site of the ligamentum flavum angling supralaterally to the foramen on each side (Fig. 12–10).

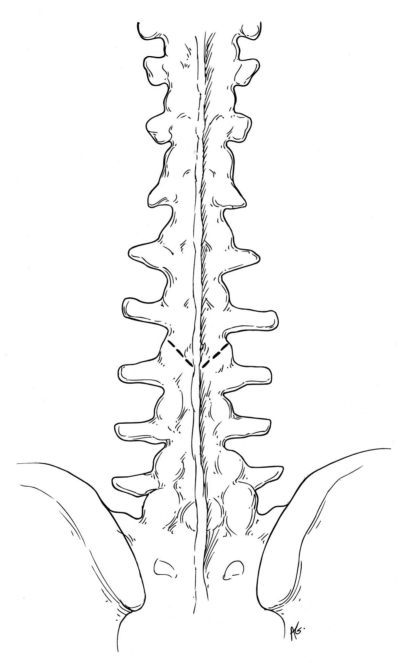

*Figure 12–10*

### HOOK PLACEMENT

Once the spine is exposed and the site of the osteotomy determined, the hooks or screws for the closure of the wedge are inserted. The hook sites are over the lamina or transverse processes in the thoracic area or under the lamina in the lumbar area. Using a gouge or dental burr in the midline, the fused ligamentum flavum is removed until the epidural fat is visualized. The opening is widened with a Kerrison rongeur so a hook can be placed over (or under) the lamina. Depending on the instrumentation to be used, all the hooks can be placed in compression, with the hooks above the osteotomy in the supralaminar position and below in the infralaminar position. An alternative hook system is to use one to two claws (transverse process/laminar or laminar/laminar) cranial to the osteotomy with one to one and one-half claws (laminar/laminar) below the osteotomy (Fig. 12–11).

An alternative method to close the osteotomy is using the Zielke screws. The sites of the pedicle are determined using the transverse processes, and a dental burr is used to start the hole into the pedicle. Temporary screws are inserted using small cortical screws and an anteroposterior and lateral x-rays are taken to ensure that the screws are correctly placed in the pedicle (see page 444 for screw placement). Three to four Zielke screws are inserted above and below the osteotomy on each side.

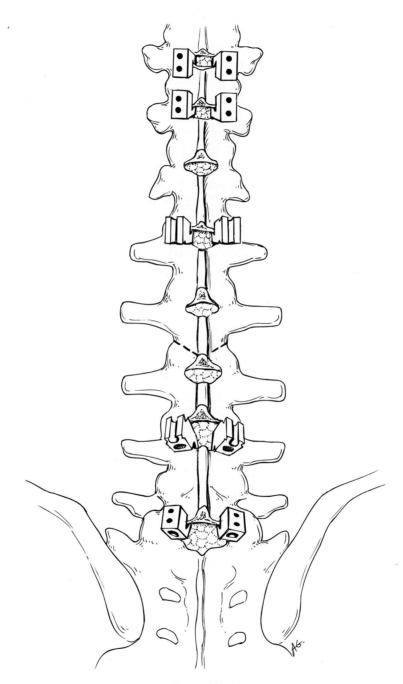

*Figure 12–11*

## OSTEOTOMY

Using a large, double-action rongeur, the bone in the midline of the ossified interspinous/supraspinous ligament and a portion of the spinous process cranial and caudad to it are removed. A rongeur is used in the midline interlaminar space to remove the ossified ligamentum flavum so the epidural fat is visible in the midline (Fig. 12–12A). Using a Kerrison rongeur, the small hole in the midline is widened, removing bone laterally and angling a little superiorly so a large enough opening is made to insert an Olivecrona dissector (Fig. 12–12B). With the Olivecrona dissector, the pedicles and foramina superior to them are felt. The direction and site of the foramen determine the area of bone to be removed. Bone removal is done using a double-action Leksell rongeur and a Kerrison rongeur or a burr and Kerrison rongeur. Using the double-action rongeur, the lamina in the direction indicated by the Olivecrona is thinned so the bone is more easily removed with a Kerrison rongeur (Fig. 12–12C). A portion of bone one-quarter to one-half inch wide (6 to 12 mm) is removed. Once the bone is removed, a Kerrison rongeur is inserted from the midline and the inner cortex is removed (Fig. 12–12D), the spinal canal contents being protected with a Cottonoid inserted in the midline and displacing the dural sac and epidural fat. Once the bone is removed on the one side, a similar removal is performed on the opposite side. Often when completed, the osteotomy starts closing because of the patient positioning.

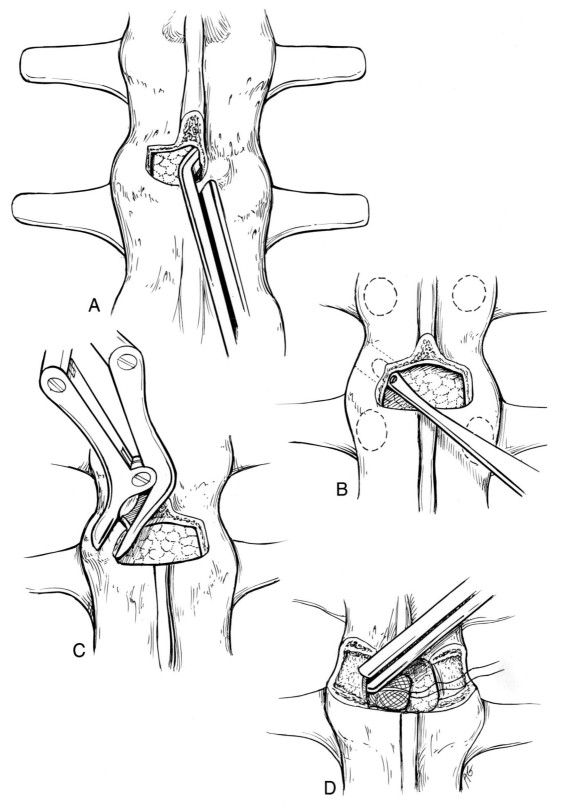

*Figure 12–12*

When using a burr to remove the bone, a medium size bit is used to thin the cortex until the inner cortex remains. The Kerrison rongeur is used to remove the inner cortex (Fig. 12–13).

Once the osteotomy has been completed on both sides, it is modified to prepare for complete closure. On the deep surface of the osteotomy any small spikes of bone are removed so the two osteotomy edges are completely flat. This is especially important laterally so there is no bone projecting into the intervertebral foramina. Using the Kerrison rongeur at an angle, the underside of each osteotomy is beveled and undercut so on closure they will not pinch and trap the contents of the spinal canal or the intervertebral foramina. The superficial surface of the osteotomy is widened, removing additional bone from the spinous processes and lamina with a rongeur or dental burr, so the two surfaces are in contact on closure. The angle of the two osteotomy walls is such that they are projected in the surgeon's eye to meet at the anterior margin of the spinal canal at the posterior longitudinal ligament.

### Osteotomy Closure/Instrumentation

The osteotomy is closed by inserting the appropriate rods—Harrington compression, C-D, or Zielke rods. The two rods are inserted and alternately tightened with appropriate in situ recontouring to allow closure of the osteotomy. During closure of the osteotomy, the depths are constantly palpated with an Olivecrona to ensure that no canal contents are pinched between the osteotomy edges and that the two walls of the osteotomy are closing equally with no bony ridges, preventing bone to bone contact. It is often found that bone removal was inadequate and additional bone is removed so complete closure and bone to bone contact are obtained. When the osteotomy is completely closed and bone to bone contact throughout the whole length of the osteotomy exists, the bone adjacent to the osteotomy on each side is decorticated with a rongeur, gouge, or burr. Bone removed from the osteotomy augmented with autologous iliac bone is packed around the osteotomy for the arthrodesis.

If the osteotomy has partially closed, a bone spreader, for example, a baby Inge, may be used to gain access to the osteotomy edges.

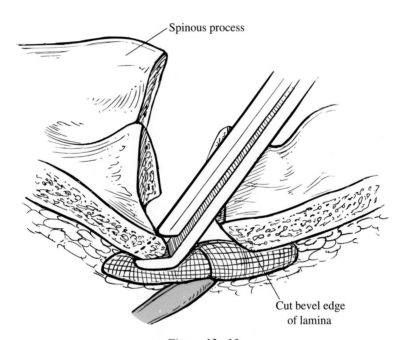

Spinous process

Cut bevel edge
of lamina

*Figure 12–13*

# "FLATBACK SYNDROME"

When there is loss of lumbar lordosis (flatback syndrome), correction of the deformity is by a posterior, closing wedge lumbar osteotomy. This correction is best obtained with an anterior opening wedge osteotomy and posterior closing wedge osteotomy to restore normal lumbar lordosis. Often this problem is part of multistage corrective surgery with the repair of a pseudarthrosis at the thoracolumbar or lumbosacral level or to correct scoliosis. With this reconstructive surgery, the previous instrumentation is removed at the posterior stage as part of the reconstruction.

## Anterior Stage

A retroperitoneal approach is made to the lumbar or lumbosacral spine (depending on the presence of lumbosacral pseudarthrosis). (See page 382 for discussion of exposure.) Even if a single osteotomy is planned, multilevel diskectomies are performed to ensure that the diskectomy is at the correct level and in case more than one lumbar osteotomy is necessary to correct the flatback syndrome. (See page 382 for discussion of multilevel diskectomies.) The only variation in the technique is that in the exposure the dissection is carried around the anterior longitudinal ligament so a Chandler elevator can be placed in this area, and the anterior annulus and anterior longitudinal ligament are removed to allow complete release and opening of the disk space anteriorly with closure of the wedge posteriorly. After decortication of the end plates with an osteotome or burr, the disk space is packed with bone, usually allograft croutons. Tight packing is essential because with correction of the deformity the disk space opens anteriorly and sufficient bone graft must be present to allow a solid arthrodesis to occur.

## Posterior Stage

The patient is placed on a four-poster frame and the thighs are positioned on large foam blocks so the hips are in extension with the knees in slight flexion. This places the body in an anatomic position in which spontaneous closure of the osteotomy will occur when the osteotomy is completed (Fig. 12–14).

The spine is exposed using the previous skin incision, and the previous fusion mass is exposed, removing any instrumentation that may be present. Additional fusion mass is exposed cranially and caudally as is necessary to obtain adequate fixation into the spine in these two areas to provide stable instrumentation and when there are pseudarthroses present or when other procedures are necessary as part of the reconstruction. The fusion mass is exposed to the irregular lateral contour. All soft tissue is removed using a curette. The osteotomy level (usually L2, L3) is identified with intraoperative x-ray or by the lumbosacral area and alae and counting upwards. The lateral aspect of the fusion mass is sinuous. In the lumbar area, the indentations correspond to the level of the pars interarticularis and the intervertebral foramina and the protrusions correspond to the fused facet joints. The site of the osteotomy is at an intervertebral foramen, that is, an indentation of the lateral aspect of the fusion.

476

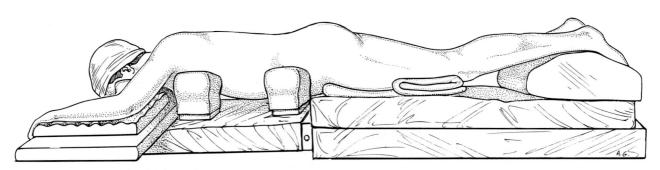

*Figure 12–14*

# SPONDYLOLISTHESIS AND OSTEOTOMY SURGERY

## HOOK INSERTION

Once the previous fusion is completely exposed and the level of the osteotomy chosen, the instrumentation levels are planned and the hooks inserted. Hook sites are made above and below the level of the osteotomy with at least three to four hooks placed above and three hooks below the osteotomy on each side. In long fusions, adequate fixation to the fusion mass cranial to the osteotomy is necessary to ensure rigid fixation. In these cases additional hooks in the fusion are necessary.

A solid fusion consists of a posterior cortical layer, a central cancellous area, and a deep cortical layer with the thickness of the fusion varying, being thicker on the concavity of a scoliotic deformity. In addition the outer cortex may be very thick with the cancellous area being small. The outer cortex is removed with an osteotome and gouges or with a dental burr; a rectangle of bone is removed for hook insertion. The cancellous bone is removed with a curette. If the fusion is thick, the hook is placed in the fusion mass, this being the usual placement. Additional deep bone is removed (with a curette or burr) to aid in the placement of the blade of the hook. The hook is inserted in the fusion securely seated on the posterior cortex. If the fusion is thin, the hook is placed around the whole fusion, for example, superficial and deep cortices. The deep cortex is thinned with a curette (or burr) until a small hole is present which is then enlarged to receive a Kerrison rongeur. This hole is widened for the blade and the hook is inserted.

## OSTEOTOMY

The line of the osteotomy in the posterior cortical layer is made with a straight osteotome and the posterior cortex removed with a gouge. A burr can be used to remove the bone, but less bone graft is available. It is advantageous to use osteotomes, rongeurs, and curettes to save the osteotomy bone for bone graft for the fusion.

Once the posterior cortex has been removed and the cancellous bone exposed, all the cancellous bone is removed using a curette so the deep cortex and lateral walls of the fusion mass remain. In the center of the fusion mass, the deep cortex is thinned so a hole is made in the fusion exposing the fat of the epidural space. This bone removal can be with a sharp curette or a burr, the deep cortex being thinned using a gouge and rongeurs or a burr.

Once the deep cortex has been removed in the midline exposing the epidural fat, a Kerrison rongeur is used to enlarge the hole so a Cottonoid can be placed in the epidural space displacing the epidural fat and dural sac. An Olivecrona is used to explore the epidural space and locate the pedicles so the osteotomy can be directed to the foramen on each side. A Kerrison rongeur is used to remove the bone, working from the midline towards the lateral aspect of the fusion mass. The Cottonoid is continually repositioned as additional bone is removed. Often the thickest part of the deep cortex is the lateral wall of the fusion mass. This bone is removed using a combination of a double-action Leksell rongeur and the Kerrison rongeur. Once the osteotomy has been completed on one side, the same procedure is performed on the opposite side, removing all the deep cortex and completing the osteotomy.

The osteotomy is now undercut using the Kerrison rongeur. Using a 45 degree angled Kerrison rongeur the deep cortex is beveled to prevent any trapping of epidural fat, dura, or nerve root with closure of the osteotomy. More bone is removed posteriorly using a double-action rongeur or burr so the osteotomy will close posteriorly. The wedge is planned so the apex of the wedge is at the posterior longitudinal ligament and posterior aspect of the vertebral bodies. As this bone is gradually removed, the osteotomy closes. Additional bone is often removed to allow additional correction. With closure of the osteotomy, creation of lumbar lordosis occurs.

Closure of the osteotomy is made using compression instrumentation (large Harrington compression rods or C-D system loaded in compression). The instrumentation is inserted and compression applied. Both rods are inserted and correction applied on each rod consecutively to gradually close the osteotomy equally, not giving lateral angulation of the spine after closure. During tightening of the instrumentation, the osteotomy is constantly checked using an Olive-crona to ensure that it closes equally on both sides and there are no areas of bone impingement preventing complete closure. In addition, appropriate in situ rod bending is often necessary to allow closure and bone to bone contact. If this is the case, additional bone needs to be removed using a Kerrison or double-action rongeur to allow equal closure of the osteotomy. When closure has occurred and secure fixation obtained, the spine in the area of the osteotomy is decorticated using a rongeur and/or gouge and local bone is augmented by iliac bone and allograft croutons added for the bone graft (Fig. 12–15).

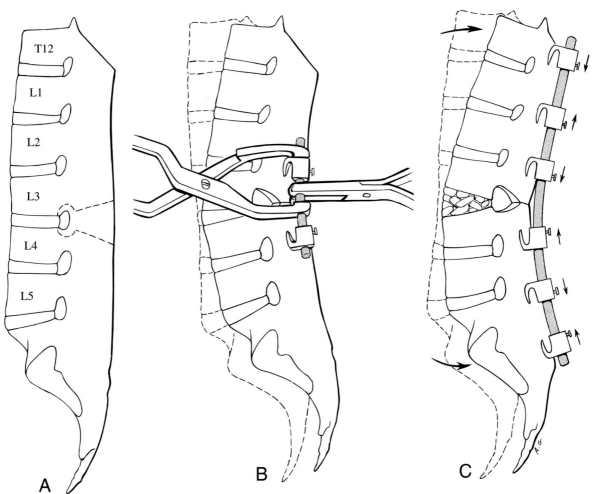

*Figure 12–15*

# SCOLIOSIS RECONSTRUCTION

In recorrection after a previous spinal fusion, it is often necessary to obtain correction in the area of the previous fusion with osteotomies. This is accompanied by an anterior fusion to allow more correction by creating closing wedge osteotomies on the convexity of the curve and to ensure a solid arthrodesis. The osteotomies are thus a part of a single or multistage procedure, the number of stages depending on the choice of the surgeon. A single-stage correction is a combination of (a) anterior osteotomies and fusion and (b) posterior osteotomies plus reinstrumentation and bone grafting. Two-stage procedures can be posterior osteotomies performed at one stage and the reinstrumentation and bone grafting at the second stage or the first stage is the anterior wedge osteotomies and fusion, with posterior osteotomies and reinstrumentation and bone grafting at the second stage. In the three-stage procedure, the three parts, namely, the anterior wedge osteotomies and fusion, posterior osteotomies, and the reinstrumentation and bone grafting, are done separately. In any staged procedure, the patient is placed in longitudinal traction (either halo femoral or halo gravity) to obtain the correction. The tendency today is to use a one- or two-stage approach.

The previous fusion is exposed throughout its length including unfused additional spine that is to be added to the previous fusion cranially and/or caudally. The exposure is the same as previously described (see page 74). In the line of the previous fusion, the incision is made down to the fusion mass and, with careful subperiosteal dissection, the periosteum is dissected off the fusion mass bilaterally. The whole width of the previous fusion is exposed so the lateral borders are well visualized. In addition, the transverse processes are exposed lateral to the fusion mass when there is no fusion overlying them. Often because of the tight scar tissue present, exposure on the convexity is difficult and a releasing incision is made through the previous scar tissue and muscle.

After exposure of the fusion mass, the site of the osteotomy is planned. The osteotomy is usually placed at the apex of the deformity with additional osteotomies cranial and caudal to this. The exact site is through the intervertebral foramina on each side. The site of the intervertebral foramina is visualized by the lateral aspect of the fusion mass. In the thoracic area, the intervertebral foramina will lie between the transverse processes. In the lumbar area, the lateral aspect of the fusion mass is usually undulating, the projections corresponding to the previous fused facet joints (Fig. 12–16). Between these projections lie the intervertebral foramina, the site of the osteotomy (Fig. 12–17). Two appropriate intervertebral foramina indentations in the lateral aspect of the fusion mass are identified and an osteotome used to mark out the line of the osteotomy. Two parallel cuts are made usually approximately one-half inch (12 mm) apart. The advantage of using an osteotome at this stage is that all the removed bone can be saved. A dental burr can be used for this stage but all the bone removed is lost.

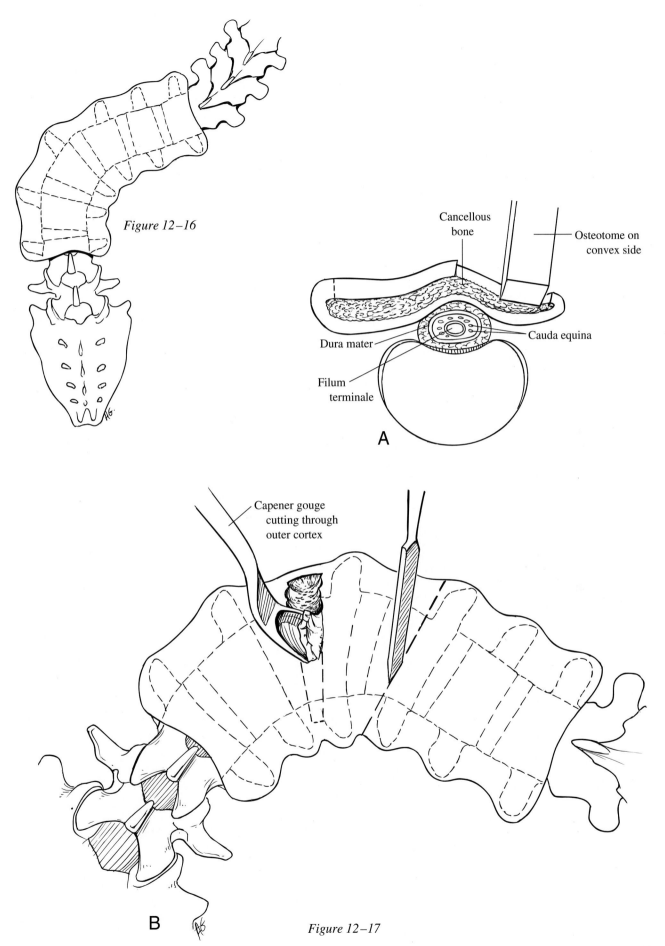

*Figure 12–16*

Cancellous
bone

Osteotome on
convex side

Dura mater

Cauda equina

Filum
terminale

A

Capener gouge
cutting through
outer cortex

B

*Figure 12–17*

The anatomy of the fusion mass is such that a solid fusion consists of three layers, a posterior cortex, a central cancellous bed, and a deep cortex (Fig. 12–18). The thickness of these three layers varies, but they are usually thickest on the concavity of the curve. In addition, in the foramen, the two cortical layers join at the lateral wall of the fusion mass, which can be very thick on the concavity of the scoliosis.

The outer cortex is removed with a combination of osteotomes and gouges exposing the cancellous central portion of the osteotomy. This is removed with a curette leaving the cortical bone of the lateral walls and deep cortex (Fig. 12–19).

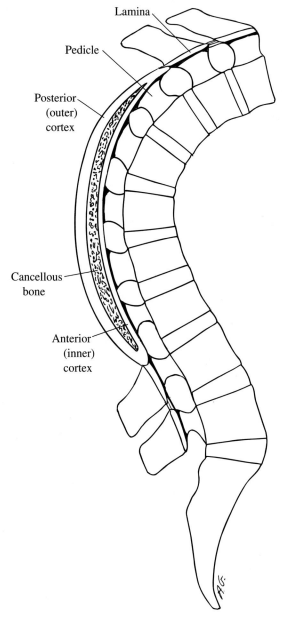

*Figure 12–18*

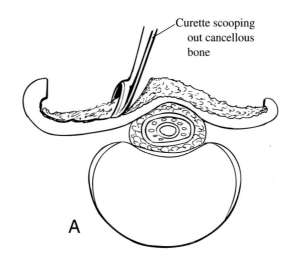

Curette scooping
out cancellous
bone

A

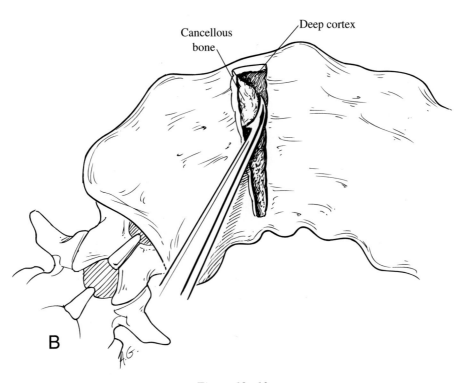

Cancellous
bone

Deep cortex

B

*Figure 12–19*

The central portion of the osteotomy is thinned using a sharp curette gradually removing the bone until the epidural fat at the center of the canal is seen (Fig. 12–20A,B). The hole is enlarged with a Kerrison rongeur until a Cottonoid can be placed deep in the spinal canal, displacing the dural sac (Fig. 12–21A). Bone is gradually removed on the convexity of the osteotomy first since the spinal cord is applied to the concavity of the curve (Fig. 12–21B). Once a portion of bone has been removed, an additional Cottonoid is inserted to displace the contents of the spinal canal. An Olivecrona is used to feel the undersurface of the fusion mass, identifying the pedicle and guiding the osteotomy into the intervertebral foramen (Fig. 12–22A). Bone is gradually removed with Kerrison rongeurs working laterally towards the convexity of the curve. The lateral margin of the osteotomy remains and this is cleared of all periosteum on its outer surface using a periosteal elevator and the Olivecrona. The bone is gradually removed using a double-action Leksell rongeur and a Kerrison rongeur until all the bone has been removed and the osteotomy completed on the convexity (Fig. 12–22B,C).

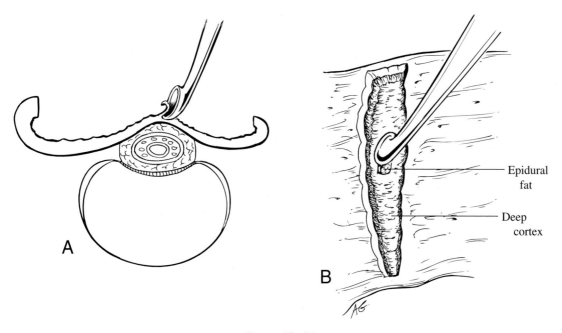

*Figure 12–20*

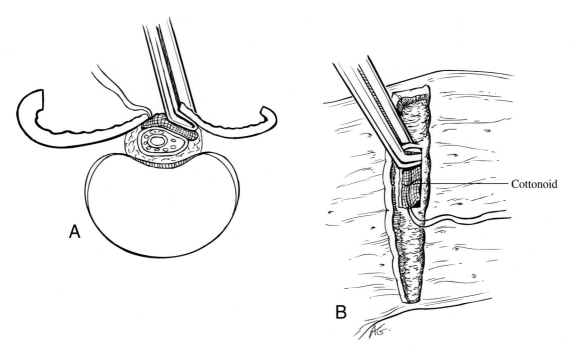

Cottonoid

**Figure 12–21**

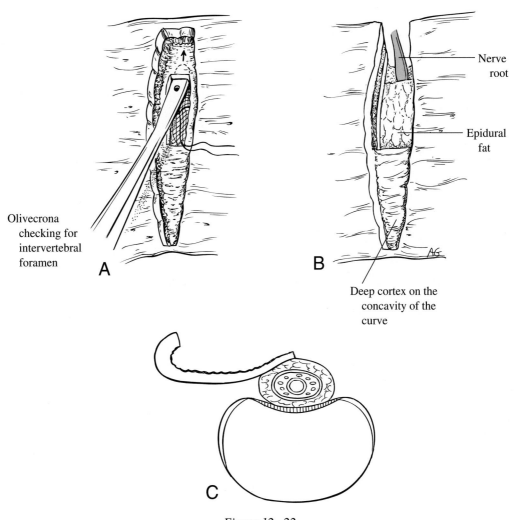

Olivecrona
checking for
intervertebral
foramen

Nerve
root

Epidural
fat

Deep cortex on the
concavity of the
curve

**Figure 12–22**

A similar removal is performed on the concavity. The lateral margin of the osteotomy is often difficult to remove because it is very thick and has to be thinned with an osteotome, gouge, or rongeur so the remaining bone can be removed with a double-action Leksell and/or Kerrison rongeur. The osteotomy is completed so no bone remains between the two surfaces, and motion can be demonstrated with a Blount spreader.

To prevent trapping the spinal canal contents between the two bone surfaces of the osteotomy during closure, the osteotomy edges are undercut. Using the 45 degree Kerrison rongeur at an angle, the deep surface of the osteotomy is beveled in the foramen on each side to ensure that there is enough space in the foramen for osteotomy closure and to prevent trapping the exiting spinal nerve between the osteotomy edges (Fig. 12–23).

An alternative method to perform the osteotomy is using a burr. The outer cortex and cancellous bone are removed exposing the deep cortex (Fig. 12–24). The deep cortex is thinned with the burr, the epidural space is entered, and bone removal is with a Kerrison rongeur as above.

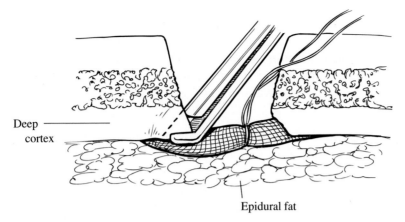

Deep cortex

Epidural fat

*Figure 12–23*

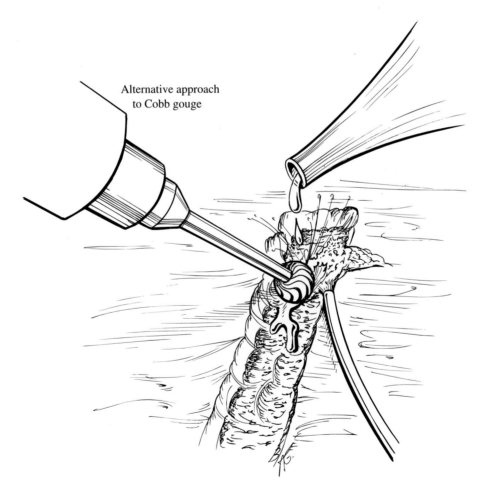

Alternative approach to Cobb gouge

*Figure 12–24*

The osteotomy edges are shaped depending on the correction to be obtained. With correction of scoliosis, the osteotomy tends to be wider on the convexity than concavity to allow correction with a closing wedge osteotomy on the curve's convexity. In kyphosis correction, the osteotomy is wider posteriorly to allow closure posteriorly and correction of kyphosis. When both scoliosis and kyphosis are corrected at the same time, the osteotomy is trapezoidal, narrower on the concavity and deep surface and wider on convexity and posteriorly (Fig. 12–25).

Reinstrumentation is performed for correction and stabilization of the osteotomy. If traction is used, reinstrumentation will usually consist of maintenance of curve correction. If correction is performed intraoperatively, this consists of compression on the convexity of the curve combined with distraction on the concavity. It is safer to obtain the correction with compression and closing wedges than distracting the concavity, which puts tension on the spinal cord and canal contents. The hooks are placed in the fusion mass. Wherever possible, the hook sites are made prior to performing the osteotomies. Compression instrumentation on the convexity is applied first, followed by distraction instrumentation on the concavity.

The spine is now decorticated using a rongeur, gouge, or burr. Bone graft is added consisting of bone removed during the osteotomies plus autologous iliac bone augmented by allograft when insufficient local and iliac bone are present.

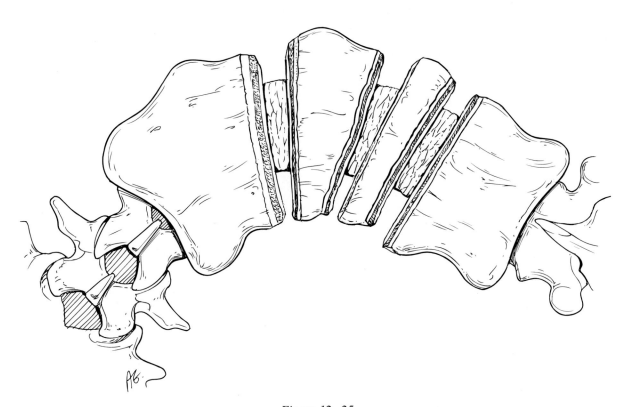

*Figure 12–25*

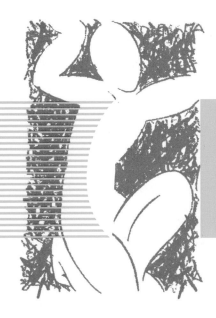

# 13

# POSTERIOR LONG FUSIONS TO THE SACRUM

# Basic Luque-Galveston Technique

The long Luque-Galveston fusion to the sacrum usually involves a fusion of T2 to the sacrum using Luque rods with Galveston pelvic fixation.

In any long fusion to the sacrum, patient positioning is important. With long fusions in ambulatory patients, it is essential to maintain a normal sagittal contour to the spine and to prevent loss of lumbar lordosis with forward tilt of the torso and its accompanying problems. The patient is placed in a prone position on a Relton-Hall frame with foam pads under the thighs to extend the hips. The spinal contour is as if the patient is standing, with maintenance of the normal lumbar lordosis (Fig. 13–1).

In nonambulatory, neuromuscular patients, positioning is with the hips flexed. When marked hip flexion contractures are present, positioning on the Relton-Hall frame is modified in the following manner: (a) the lower posts are placed at the lower edge of the frame; (b) the patient's hips are flexed to a range beyond the hip flexion contracture; (c) the lower end of the frame is raised so with the hip flexion the knees do not rest on the operative table and foam pads are placed under the knees; (d) pillows are placed under the feet and lower legs to flex the knees (Fig. 13–2A); and the operating table is placed in a reverse Trendelenburg position so the back is horizontal (Fig. 13–2B). If the contractures are less severe, the patient can be positioned as shown in Figure 13–2C.

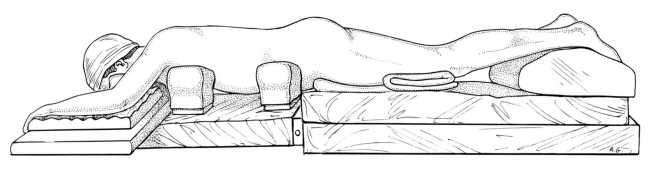

*Figure 13–1*

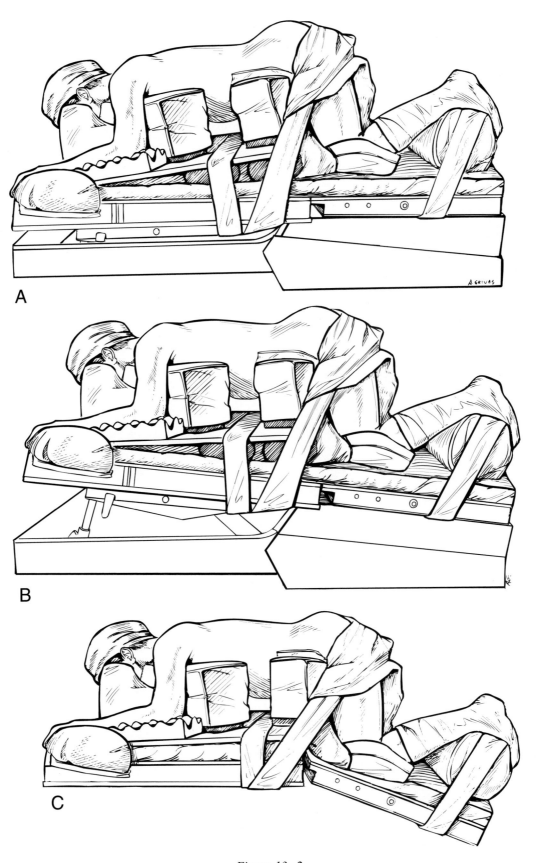

*Figure 13–2*

# POSTERIOR LONG FUSIONS TO THE SACRUM

The spine is exposed with subperiosteal dissection to the tips of the transverse processes throughout the area to be fused with all facet joint capsules being removed with a curette. The sacrum is exposed for approximately three segments dissecting lateral to the sacral foramina. In the lumbosacral area the tips of all the transverse processes and the sacral alae are exposed bilaterally (Fig. 13–3).

Once the spine, sacrum, and lumbosacral area are exposed the best sequence to minimize blood loss is:

preparation of ilium for pelvic pin insertion

rod bending

excision of ligamentum flavum and facet excision

wire insertion on first side

insertion of first rod

wire tightening

insertion of wires on second side

insertion of second rod

wire tightening

insertion of cross-connecting devices

decortication

closure

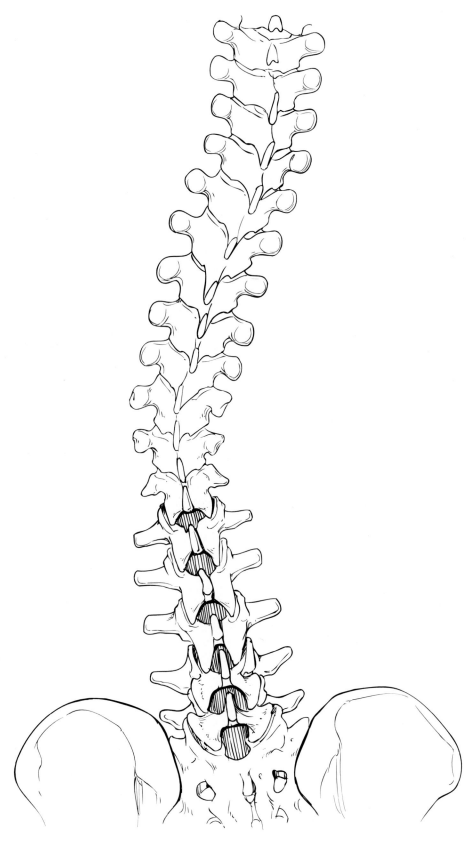

*Figure 13–3*

## Preparation of Pelvic Insertion Site

The Luque rod with Galveston pelvic fixation has three portions—spinal, sacral, and pelvic. After the spine and sacrum are exposed, the posterior ilium is exposed for the insertion of the pelvic portion of the rod. Towel clips are used to approximate the lumbar deep fascia. Dissection is carried out in the plane superficial to the fascia exposing the posterior iliac crest. The cartilage cap of the crest is incised and dissection is carried out subperiosteally on the outer aspect of the ilium, exposing the portion of the ilium superior to the greater sciatic notch. A ridge of bone extending from the posterior superior iliac spine area above the notch is often present; this ridge of bone and the notch are exposed. Dissection is then carried out on the inner aspect of the ilium toward the sacrum, exposing the posterosuperior iliac spine medially and laterally. On the inner aspect of the crest, dissection is toward the sacrum under the muscle mass so that the area of dissection medial to the crest communicates with the main posterior dissection. At times increased mobility of the paraspinal muscles is necessary and this is obtained with releasing incisions in the posterior fascia in the midline and in the crest area.

A notch is made on the inner aspect in the posterior crest in line with the ridge in the ilium to allow the Luque rod to lie on the sacrum and enter the ilium in this area (Fig. 13–4A). A drill is then used to create a channel in the ilium. A 1/4-inch (6.4 mm) drill is used for the larger Luque rod and a 3/16-inch (4.8 mm) drill for the smaller rod. The drill and rod size are chosen depending on the thickness of the iliac crest. Drilling is from the posterosuperior iliac spine through the ridge of bone just above the sciatic notch. When there is no bony ridge, drilling is 1.5 cm above the iliac notch, which is visualized to ensure correct drill direction. The drill hole is parallel to the outer cortex of the ilium, thus maintaining its path between the two cortices of the ilium (Fig. 13–4B). The total distance drilled varies with the size of the pelvis but is between 2 1/2 and 4 inches (6.5 and 10 cm) generally being 3 to 3 1/2 inches (7.5 to 9 cm). A Steinmann pin is passed down the channel to ensure that the base of the hole is solid bone, that is, no penetration of the supra-acetabular portion of the ilium has occurred (Fig. 13–4C). The portion of the Steinmann pin that is in the ilium is measured; this represents the pelvic portion of the Luque rod. In addition, the distance between the hole in the ilium and the midpoint of the sacral lamina is measured; this represents the sacral portion of the rod. The same procedure is carried out on the other side.

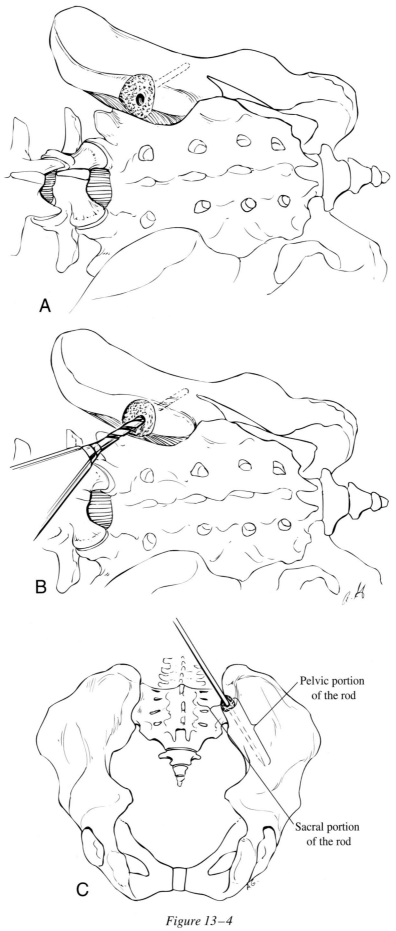

A

B

C

Pelvic portion
of the rod

Sacral portion
of the rod

*Figure 13–4*

497

## Rod Bending

The first bend in the rod is between the spinal and sacral portions. A tubular Luque rod bender is placed on the long end of the Luque rod and the portion outside the bender is measured (Fig. 13–5A). This portion is made up of the measured intrapelvic portion of the pin inserted in the pelvis plus the distance from the posterior crest to the middle of the sacral lamina plus an amount for the two bends in the rod. On an average, this is 3 to 3 1/2 inches (7.5 to 9 cm) for the intrapelvic portion plus 3/4 to 1 inch (2 to 2.5 cm) for the sacral portion. To this is added 1/4 inch (6 mm) for the two bends in the rod. The tubular bender is locked on the rod. A second rod bender is placed on the end of the rod, leaving a small distance between the two benders to allow for bending (Fig. 13–5B). The long end of the rod is placed on the straddle table and held in place, and the proposed area of the bend is placed at the edge of the table. While grasping the one rod bender and holding it to the table, the rod is bent over the end of the table into a 90 degree bend (Fig. 13–5C,D). The rod bender is removed from the short end of the rod, and a large vice grip is placed on the sacral portion of the rod at the right angle bend so that the portion of the rod remaining is equal to the proposed intrapelvic portion of the rod plus 1/8 inch (3 mm) for the bend (Fig. 13–6A). The rod is placed along the edge of the straddle table with the point of the vice grip positioned at the end of the table and the second rod bender is placed on the short end of the rod (Fig. 13–6B). While grasping the vice grip and holding the rod and rod bender stable on the straddle table, a second bend is placed between the sacral and pelvic portions of the rod (Fig. 13–6C). An assistant can help stabilize the tubular rod bender and vice grip on the straddle table. The angle of this bend is compared to the Steinmann pin, which is placed in the pelvis, so that with the sacral portion of rod horizontal, the pelvic portion is in the same direction as the Steinmann pin (Fig. 13–6D). The rod bending is complete, resulting in a 90 degree bend between the spinal and the sacral segments and an angulation for the pelvic portion (Fig. 13–7). If the rod is laid along the spine, the pin in the pelvis and the pelvic portion of the rod will be at different angles (Fig. 13–8A). The lordosis is placed in the rod using the French rod bender. With the addition of the lordosis, the pelvic portion of the rod lies parallel to the Steinmann pin in the pelvis. The rod is contoured for the lumbar lordosis, thoracic kyphosis, and any necessary scoliosis (Fig. 13–8B). The rod is underbent to the best correction of the scoliosis, that is, the correction of the spine with convex pressure on the apex of the scoliosis. This is to allow the spine to be approximated to the rod, using the concave correction technique as described in Figure 13–13. The second rod is also bent as described, the rod contouring for lordosis, kyphosis, and scoliosis being performed only after insertion of the concave rod.

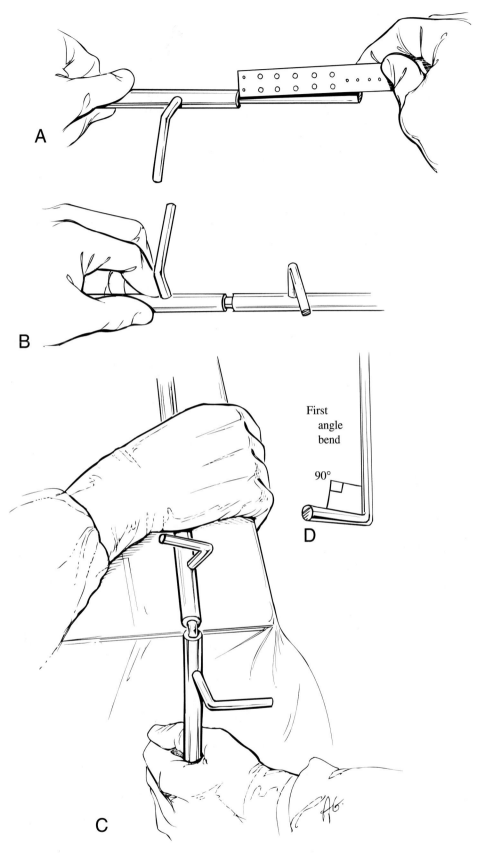

A

B

First
angle
bend

90°

D

C

*Figure 13–5*

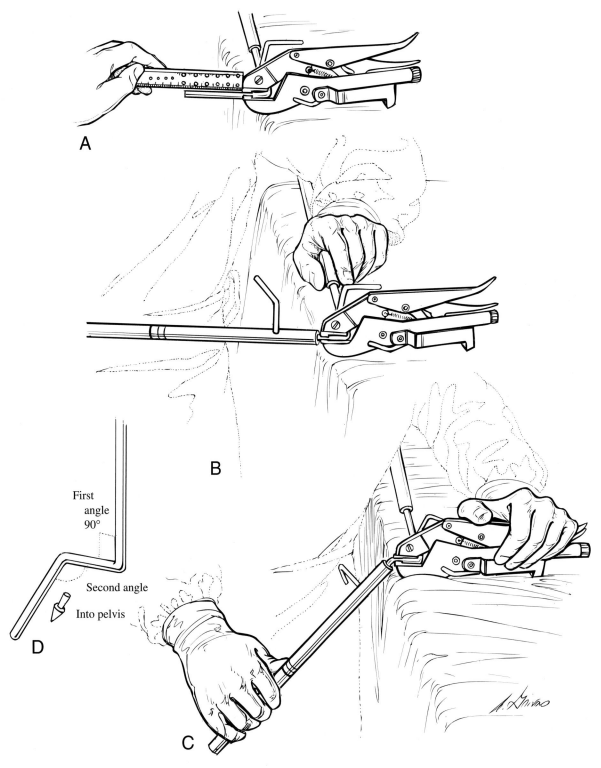

First
angle
90°

Second angle

Into pelvis

A

B

C

D

*Figure 13–6*

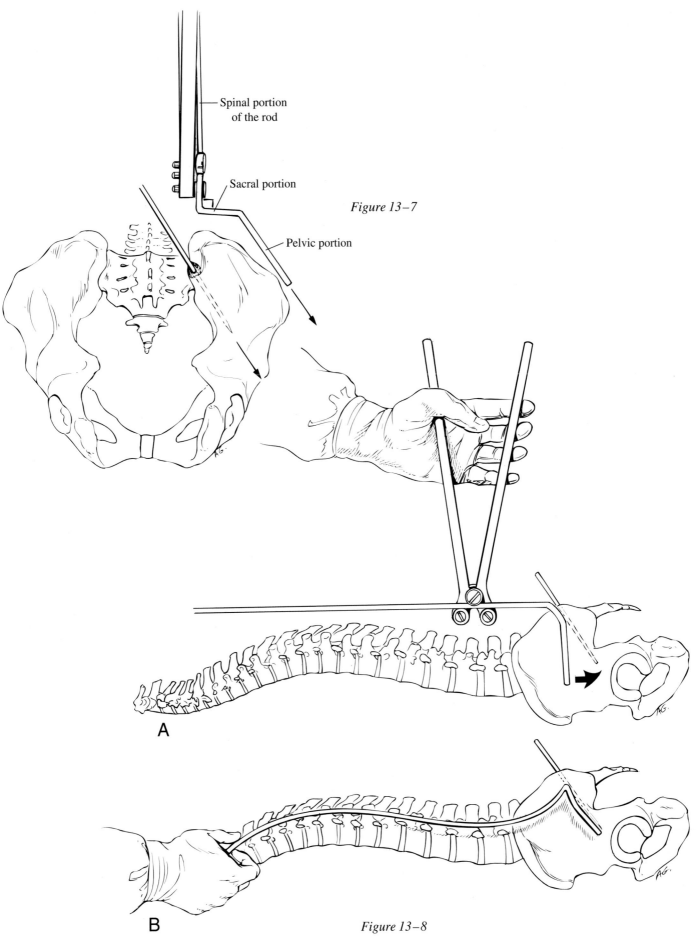

Spinal portion of the rod

Sacral portion

Pelvic portion

*Figure 13–7*

A

B

*Figure 13–8*

## Excision of the Ligamentum Flavum

Laminotomies are performed at all the levels, usually from T1-T2 to L5-S1 for a T2 to sacrum fusion. All the facets are excised prior to doing the laminotomies. The laminotomy technique is shown in Figures 7–34 and 7–35.

## Wire Passage

A double strand of #16 wire (1.2 cm) is passed at each level as shown in Figures 7–36 and 7–37. The wires are bent over the laminae with one wire placed on the concavity and one on the convexity of the curve (Fig. 13–9).

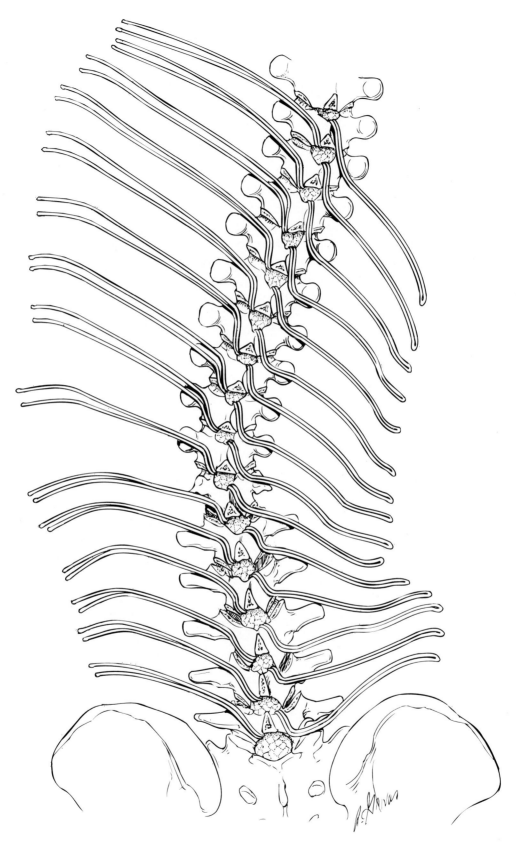

*Figure 13–9*

503

## Rod Insertion

The Steinmann pin is inserted in the pelvic hole from the medial to the paraspinal muscles, that is, the muscles lie over the entrance of the pin into the iliac crest. The contoured Luque rod is held with the main portion of the rod pointing away from the back and the pelvic portion of the rod parallel and next to the Steinmann pin (Fig. 13–10A). The Steinmann pin is removed and the pelvic portion of the rod is advanced into the hole maintaining the direction of the Steinmann pin (Fig. 13–10B). Once the rod has been inserted as far as possible (Fig. 13–10C), it is rotated toward the spine ensuring that it passes between the previously inserted wires (Fig. 13–10D). Once the rod is rotated so it lies alongside the spine, it is fully seated in the pelvis using an impactor or rod inserter at the junction of the spinal and sacral portions of the rod (Fig. 13–11). By using this site on the rod, the impaction overcomes the force of muscle overlying the rod and the rod is well-seated. Any final adjustment to the lumbar lordosis, thoracic kyphosis, or scoliosis is made using in situ rod-bending irons. The C-D in situ benders are ideal for this purpose. The final adjustment to the rod contour is made immediately or after tightening 2 or 3 of the caudal wires. During the rod bending, the portion of the rod near the pelvis is grasped and controlled with a rod holder to prevent any force from being transmitted to the inserted pelvic portion.

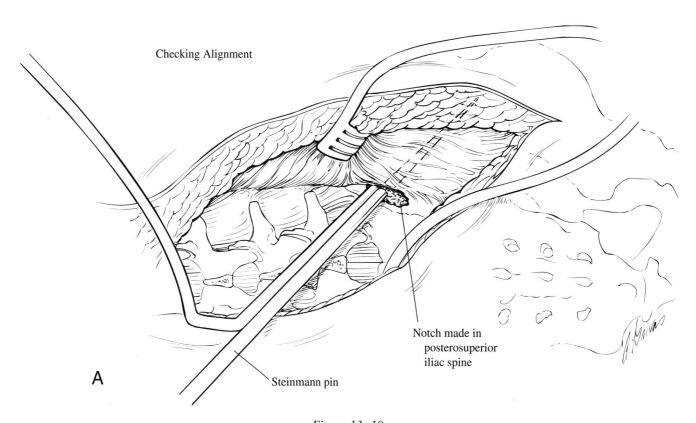

Checking Alignment

Notch made in posterosuperior iliac spine

A

Steinmann pin

*Figure 13–10*

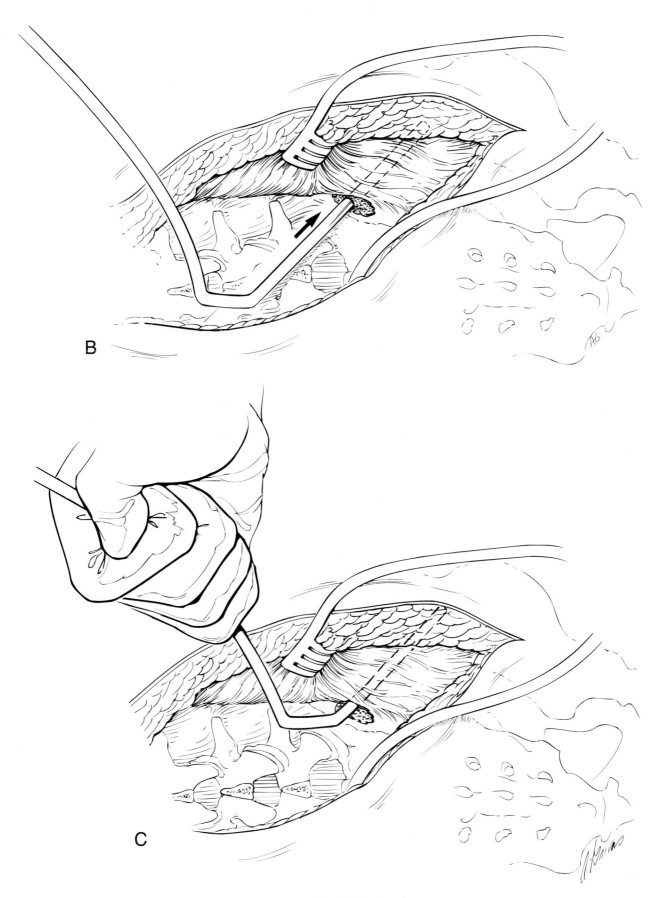

B

C

*Figure 13–10 Continued*

505

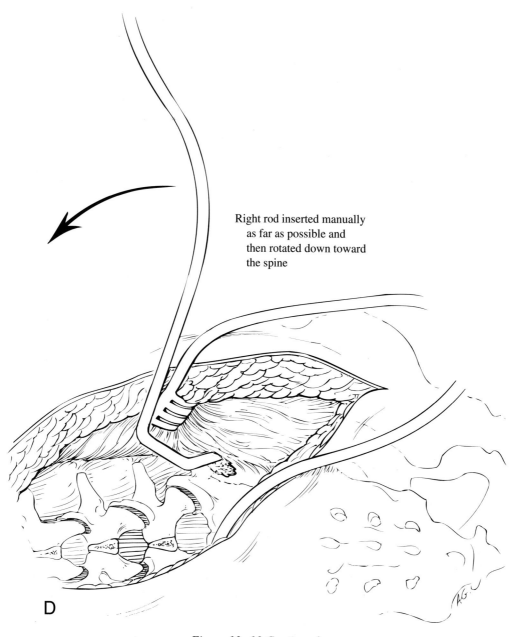

Right rod inserted manually
as far as possible and
then rotated down toward
the spine

D

*Figure 13–10 Continued*

506

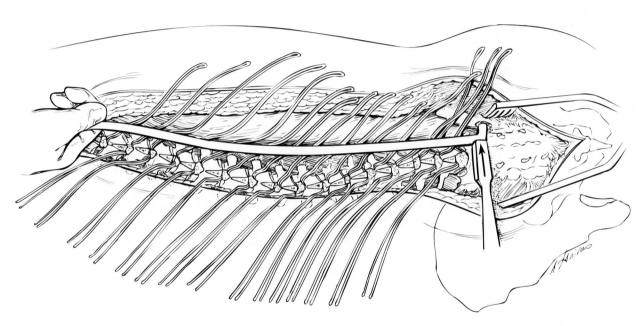

*Figure 13–11*

507

The wires are tightened starting at the opposite ends of the curve and working toward the apex of the curve. The wires initially tightened are on L5 and L4 and on T2 and T3 (Fig. 13–12). As the wires are tightened, those at the ends become loose. The wires are again tightened working from the ends of the curve toward the apex until the rod lies in direct contact with the bone. During tightening of the apical wires, pressure is placed on the convexity of the curve to approximate the spine to the rod making wire tightening easier. Once all the wires are tightened, they are bent toward the right side (for a right rod insertion) and a towel is placed over the wires; the towel is held in place with towel clips (Fig. 13–13).

The convex wires are now inserted followed by insertion of the convex rod, which has been bent for lordosis, kyphosis, any residual scoliosis, and matching the convex curve of the spinal contour (Fig. 13–13). The convex wires are tightened. All the wires are cut leaving approximately 5/8 inch or 1.5 cm of wire, which are bent toward the spine. Two cross-connectors are added, the upper stabilizing the two rods and the lower placed in distraction to keep the rods well-seated in the pelvis (Fig. 13–14).

The laminae in the midline and the transverse processes are decorticated. In the lumbar and lumbosacral areas, the transverse processes, lateral aspect of the superior articular processes, and the sacral ala are carefully decorticated. Because pseudarthroses are more common in the lumbosacral area, all the local bone (spinous processes, decorticated bone) is placed in the lumbosacral area. Allograft bone is used for the fusion in the lumbosacral gutters over the patient's bone and cranially in the lumbar gutters and over the thoracic transverse processes. Another common site of pseudarthroses is the thoracolumbar junction area; therefore, this area should be adequately decorticated and allograft bone inserted.

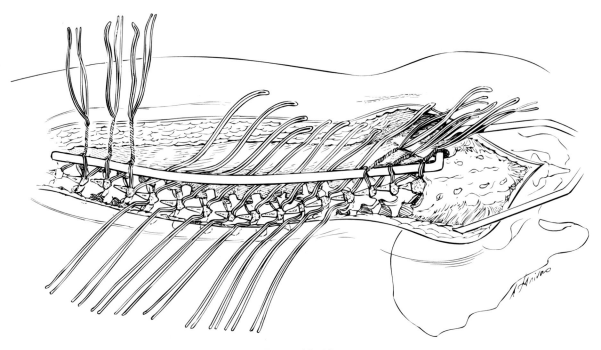

*Figure 13–12*

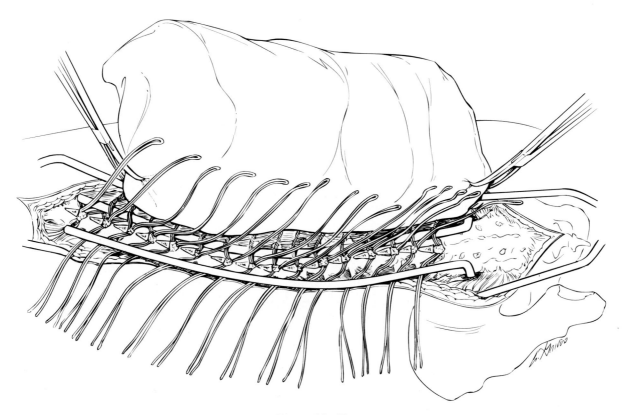

*Figure 13–13*

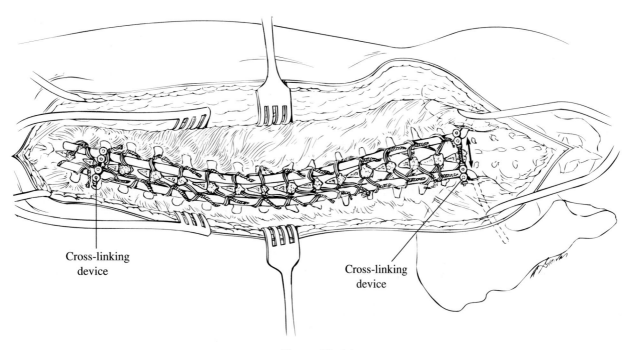

Cross-linking device

Cross-linking device

*Figure 13–14*

# Luque-Galveston with Harrington Distraction Instrumentation

With a very stiff lumbar curve, it is often necessary to obtain distraction correction in the lumbar area. This is best achieved using a Harrington distraction rod wired to the spine for stabilization.

Following exposure of the spine from T2 to the sacrum, as described under the Basic Luque-Galveston technique, the hook sites for a single Harrington distraction rod, usually from the lower thoracic area to L4 or L5, are prepared. (For hook insertion see Chapter 7, Harrington Instrumentation.) The Harrington rod is contoured so that with correction it lies along the laminae to be secured with sublaminar wires.

The laminotomies are performed throughout the extent of the fusion and the wires are passed on the concavity of the curve in the area where the Harrington rod is to be inserted. The rod is inserted and distraction applied, and then the rod is secured to the spine with the sublaminar wires. This allows initial correction of the apex of the scoliosis and also helps maintain the correction. The remainder of the Luque-Galveston procedure is followed, as previously described, with the exception that the concave rod is contoured to lie lateral to the Harrington rod and is wired to the Harrington rod rather than to the spine. The sacral portion of the concave rod is shorter and lateral to the Harrington rod.

# C-D Sacral Fixation

In a long C-D instrumentation to the sacrum, the following alternatives can be used for the sacral fixation: (1) C-D instrumentation with Galveston pelvic fixation, (2) C-D instrumentation to L3 or L4 with C-D rods fixed to the pelvis using the Galveston technique and attached to the spinal C-D instrumentation, and (3) C-D instrumentation using sacral screws. In these techniques an anterior lumbosacral procedure (from T10 to S1) for diskectomies and fusion is performed first, either as a separate procedure or as a combination procedure under the same anesthetic.

## C-D Instrumentation with Galveston Technique

The spine from T2 to the sacrum with the alae is exposed, as previously described under the basic Luque-Galveston technique. The hooks are inserted using the routine C-D technique with the exception that all the hooks are open to allow insertion of the C-D rod once the sacral fixation has been performed (see Chapter 7, Cotrel–Dubousset Instrumention).

The C-D rod is contoured for the Galveston pelvic fixation consisting of pelvic, sacral, and spinal portions. The rod is inserted using the usual Galveston technique.

For the C-D technique to L3 or L4, a shorter C-D rod is contoured for the Galveston pelvic fixation and inserted lateral to the previous C-D rod. Dominoes are placed on the rods prior to insertion so they can be used on each rod. The best method is to apply an open-closed or closed-closed domino on the C-D rod. The domino is fixed to the Galveston rod. In addition, a second domino is placed on the Galveston rod caudally and is slid onto the protruding end of the C-D rod below the lowest hook. The C-D rods are longer than normal allowing an extra section for attachment to the Galveston rod. Once the Galveston portion has been adequately inserted into the pelvis, it is contoured with in situ benders to lie adjacent and lateral to the C-D rods and fixed to the C-D rods with the two dominoes. Remember to do a thorough posterolateral fusion to the sacrum.

# Long C-D Instrumentation with Sacral Screws

In a long fusion to the sacrum with sacral screws, anterior and posterior approaches are used. The anterior approach is the same as previously described with multiple diskectomies and anterior fusion. To help stabilize the lumbosacral area at L4–L5 and L5–S1, tricortical plugs are used.

For the posterior approach, a routine C-D fixation is used proximally for the scoliosis or kyphosis and extended distally with C-D screws inserted in the sacrum and in the pedicles of L4 and L5. A single C-D rod is inserted and passed caudally into the sacral screws providing the sacral fixation.

In cases where the sacral screw fixation is not as secure as wished, or additional lumbosacral stability is desired, a Galveston rod can be added. The additional rod is inserted with the spinal portion lateral to the inserted C-D rod and secured to the C-D rod with two open-closed dominoes, placed on the rod prior to insertion.

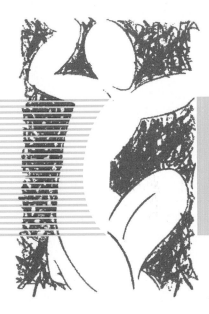

# 14

# MYELOMENINGOCELE SURGERY AND SACRAL AGENESIS

# *Late Kyphosis Surgery*

## Sac Excision

In cases of myelomeningocele kyphosis there is usually a sharp, angular kyphotic deformity, although on occasion the deformity may be round. In either situation the goal is to achieve correction of the deformity and solid arthrodesis. To achieve solid arthrodesis, interbody fusion is absolutely necessary since there are totally inadequate posterior elements for a fusion. It is relatively easy to dissect the sac if the patient is paraplegic and exposure of the disks and intervertebral body areas can be posterior rather than anterior.

In order to resect the sac, the spine is exposed from well up into the normal area, and the incision is carried down posteriorly to the low sacrum. This is a posterior midline incision but is always tempered by the previous incisions and scars resulting from sac closure in the newborn plus any rotational flaps or other surgical procedures which might have been done. Thus, the surgeon usually follows some previous curvilinear posterior scar. The better the skin obtained from the closure in the neonatal period, the easier the surgery at the time of kyphosis reconstruction. The skin flaps are injected with dilute 1:500,000 adrenalin solution, which is not only good for reduction of blood loss but also helps in the dissection. The flaps are very carefully dissected from the sac leaving the flap as thick as possible to avoid later skin necrosis. The object is to make the dissection immediately outside of the sac but not penetrate it. Use the fingertips to feel for the ridges of bone lateral to the sac. These are the everted laminae (not the pedicles). Once the everted laminae are identified on each side, indicating a lateral position to the sac, the dissection becomes easier. Dissection is then carried down the dorsal or lateral surface of the laminar stub to the end of the laminae on which there will be a rudimentary facet joint; then proceed laterally and deeper to the transverse processes. All lateral dissection is carried out prior to entering the canal itself (Fig. 14–1A).

The canal is entered by dissecting subperiosteally down the medial walls of the laminar stubs outside of the sac. There is usually very little difficulty until the nerve root in the foraminal area is located. At the junction of the healthy laminae and the sac there will be a sharp division from one to the other. This area must be identified and dissection carried up into several healthy laminae proximally. Distally, dissection is carried down inside the canal to the sacrum.

At the level of the kyphotic apex, the sac is usually adhered against the bone, is scarred, and usually very flat. Transection of the sac at this level is quite easy and there is usually little bleeding or spinal fluid leakage owing to the scarring. The sac is then dissected distally. There is one small artery and usually two veins exiting each neural foramen along with the nerve root. The nerve root is transected by electrocautery and the vessels carefully cauterized at each foramen. There may be bleeding from venous sinuses in the posterior aspect of the vertebral body and these can be stuffed with bone wax. Working carefully at one level at a time and controlling blood loss, the sac is dissected from above downward, the sacral roots are transected, and the sac is removed and discarded (Fig. 14–1B). At the level where the sac was transected, one usually wishes to go a little more proximally and the dissection is then carried out in this area outside of the sac, lifting it up and cutting two or three roots and controlling blood loss. At this point the sac is usually opened; the cord may be identified. It is transected separately and the sac is closed, taking care to leave the central canal of the spinal cord, which is usually fairly large, open to communicate with the subarachnoid space. It is not desirable to seal off the end of the cord as this may cause acute hydrocephalus (Fig. 14–1C,D).

## Sac Reflection

It is not always necessary to resect the sac. The sac can be dissected starting distally at the sacrum and, in the manner described above, transect each root and cauterize the segmental vessels, gradually lifting the sac upward until the apex of the kyphos is reached. Dissection is carried past the apex, usually two or three vertebral bodies, and the sac is reflected proximally (Fig. 14–1E).

There are two advantages to this procedure over sac transection and removal: (1) the sac is left intact and, therefore, hydrocephalus and CSF communication problems are apparently reduced; (2) the sac, which usually has a very good blood supply, can be laid back down over the fusion and instrumentation as a protective soft tissue barrier with skin closure above it providing better protection of the internal fixation.

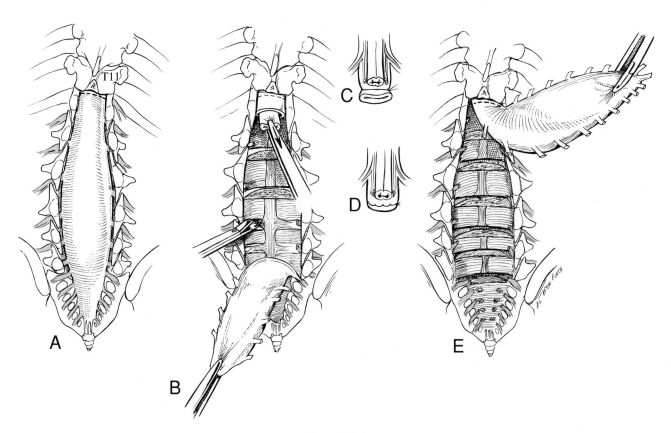

*Figure 14–1*

## Multiple Level Disk Resection and L Rods

After sac reflection or sac excision, the posterior aspect of the vertebral bodies and disks in the area of the spina bifida are exposed. There are no neurologic tissues remaining. This allows the surgeon to incise and remove the disks from the back leaving the anterior longitudinal ligament intact. This is done at every level in the fusion from the sacrum up to the point where the sac was transected or reflected. This will provide considerably more mobility to the spine; and in cases of round kyphosis, the amount of mobility is such that full correction can be obtained.

To test the correction, push forward on the apex of the kyphosis with the fingertip and the amount of correction achieved can be easily observed. Continue removing bone until this is easily accomplished. At this time, the hips should also always be in an extended position or as much as the hip flexion contractors allow so that the pelvis tilts in the desired alignment. Once adequate disk and/or bone has been resected, the next step is internal fixation. For the round kyphosis after diskectomy, L rods are used. The rods are placed inside the spinal canal medial to the everted laminae and pedicles and then wired to the pedicles or laminar stumps. Distally the rods are secured to the sacro-pelvis, which has been a challenge particularly because of the thin iliac wings of the myelomeningocele patient.

Dunn has devised a technique where the rods are precontoured to pass laterally around the L5 pedicle and then wrap forward around the front of the ala. Because of the complexity of the bend, contouring should be done in the machine shop ahead of time. The most distal part of the rod must go down the front of the sacrum for an adequate distance to provide a decent grip. For these cases the round, nonsharp part of the rod should be placed in this area. The Dunn technique is particularly apropos for kyphosis problems but is not as appropriate for scoliosis.

An alternative to this technique is the Galveston technique described previously. This is appropriate when the interior laminar space in the ilium is adequate for the insertion of the Galveston portion of the Luque rod.

## Posterior Wedge Osteotomy for More Angular Kyphosis

For more angular kyphosis simply removing the disks in the spina bifida area is not adequate to achieve correction. One to three vertebral bodies must be fully removed in order to obtain adequate posterior shortening. These are not the three apical vertebrae but the vertebrae between the apex of the lumbar kyphosis and the apex of the thoracic lordosis. This allows the posterior translation of the thorax placing the lower lumbar spine and pelvis in the proper relationship. The anterior longitudinal ligament and annulus are usually preserved. The bone is removed from within this fibrous envelope. When sufficient bone is removed, the spine is placed in alignment and the rods are inserted as mentioned previously. Any bone removed should, of course, be replaced as an autogenous bone graft (Fig. 14–2).

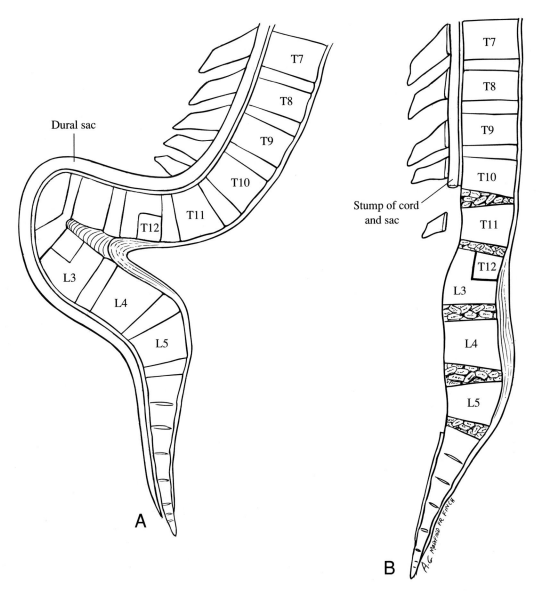

T7
T8
Dural sac
T9
T10
T11
T12
L3
L4
L5
A

T7
T8
T9
T10
Stump of cord
and sac
T11
T12
L3
L4
L5
A.G. MANFRID FR FINCH
B

*Figure 14–2*

It may be tempting to use an anterior approach releasing the anterior ligaments allowing lengthening of the front of the spine. It must be remembered that in cases of myelomeningocele kyphosis, the aorta is very short and does not permit the lengthening desired. It is best, therefore, to use the soft tissue as the anterior tethering hinge, which is the anterior ligament as well as the aorta, and do the necessary shortening posteriorly (Fig. 14–3).

These patients often have a major amount of thoracic lordosis. Depending on the individual situation, it may be necessary to do a preliminary anterior transthoracic diskectomy of the lordotic area. This allows the lordotic thoracic spine to be pulled back to the kyphotically contoured Luque rods to reshape the thorax into kyphosis as the lumbar kyphosis is reduced to a straight or lordotic lumbar spine. This can be quite important for the respiratory function of the child.

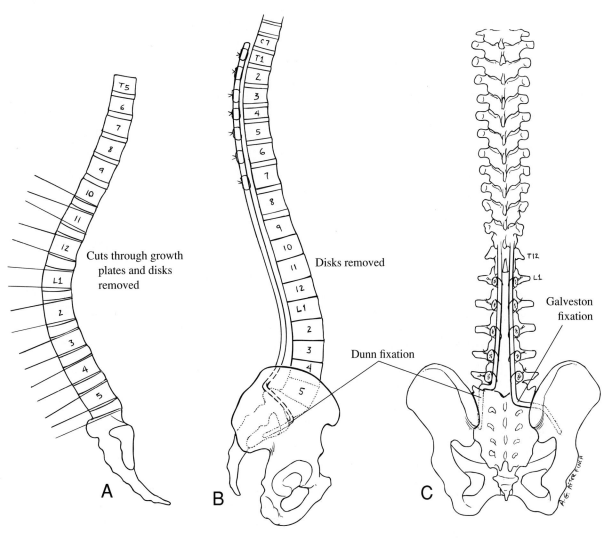

Cuts through growth
plates and disks
removed

A

Disks removed

Dunn fixation

B

Galveston
fixation

T12
L1

C

*Figure 14–3*

# Distal Spinal Agenesis (Sacral Agenesis)

In situations of caudal regression, children are often born with absence of the sacrum and one or more lumbar vertebral bodies. If more than two vertebral bodies are missing in addition to the sacrum, there can be a spinal pelvic instability problem where the pelvis flexes anteriorly relative to the rest of the spine and the child sits on the back of the sacrum pushing the internal organs up into the chest and severely compromising renal function. In situations of spinal pelvic instability, the desire is to gain a spinal pelvic stabilization in a decent alignment. If there are absent lumbar vertebrae with a gap between the thoracic spine and the pelvis, this gap must be reconstructed with some type of bone and metallic structure.

The spine is exposed posteriorly from well up into the thoracic spine down to the common sciatic notch. (There is no sacrum and the two iliac wings butt against each other.) The common sciatic notch is squared off using a Kerrison rongeur to insert hooks on each side facing upward; a second hook is placed facing downward on the top of the iliac crest or into the top of the iliac directly above the previous hook. This provides a "claw" configuration. A rod is passed through the two hooks and the claw is established. Two long rods running upward are brought against the back of the normal spine. Distraction hooks are placed in the upper end of the area and the rods are anchored to the hooks. Distraction force is applied to elongate the area between the pelvis and the intact spine to lengthen the lumbar spine as much as possible. This rod is then secured in place with additional hooks and/or wires. The distance between the end of the regular spinal vertebral body and the iliac wings is measured and a bone graft is obtained to span this distance. There are several choices. If leg amputation or knee disarticulation is anticipated, the tibia and fibula should be saved to be used to fill the gap between the thoracic spine and pelvis. If amputation is not anticipated, fibular grafts obtained bilaterally, autogenous tibial grafts, and ribs can be used. The rib grafts can be swung down on a vascular pedicle so that the bone remains viable (see Chapter 6, page 190). Allograft can be used but is highly likely to undergo lysis, and autograft is highly desirable in this situation. The spine is immobilized until total union and revascularization have been accomplished, which can take a considerable period of time since these bone grafts are not surrounded by muscle tissue.

If pseudarthrosis is detected on x-rays in the postoperative period, immediate repair should be accomplished. Failure to repair the pseudarthrosis will result in breakage of the instrumentation and loss of all fixation.

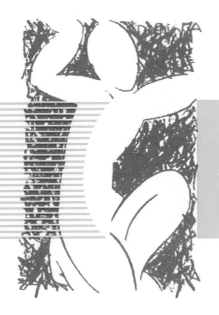

# TAKING BONE GRAFTS

# *Iliac*

## Posterior Grafts

Posterior iliac grafts are obtained from the posterior iliac crest where the ilium is thicker. The posterior crest is usually identified by palpation of the crest and tubercle, which lie approximately 4 to 6 cm lateral to the midline.

The incision is at the lower end of a midline spine or 3 to 4 inches (7.5 to 10 cm) vertical just lateral to the palpable iliac crest (Fig. 15–1A). The dissection is extended superficially to the iliolumbar fascia to the iliac crest, visualizing the interval between the lumbar fascia medially and the gluteus maximus muscle laterally, and extended inferiorly through the fibers of the gluteus maximus (Fig. 15–1B). In children, the incision is through the iliac crest cartilaginous apophysis; in adults, through the periosteum. Using subperiosteal dissection starting posteriorly, the periosteum and gluteus maximus are elevated from the iliac crest. Dissection continues to the iliac ridge between the attachments of gluteus maximus and gluteus medius and continues deep to gluteus medius. In children with a thick cartilaginous iliac crest apophysis and thick periosteum, it is often necessary to make releasing incisions anteriorly and posteriorly to allow for subperiosteal dissection. The inferior exposure is directed away from the sciatic notch.

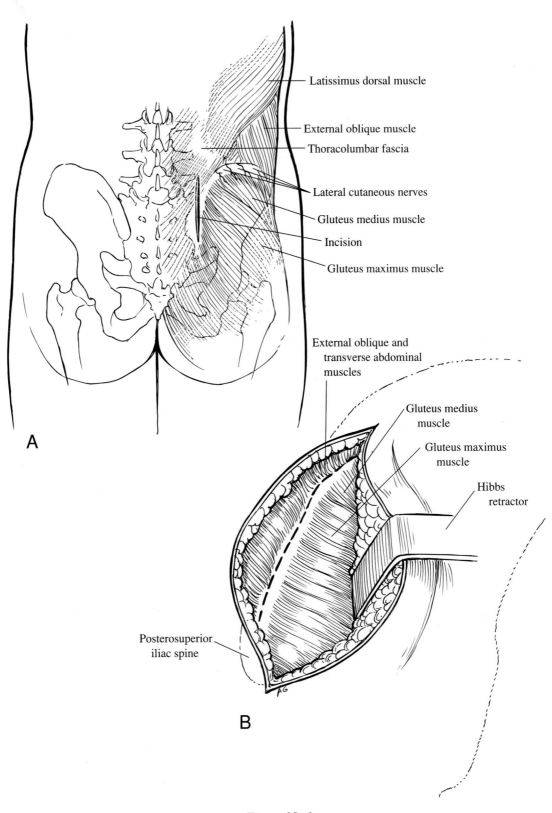

Latissimus dorsal muscle

External oblique muscle

Thoracolumbar fascia

Lateral cutaneous nerves

Gluteus medius muscle

Incision

Gluteus maximus muscle

External oblique and transverse abdominal muscles

Gluteus medius muscle

Gluteus maximus muscle

Hibbs retractor

Posterosuperior iliac spine

A

B

*Figure 15–1*

Once the outer aspect of the iliac crest has been exposed, a Taylor retractor is placed in the incision to retract the glutei and provide adequate exposure of the outer aspect of the iliac crest (Fig. 15–2A). Using a large Cobb gouge, strips of corticocancellous bone are taken starting at the posterior spine and proceeding anteriorly. The first strip is taken parallel to the iliac crest with each subsequent strip deeper to this, removing the cortex on the outer aspects of the iliac crest (Fig. 15–2B). A medium Cobb gouge is used to remove slivers or larger cores of cancellous bone for facet fusions (Fig. 15–3A). Thin slivers of bone are then removed with a Cobb or Capener gouge until the inner aspect of the iliac crest is approached. Using a large curette, the remainder of the cancellous bone is removed from under the iliac crest, between the two layers of the cortex in the depth of the wound, and in the posterior spine area where the crest is thick and there is usually a large amount of cancellous bone (Fig. 15–3B).

Following the removal of all the cancellous bone, a large piece of Gelfoam soaked in thrombin is placed in the iliac defect, and an abdominal sponge is packed in the wound before removal of the Taylor retractor.

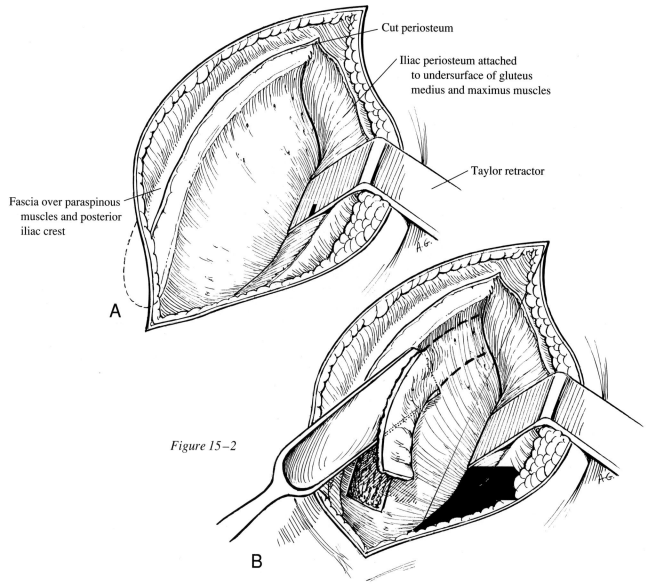

Cut periosteum

Iliac periosteum attached
to undersurface of gluteus
medius and maximus muscles

Taylor retractor

Fascia over paraspinous
muscles and posterior
iliac crest

A

*Figure 15–2*

B

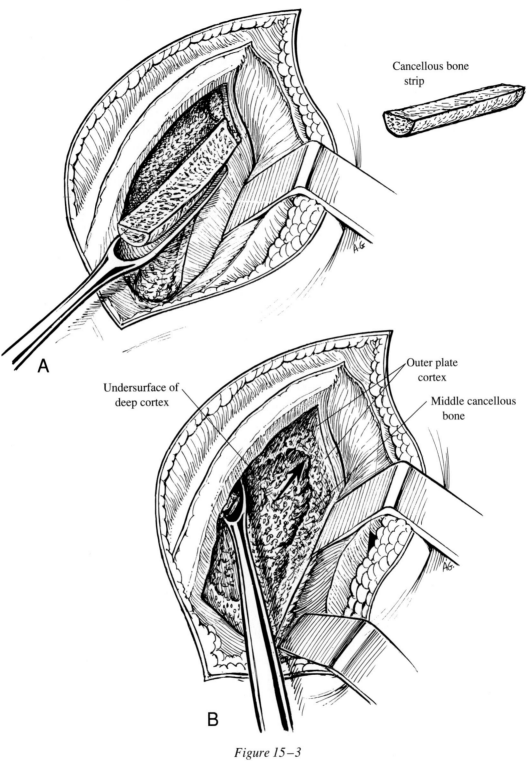

Cancellous bone strip

A

Undersurface of deep cortex

Outer plate cortex

Middle cancellous bone

B

*Figure 15–3*

## Anterior Graft

Anterior iliac grafts are obtained from the iliac crest posterior to the anterosuperior iliac spine. The patient is positioned supine for cervical surgery or in a lateral position for anterior lumbar surgery.

The anterior iliac crest is palpated and an incision is made directly over it. With subcutaneous dissection, the iliac crest is visualized in the gap between the oblique abdominal muscles superiorly and the tensor fascia lata and gluteus medius muscles inferiorly. An incision is made over the iliac crest in this interval and carried on the outer aspect of the crest, stripping off the tensor fascia lata and gluteus medius muscles. A sponge is packed in the depths of the incision. Dissection is carried over the top of the iliac crest stripping off the external abdominal, transverse abdominal, and the iliac muscles. The iliac crest is exposed with the ridge of the crest and the inner and outer tables visualized. Taylor retractors are now placed in the two areas on the inner and outer aspects of the crests so that good visualization of the crest can be maintained (Fig. 15–4). The size of the required graft is measured.

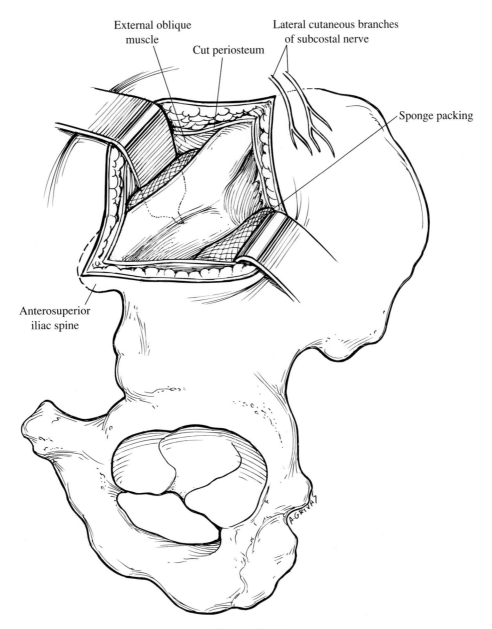

External oblique muscle

Cut periosteum

Lateral cutaneous branches of subcostal nerve

Sponge packing

Anterosuperior iliac spine

*Figure 15–4*

## Small Tricortical Grafts

With the crest exposed, the retractors placed, and the size of the graft measured, the crest is measured and marked in length and depth for harvesting of the graft (Fig. 15–5A). It is essential to make the harvested piece larger than the piece required. After harvesting, the graft is trimmed for final size and fit.

Using an osteotome or a power saw with an Army/Navy retractor placed at the end of the incision to protect the soft tissue, cuts are made in the ilium at right angles to the crest to the required depth (Fig. 15–5B). After the anterior and posterior cuts are made, the transverse cut is made, again using an osteotome or the power saw, taking care to protect the soft tissues and muscle on the side of the osteotome or saw and the opposite side of the crest (Fig. 15–5C).

A single long piece of the crest is taken to reconstruct defects from a corpectomy (Fig. 15–5D). Individual pieces can be cut from the crest for anterior cervical fusions or a larger piece can be cut into smaller pieces for each disk space.

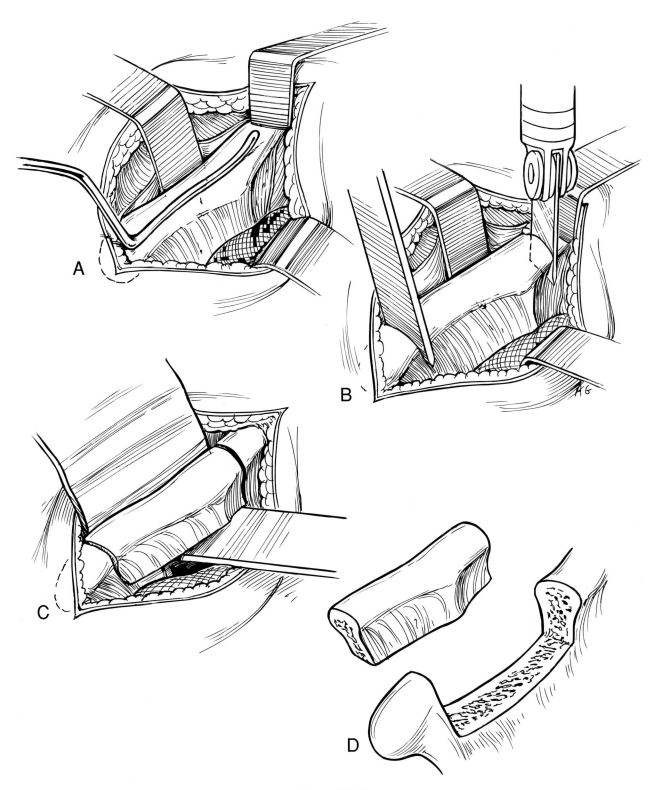

A

B

C

D

*Figure 15—5*

## Crest-Sparing Graft

When bicortical grafts are required, usually for anterior cervical surgery, they are taken from the ilium using a power saw leaving the iliac crest intact and removing the bicortical bone from below the crest.

## Iliac Crest Reconstruction

When large tricortical iliac grafts are obtained, a defect is left in the iliac crest that can cause a problem cosmetically and is often painful. The iliac crest can be reconstructed using allograft fibula or rib. A curette is used to remove the cancellous bone in the iliac crest area on both sides of the defect. The fibula or rib is cut approximately 1 to 1.5 cm longer than the gap. It is then placed into the iliac crest on one side of the defect and then into the opposite side of the defect, bridging the defect (Fig. 15–6). The periosteal muscles are very carefully closed over the crest with a continuous closure followed by subcutaneous skin closure over a Hemovac tube in the subcutaneous layer.

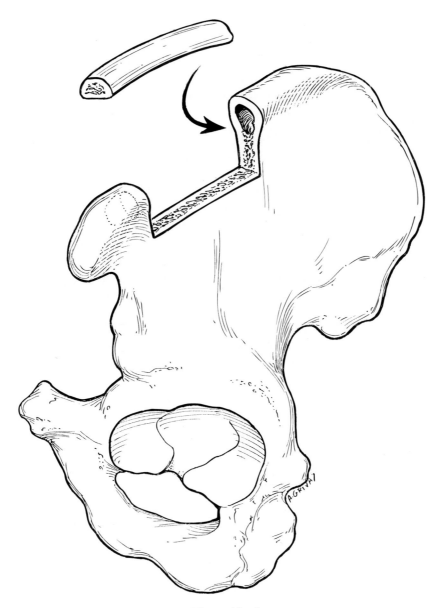

*Figure 15–6*

# *Fibula Graft*

Bone is harvested from the fibula for anterior strut grafts in the cervical or thoracolumbar spine. In general, the middle third to half of the fibula is harvested, preserving the distal third to maintain the integrity of the distal tibia-fibula joint and the ankle mortise.

The patient is placed in a lateral position for anterior thoracolumbar surgery or supine for anterior cervical surgery. An appropriately sized tourniquet is placed around the thigh and the lower leg is prepped and draped free. When the appropriate anterior surgery has been performed and the length of the fibula required has been measured, the graft is taken.

The leg is exsanguinated with an Esmarch bandage and the tourniquet inflated. The upper and lower ends of the fibula, that is, the fibular head and lateral malleolus, are palpated and the incision is made in a line joining these two bony prominences over the middle half of the fibula (Fig. 15–7A). The skin and subcutaneous tissue are divided exposing the fascia of the lower leg. The tendon of the long peroneal muscle overlies the other peroneal muscles in the lower part of the incision. The fascia is incised posterior to the peroneal muscles and tendons in the line of the separation of the anterior peroneal and the posterior soleus muscles (Fig. 15–7B). Dissection is carried out in this plane exposing the posterior crest of the fibula which lies between the peroneal muscle anteriorly and flexor hallucis longus muscle posteriorly (Fig. 15–8). An incision is made between these latter muscles over the posterior crest of the fibula. With careful subperiosteal dissection the muscles are stripped off the fibula, starting distally and extending proximally because of the oblique muscle attachments (Fig. 15–9A). Dissection is carried around the fibula and using a right angle clamp, a sponge is passed around the fibula distally. Using the sponge the periosteum and muscles on the third surface of the fibula are dissected free (Fig. 15–9B,C). This sponge is placed superiorly and a new sponge inserted inferiorly. The section of fibula to be removed is measured and marked (Fig. 15–9D).

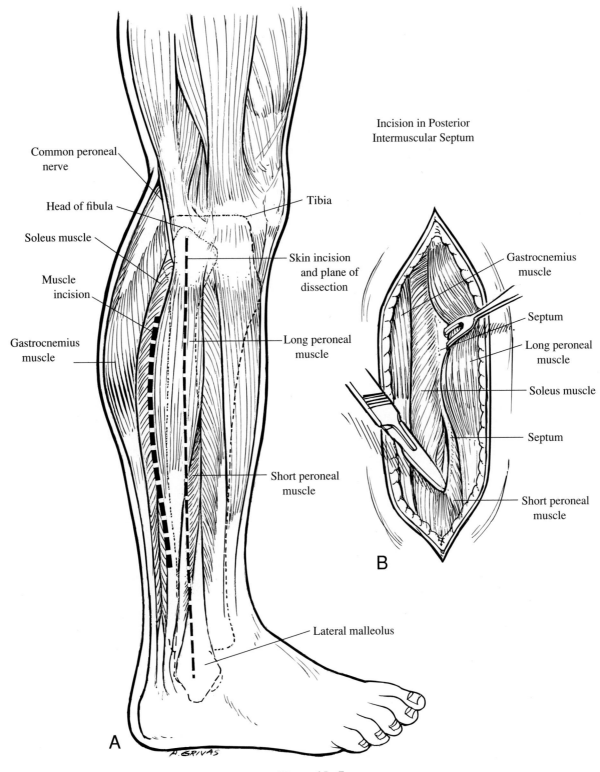

Common peroneal nerve

Head of fibula

Soleus muscle

Muscle incision

Gastrocnemius muscle

Tibia

Skin incision and plane of dissection

Long peroneal muscle

Short peroneal muscle

Lateral malleolus

A

A. GRIVAS

Incision in Posterior Intermuscular Septum

Gastrocnemius muscle

Septum

Long peroneal muscle

Soleus muscle

Septum

Short peroneal muscle

B

*Figure 15–7*

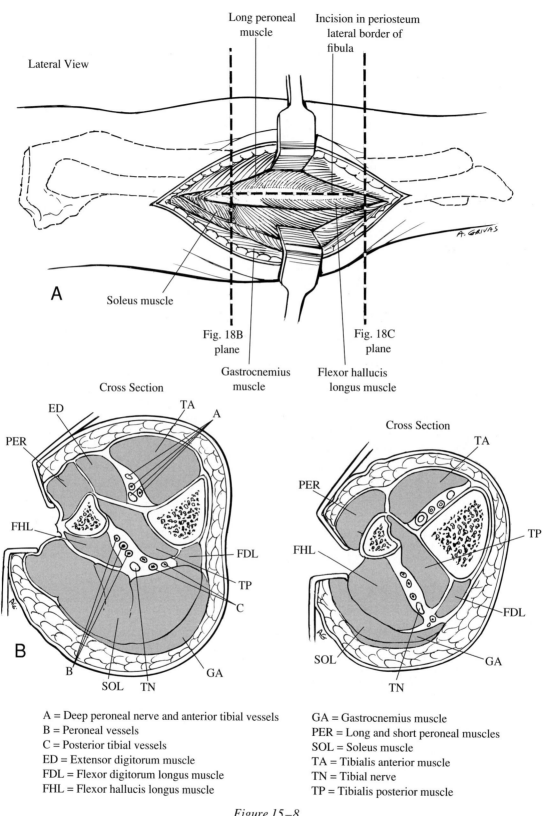

Lateral View

Long peroneal
muscle

Incision in periosteum
lateral border of
fibula

A

Soleus muscle

Fig. 18B
plane

Fig. 18C
plane

Gastrocnemius
muscle

Flexor hallucis
longus muscle

Cross Section

ED

TA

A

PER

FHL

FDL

TP

C

B

B

SOL

TN

GA

Cross Section

TA

PER

TP

FHL

FDL

SOL

GA

TN

A = Deep peroneal nerve and anterior tibial vessels
B = Peroneal vessels
C = Posterior tibial vessels
ED = Extensor digitorum muscle
FDL = Flexor digitorum longus muscle
FHL = Flexor hallucis longus muscle

GA = Gastrocnemius muscle
PER = Long and short peroneal muscles
SOL = Soleus muscle
TA = Tibialis anterior muscle
TN = Tibial nerve
TP = Tibialis posterior muscle

*Figure 15–8*

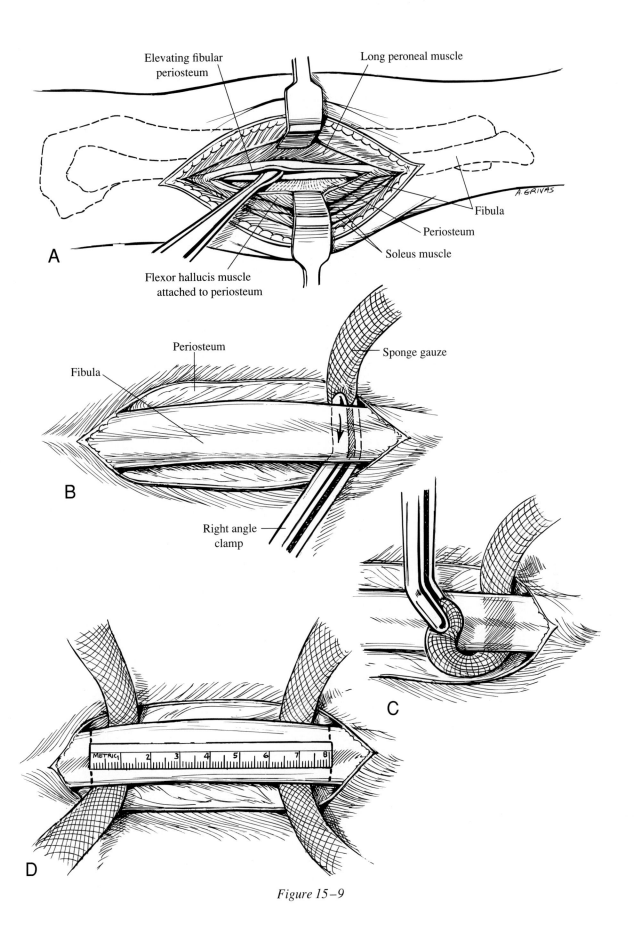

A

Elevating fibular
periosteum

Long peroneal muscle

Fibula

Periosteum

Soleus muscle

Flexor hallucis muscle
attached to periosteum

B

Periosteum

Fibula

Sponge gauze

Right angle
clamp

C

D

*Figure 15–9*

535

Using a power saw a portion of fibula is resected. A periosteal elevator or small malleable retractor is placed adjacent to the area of dissection to hold soft tissues away from the fibula preventing damage to these tissues by the saw (Fig. 15–10). The section of fibula is removed and the wound is irrigated with saline. The periosteal sheath remains in the fibular bed. The fascia is approximated with a few interrupted sutures. Complete fascial closure is not performed in order to prevent a compartment syndrome. Subcutaneous tissue and skin are closed in layers. After application of a dry sterile dressing and Ace bandage, the tourniquet is released.

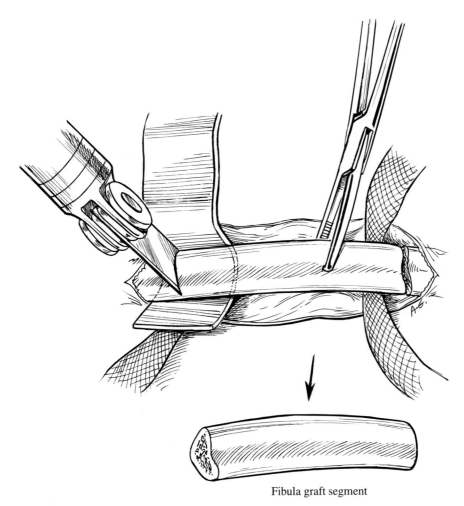

Fibula graft segment

*Figure 15–10*

537

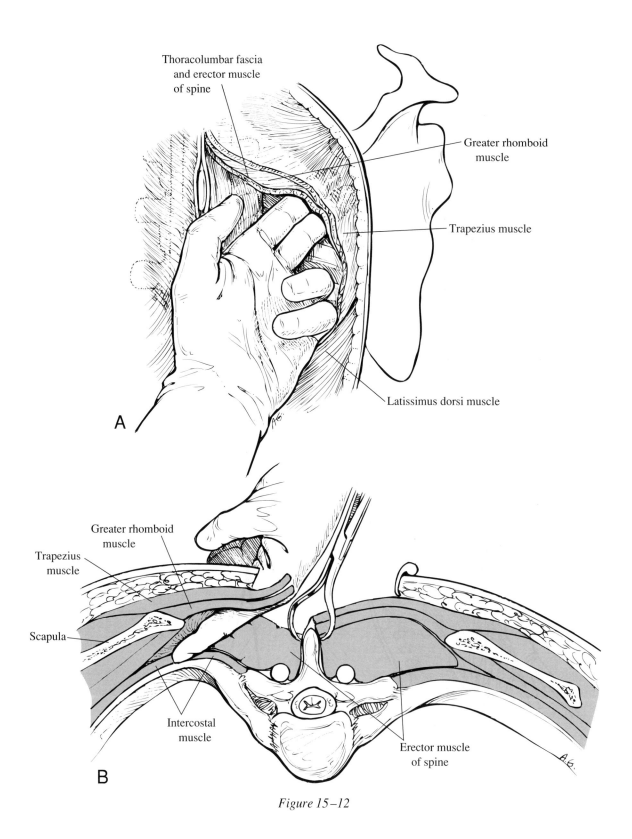

*Figure 15–12*

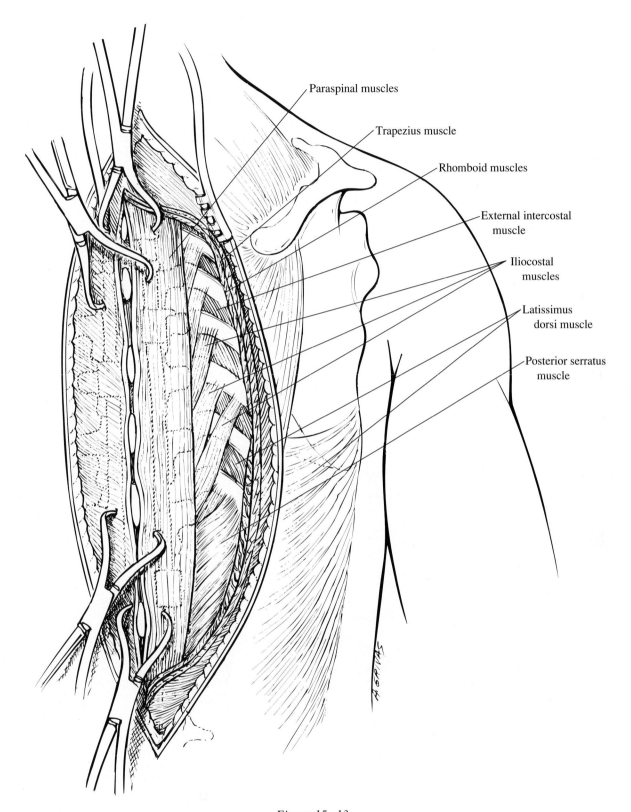

Paraspinal muscles

Trapezius muscle

Rhomboid muscles

External intercostal
muscle

Iliocostal
muscles

Latissimus
dorsi muscle

Posterior serratus
muscle

*Figure 15–13*

541

The rib medial to the prominence is identified and an incision made through the periosteum using cutting cautery. All bleeders are coagulated. Using a periosteal elevator, the periosteum is dissected from the superficial surface of the rib and then from the superior, inferior, and deep surfaces of the rib. It must be remembered that during dissection on the superior and inferior edges of the rib, the plane of dissection is toward the spine on the inferior edge and away from the spine on the superior edge (Fig. 15–14). Alternative instruments for dissection of the periosteum are the Alexander periosteal elevator and Doyen periosteal stripper (Fig. 15–15). Once the periosteum is dissected off the deep surface of the rib, a sponge is placed around the rib using a right angle clamp. The sponge is used to dissect any residual periosteum from the rib in the area of the rib to be excised (Fig. 15–16). Depending on the nature of the rotational prominence and its sharpness, 3 to 8 cm of the rib need to be removed for adequate thoracoplasty. The amount will depend on the anatomy of the prominence and whether it is sharp or gradually rounded.

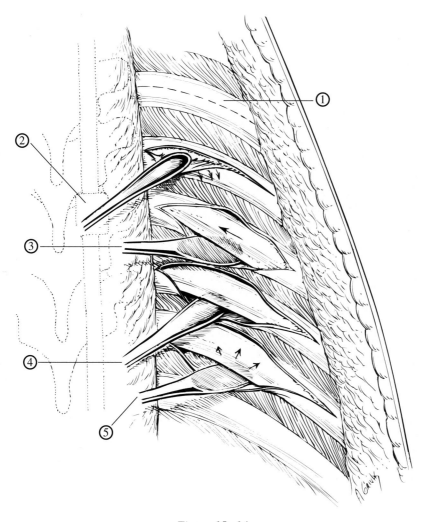

*Figure 15–14*

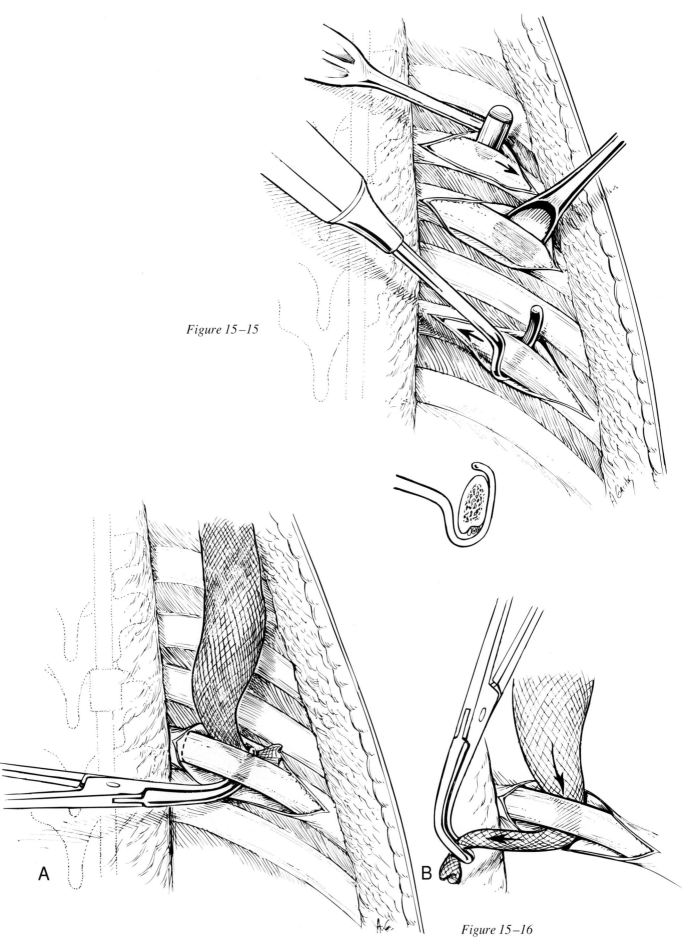

*Figure 15–15*

*Figure 15–16*

A

B

Using a rib cutter, the rib is first cut laterally. During the cutting, the sponge is placed under the lateral end of the rib to protect the deep periosteum and pleura (Fig. 15–17A). The sponge is moved medially and the rib cut holding it with a Kocher clamp (Fig. 15–17B). The ends of the cut rib are felt to ensure that there are no sharp spikes of bone. Any sharp spikes are removed with a large double-action rongeur. During this process, the rib end is elevated to avoid any possible damage to the periosteum and pleura (Fig. 15–18). Often, in cases of a very sharp rotational prominence, the cut medial stump of the rib is now prominent. A periosteal elevator is used to strip the periosteum from the medial stump, and a double-action rongeur is used to remove additional rib. The deep periosteum and pleura are protected with a curved Matson periosteal elevator, which fits well in this area as the bone is removed. A sponge is placed in the bed of the removed rib. A similar procedure is performed on the ribs cranially, removing sections of at least five to six ribs for adequate thoracoplasty.

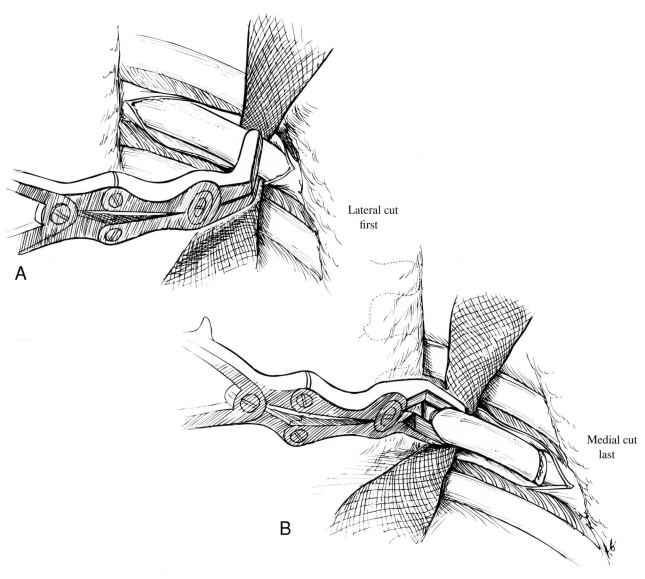

Lateral cut
first

A

Medial cut
last

B

*Figure 15–17*

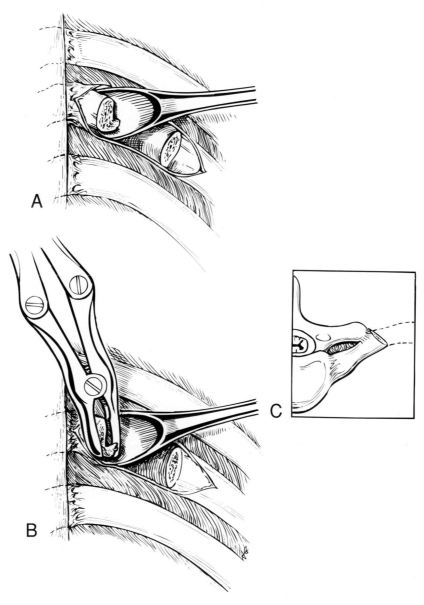

*Figure 15–18*

Once the ribs are removed, the retractors are taken out of the incision and the rotational prominence palpated through the skin to make sure that (a) an adequate number of ribs have been removed and (b) there is no bony stump remaining that is now prominent (Fig. 15-19). This is more common on the medial rib stump, especially if there is marked vertebral rotation where the neck of the rib and transverse processes are now prominent. In such cases, additional bone is removed, while protecting the deep periosteum and pleura.

Once hemostasis is obtained, the incision is irrigated and the anesthesiologist forcibly expands the lungs to ensure that there is no air leak from the thoracoplasty (Fig. 15-20). When an air leak does occur, a chest tube is inserted to prevent a pneumothorax.

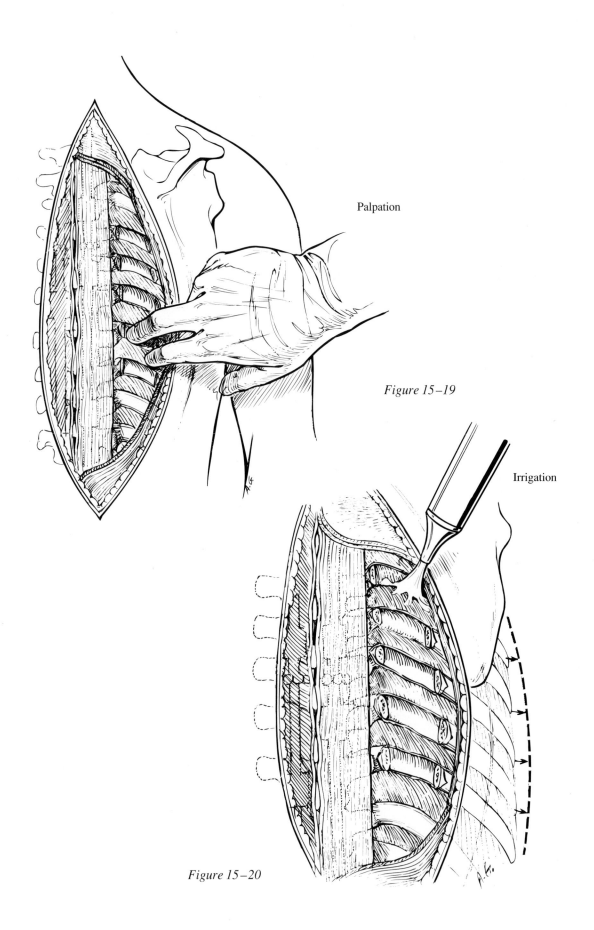

Palpation

Figure 15–19

Irrigation

Figure 15–20

547

### Anterior

Anterior ("Internal") thoracoplasty can be done when an anterior approach to the spine is used for diskectomy and fusion. This approach may be required because of the severity and rigidity of the curve or the patient is young and postarthrodesis bending of the fusion ("crankshaft" effect) is feared. Usually the rib leading to the superior end of the area to be fused anteriorly is resected for a standard thoracotomy approach (Fig. 15–21A). After the chest is opened, the periosteum of the remaining portion of this rib is incised along its length, connecting to a longitudinal division of the parietal pleura of the vertebral bodies (Fig. 15–21B). Once the segmental vessels are ligated, as shown in Chapter 6, the remainder of the rib, including the neck and head, is removed by disarticulation. The flap of parietal pleura can be reflected off of the remaining distal ribs to be resected or the parietal pleura can be divided with the cautery from each rib (Fig. 15–22). The rib is cut at the point of its maximal deformity, which is usually 2 to 3 cm distal to the end of the transverse process (Fig. 15–23).

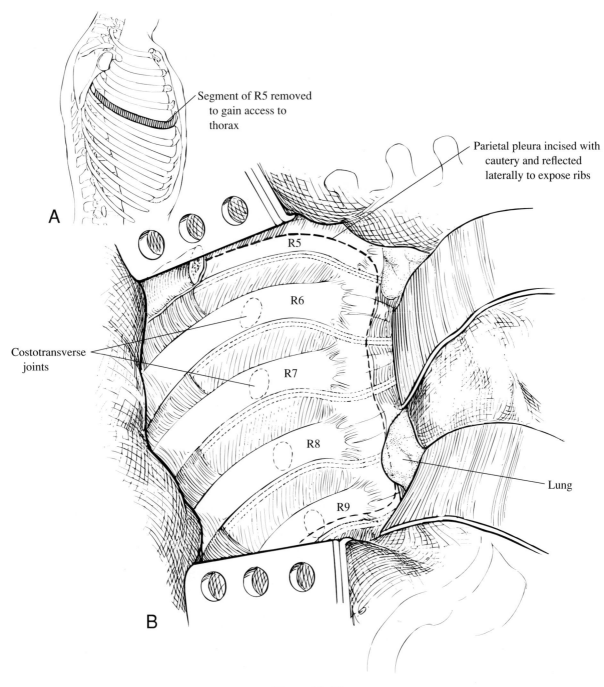

Segment of R5 removed
to gain access to
thorax

Parietal pleura incised with
cautery and reflected
laterally to expose ribs

A

R5

R6

Costotransverse
joints

R7

R8

Lung

R9

B

*Figure 15–21*

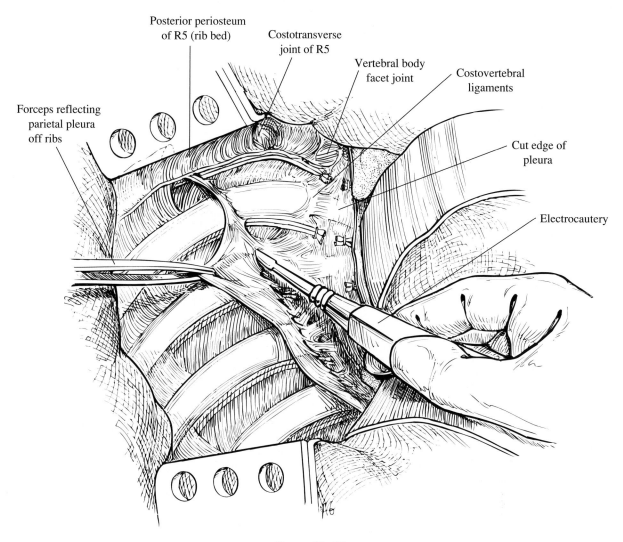

Posterior periosteum
of R5 (rib bed)

Costotransverse
joint of R5

Vertebral body
facet joint

Costovertebral
ligaments

Forceps reflecting
parietal pleura
off ribs

Cut edge of
pleura

Electrocautery

*Figure 15–22*

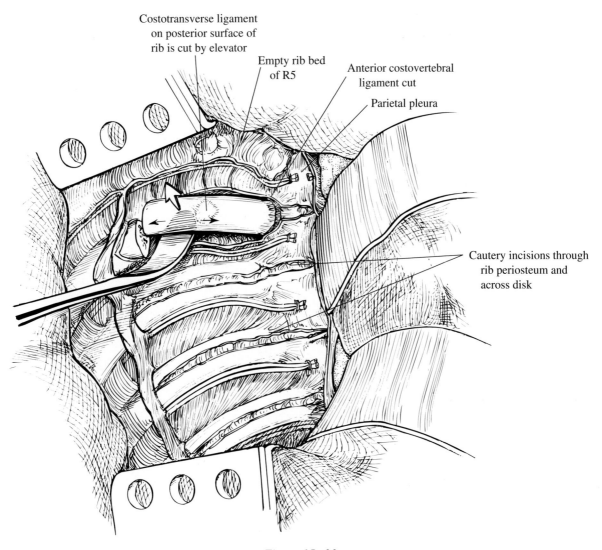

Costotransverse ligament
on posterior surface of
rib is cut by elevator

Empty rib bed
of R5

Anterior costovertebral
ligament cut

Parietal pleura

Cautery incisions through
rib periosteum and
across disk

*Figure 15–23*

The rib is grasped and stripped including dividing the ligaments of the costo-transverse joint deep to the rib, after which the rib head is disarticulated.

After five, six, or seven ribs are removed (the number removed depends on the length of the rib hump), the diskectomy and fusion are carried out. Removal of the rib head greatly facilitates removal of the disk and makes thorough lateral disk material resection possible, which makes closing the convexity of the scoliosis easier (Fig. 15–24).

When doing internal thoracoplasty, a slightly increased chest tube drainage and perhaps one day longer for chest tube placement have been noted but with no lasting complications.

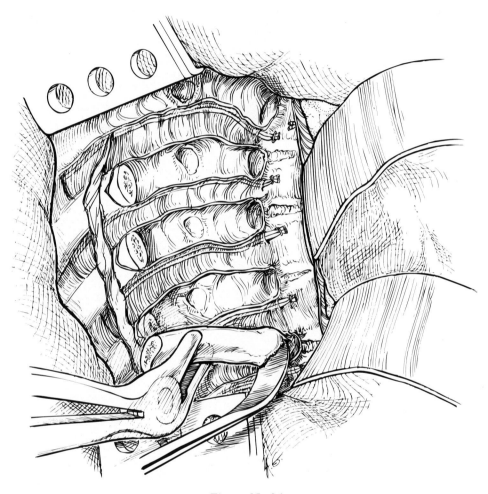

*Figure 15–24*

# Index

Note: Page numbers in *italics* refer to illustrations.

# INDEX

# INDEX

# INDEX

# INDEX

564

# INDEX

# INDEX

ISBN 0-7216-2958-X